Clinical
Neurology

Essentials of Clinical Neurology

Leon A. Weisberg, MD
Director and Professor of Neurology
Tulane University Medical Center, School of Medicine
Departments of Psychiatry and Neurology
New Orleans, Louisana

Carlos Garcia, MD
Professor of Neurology and Pathology
Departments of Neurology and Pathology
Lousiana State University School of Medicine
New Orleans, Louisiana

Richard Strub, MD
Professor of Neurology
Department of Neurology, Ochsner Clinic
New Orleans, Louisana

CONTRIBUTING AUTHOR
Elizabeth P. Bouldin, MD
Assistant Professor
Departments of Psychiatry and Neurology, Ochsner Clinic
Tulane University School of Medicine
Director, Sleep Lab
New Orleans, Louisana

THIRD EDITION

M Mosby

St. Louis Baltimore Boston Carlsbad Chicago Naples New York
Philadelphia Portland London Madrid Mexico City Singapore
Sydney Tokyo Toronto Wiesbaden

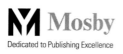

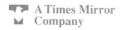

Publisher: Anne S. Patterson
Editor: Laura DeYoung
Editorial Assistant: Alicia E. Moten
Project Manager: Deborah Vogel
Editing and Production: A-R Editions, Inc.
Designer: Pati Pye
Manufacturing Supervisor: Theresa Fuchs
Cover Image: © Photographer, Science
Source/Photo Researchers

Third Edition

Copyright © 1996 by Mosby-Year Book, Inc.

Previous editions copyrighted 1983 and 1989.

Printed in the United States of America
Composition by A-R Editions, Inc.
Printing/binding by R.R. Donnelley & Sons Company

Mosby-Year Book, Inc.
11830 Westline Industrial Drive
St. Louis, Missouri 63146

International Standard Book Number
0-8151-9129-4
96 97 98 99 00 / 9 8 7 6 5 4 3 2 1

To the medical students and house officers at
Tulane University and
Louisiana State University
who have served
as an impetus and inspiration
for this book

PREFACE

This book is designed as a practical introduction to the evaluation of common neurologic diseases. It is written for the use of medical students and house officers during their initial exposure to clinical neurology and as a review for practicing physicians in primary care. In this book we intentionally stress presenting symptoms, history taking, and the neurologic examination. Differential diagnosis, neurodiagnostic investigations, and treatment of the more common neurologic conditions are also discussed.

The book is divided into three parts. The first section consists of a general discussion of history taking, neurologic examination techniques, and neurodiagnostic studies. Part II includes seven chapters, with each providing a discussion of the clinical evaluation of common neurologic disorders. Clinical features such as headache, imbalance, dizziness, and episodic loss of consciousness are explored, and a scheme for clinical and laboratory investigations is presented. This section is probably the most useful for students as they begin to see patients and to translate each patient's complaints into standard diagnostic entities. The final section is a discussion of common neurologic diseases, such as stroke, seizure disorders, brain tumors, and muscle disease. We believe that this general outline will afford the student the most practical introduction to clinical neurology. A glossary of common terms is included at the end of the book for quick reference.

In the past several years, fewer and fewer medical schools require students or house officers to rotate on neurologic services. Because of this, the general level of neurologic sophistication of graduating physicians is not as high as was previously the case. At one time a good neurology reference text could be used to supplement the clinical teaching of the faculty. However, now many students must gain all of their training in clincal neurology from text material and incidental contact with consultants on their medical services. This fact, more than any other, prompted us to tailor this book to this audience: to stress the skills of history taking, examination, and diagnosis. We hope that we have achieved this goal and that the reader will gain a solid and practical introduction to the complicated and expanding field of neurology.

L.A.W.
R.L.S.
C.A.G.

ACKNOWLEDGMENTS

We wish to thank Laura Cardin, Mary Usner, and Alison Smith for their extraordinary secretarial, editing and all other skills they devoted to the successful revision of the third edition of this book.

Our thanks to Dr. Elizabeth Bouldin for her assistance on producing the chapter on sleep.

TABLE OF CONTENTS

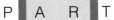

Evaluation

I

Neurologic History and Examination

1

In neurology, as in any branch of clinical medicine, a careful history and examination are critical in establishing the correct diagnosis. Many neurologic diseases do not have definitive physical findings (e.g., migraine, idiopathic epilepsy) or laboratory tests to aid in diagnosis; therefore good history-taking is critical. The student should follow a standard outline in performing the history and examination; in this way a routine will be established, and the examiner will always have a complete set of data from which to generate a diagnosis. A general outline is provided here; more specific details relating to history taking, examination, and the clinical significance of the findings are contained in Parts II and III.

▨ HISTORY

Chief Complaint

The patient's chief complaint is a short statement of the problem for which neurologic evaluation is sought, and it is best recorded in the patient's own words.

History of the Present Illness

The history of the present illness represents a spatial and temporal elaboration of the chief complaint. This is the most difficult and important aspect of the entire diagnostic process. It requires the physician to rearrange and organize the patient's symptoms into a logical historical sequence. The first step is to establish the time and character of onset (e.g., sudden, suggesting a vascular or epileptic event, or gradual, as is seen with mass or atrophic lesions). Next it is necessary to obtain a statement of the nature of the course: Is it progressive, remitting and exacerbating, or episodic such as a seizure disorder or headache? Then the actual symptoms must be detailed very carefully. The physician must not accept the patient's terminology unless it is perfectly clear; for instance, weakness or dizziness can have many meanings; therefore it is important for the physician to find out exactly what the patient means. Last, the patient is asked about any previous evaluation and treatment for the problem.

At this point the experienced examiner may have arrived at a tentative diagnosis and can expand the present illness description to include other relevant information to verify or reject that diagnosis; this skill comes with practice and with detailed knowledge of disease entities. However, the student will need to obtain a complete inventory of other neurologic symptoms, including a past history for medical illness or other conditions known to affect the nervous system.

When taking this type of detailed history, the examiner must use terms that will be understood by the patient; for example, asking an uneducated person if he has had a seizure may not elicit the proper response. A word such as *blackout, passing-out, spell,* or *convulsion* may be better. Redundancy is also helpful; using as many similar terms and descriptions as possible ensures that the patient comprehends the symptom being discussed. As in the history of the present illness, each positive symptom in the review should be explored fully. Box 1-1 presents the neurologic review of the systems, and Box 1-2 lists pertinent medical, social, and family history information.

■ NEUROLOGIC EXAMINATION

The neurologic examination is a systematic examination of the many functions of the nervous system. Because structure and function are closely related in the nervous system, the examination allows the examiner to determine both if there is dysfunction or damage of nervous tissue and also the location or structure involved. Focal, multifocal, and diffuse disease can be diagnosed. With the data from the history and examination, a logical differential diagnosis and evaluation plan can be proposed.

The following examination scheme is organized to minimize inconvenience to the patient. History and mental status examinations are carried out with the patient sitting in a chair or on the bedside; gait, strength, spine, skin, and coordination examinations are then carried out with the patient standing; the cranial nerves, carotid artery, reflexes, and sensory functions can be examined with the patient seated on the examining table or bed; and, finally, superficial reflexes, heel and shin testing, tests for meningeal irritability, and rectal examination are carried out with the patient lying down. In the following discussion, some areas are only briefly mentioned (e.g., involuntary movements, patterns of sensory loss) because these findings are discussed in the appropriate clinical chapters.

BOX 1-1 Neurologic Review of Systems

1 Headache
2 Nausea or vomiting
3 Syncope
4 Seizure
5 Pain (back, neck, muscular, radiating)
6 Paresthesias, dysesthesias, or numbness
7 Motor difficulties
   a Weakness
   b Atrophy (wasting)
   c Ataxia
   d Clumsiness
   e Involuntary movements
   f Slowed motor movements (bradykinesia)
8 Visual disturbances
   a Diplopia
   b Blurring or visual loss (general or in one field of vision)
   c Scotoma (hole in the visual field)
9 Auditory/vestibular symptoms
   a Hearing loss (bilateral or unilateral)
   b Tinnitus (noise, usually a ringing in the ears)
   c Dizziness
10 Dysphagia (swallowing difficulty)
11 Speech and language symptoms
   a Dysarthria (an articulation disturbance)
   b Dysphonia (phonation difficulty usually caused by a vocal cord dysfunction)
   c Word-finding difficulty
   d Comprehension problems
12 Mental symptoms (a history should be obtained from relatives and close associates)
   a Memory difficulty
   b General intellectual deficits (trouble at work or with finances)
   c Disorientation in the environment (e.g., getting lost)
   d Episodes of confusion or abnormal behavior (e.g., wandering at night unclothed)
   e Inattention or difficulty concentrating
   f Lethargy
   g Insomnia or excessive daytime sleepiness
   h Anxiety
   i Depression
   j Hallucinations
   k Paranoid thoughts
   l Personality change
13 Autonomic dysfunction (bowel, bladder, sexual, postural hypotension)

BOX 1-2   Pertinent Medical, Social, and Family History

1 Hypertension
2 Heart disease (e.g., chest pain, heart failure)
3 Stroke or transient ischemic attack (TIA)
4 Diabetes
5 Endocrine disease (e.g., thyroid, adrenal)
6 Other neurologic disease
7 Medical disease
8 Cancer
9 Medications
10 Alcohol or drug use; smoking history
11 Head trauma
12 Handedness (patient and family)
13 Education and vocation
14 Toxic exposure
15 Birth, development, and scholastic history (most important in epilepsy or developmental disorders)
16 Family history of pertinent medical and neurologic disease

Mental Status Examination

If the patient has any history or suspicion of behavior change, it is prudent to briefly screen mental functions. The first mental function to screen is level of consciousness (Box 1-3).

Behavioral Observations

The patient should be observed for cleanliness, evidence of depression, anxiety, confusional behavior, frontal lobe personality change (see Neurobehavioral Diseases in Chapter 14), and unilateral neglect.

Attention and Concentration

Observation and digit span (normal 7) and serial subtraction (e.g., 100 minus 7) tests are used.

BOX 1-3   Level of Consciousness

1 Alert (fully responsive, aware of the environment, and capable of responding appropriately to it)
2 Lethargic (sleepy but arousable and coherent)
3 Obtunded (very sleepy and incoherent on arousal)
4 Stuporous (requiring vigorous stimulation for arousal)
5 Comatose (unresponsive to environmental or internal stimuli such as pain)

Language

The examiner should look for evidence of aphasia (e.g., errors in syntax, word choice, comprehension), specifically test naming (objects, colors, body parts), and repetition. In language testing simple items are presented first; then difficulty is increased. Dysarthria, which is an abnormality of articulation, must be separated from aphasia, which is a language disturbance.

Memory

The most important function is recent memory or new learning ability. The patient should be asked about personal identity, place, and date. The patient is given something specific to learn, such as a name, address, and flower or four unrelated words such as brown, tulip, eyedropper, and honesty. The patient is asked to repeat the words and is then quickly asked about some recent personal information or current news items to prevent rehearsal of the items. In 5 minutes and again at the end of the examination, the examiner should ask for the information that the patient was requested to remember. A normal person should retain most of the name and address and three of the four words. Care is necessary in interpreting recent memory loss in patients with emotional problems; anxious patients are often too distracted, and depressed patients are too apathetic to perform well on learning tasks.

Drawings

The patient is asked to spontaneously draw or copy several simple drawings. Errors on this task are frequently indicative of organic brain damage, particularly dementia or parietal lobe damage. The samples and examples of errors shown in Figure 1-1 exemplify this task.

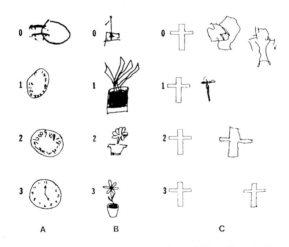

FIGURE 1-1. Illustrations of drawing ability. **A** and **B** are drawn on command, and **C** is a copy of the examiner's example. The bottom drawing in each example (*3*) is normal. The next (*2*) is good, yet mildly abnormal; this type of performance can be seen in persons with lower intelligence. The top two drawings (*0* and *1*) are abnormal and highly correlated with organic brain disease. *From Strub RL, Black FW:* The mental status examination in neurology, *Philadelphia, 1977, FA Davis. Copyright 1977 by F.A. Davis Company. Reprinted by permission.*

Abstract Reasoning

Proverb interpretation. Several examples should be used, such as "Don't cry over spilt milk," "Rome wasn't built in a day," and "People who live in glass houses shouldn't throw stones." The patients with dementia, low IQ, or schizophrenia will give concrete interpretations such as, "Rome is a big place, you couldn't build it in a day or even a month."

Similarities. These are pairs of words that have some similarity or in some way belong to the same category (e.g., banana—apple [fruit], desk—bookcase [furniture], poem—novel [literature]). The demented or retarded person either does not see any similarity or gives a very concrete association, such as "a desk and a bookcase could both be in the same room or could be associated with studying."

Calculations (written). The patient is asked to perform several complex addition, subtraction, and multiplication problems; and the examiner can observe for preservation of rote tables, arithmetic processes (borrowing, carrying), and spatial alignment.

Motor Examination

When examining a patient for motor skills, observe the following: gait, balance, involuntary movements, limb tone, strength, muscle bulk and consistency, and coordination.

Gait

- The patient is asked to stand up from the chair. Difficulty doing this can denote proximal leg weakness, which can indicate muscle disease. This difficulty can also be caused by pain (back, hip, or knee) or by poor balance.
- The patient is asked to stand and walk in a normal fashion. The normal base is 12 to 18 inches

between the inner surface of shoes or bare feet. The examiner should look for weakness, ataxia, wide-based stance, spasticity (stiffness of legs and the tendency to circumduct and scissor the legs), and arm posture (subtle flexion of one arm can indicate early hemiparesis). Patients with nerve disease (neuropathy, anterior horn cell disease) have distal weakness, with difficulty walking on heels and toes.

- The patient is asked to toe and heel walk. These maneuvers put additional demands on motor integration and balance mechanisms and bring out subtle abnormalities. Arm swing and natural hand posturing may be abnormal on the side opposite a damaged hemisphere. Toe-walking tests the strength of gastrocnemius and soleus muscles, which are primarily innervated by the S1 nerve root. Heel-walking tests the strength of foot dorsiflexors (anterior tibial muscles), which are primarily innervated by L4 and L5.

- The patient is asked to tandem walk (heel to toe on a line). This task further challenges the balance mechanism. Any tendency by the patient to fall to the side or backward should be noted.

Balance

The cerebellum, proprioceptive system, basal ganglia, and vestibular system, along with the pyramidal control of axial muscles, are the main systems responsible for maintaining proper balance. Balance is tested mainly during gait evaluation. Particular attention should be paid to performance on turns (often instability on turns is the first and only sign of imbalance). Elderly persons (usually 75 and older) have mild gait and balance problems as a concomitant of aging; therefore the examiner must adjust his or her expectations accordingly.

One useful classic clinical sign used in assessing balance is the Romberg sign. The patient stands with feet together and then closes the eyes. If the patient falls after closing the eyes, the test is considered positive. A positive Romberg sign usually indicates marked proprioceptive loss, from either peripheral neuropathy or damage to the posterior columns of the spinal cord. Patients with cerebellar disease, significant unilateral weakness, or advanced parkinsonism may fall with their eyes open, and there is little or no difference with their eyes closed.

An additional test of balance or postural stability is performed by giving a gentle push backward to the patient who is standing with feet together. The normal person will resist the push adequately or catch himself or herself by putting one foot back. In some diseases, principally Parkinson's disease, the patient cannot make proper postural adjustments and will either fall backward or start to take small rapid steps backward (retropulsion).

Involuntary Movements

The examiner should expose the patient's arms, shoulders, and upper legs and have him or her stand quietly at rest. Notation is made of any adventitious movements: tremor, chorea, athetosis, myoclonus, dystonia, hemiballism, or fasciculation (see Chapter 20 for a full description of these abnormal movements).

Limb Tone

The examiner should passively flex and extend the patient's arms and wrists in a search for increased tone: spasticity (increased tone in antigravity muscles) with clasp knife phenomenon (sudden release of increased tone in spastic limb), rigidity (increased tone in both agonists and antagonists about a joint) with cogwheeling or ratcheting (intermittent rigidity with passive movements), and decreased tone (hypotonicity or flaccidity). The examiner should also supinate and pronate the patient's wrists, as increased limb tone is often first noticed with this maneuver. Contractures represent fixed joint deformity and can develop as a consequence of neurologic disorders, for example, frozen shoulder secondary to lack of shoulder movement in hemiplegia. Any asymmetries or change in tone of isolated muscle groups should be noted.

Strength

Evaluation of muscle strength is done systematically and is designed to elicit either generalized or specific weakness. Very few neurologic conditions produce true generalized muscle weakness, with the possible exception of potassium depletion or another metabolic problem. Most diseases are somewhat selective: unilateral in central nervous system upper motor neuron lesions; proximal limb and neck muscle in myopathy, dystrophy, or myositis; distal extremity in peripheral neuropathy and amyotrophic lateral sclerosis; and in a specific muscle group as is demonstrated in a nerve root lesion with disk disease or isolated peripheral nerve lesion from entrapment, trauma, or infarction (e.g., mononeuritis multiplex caused by diabetes, collagen vascular disease). The muscles can be tested by having the patient resist the force provided by the examiner. Adequate force is needed to assess subtle weakness. In patients with a history of bilateral weakness and easy fatigability, suggesting myasthenia, the patient should repetitively exercise one muscle group in an attempt to elicit true fatigability.

Lower leg muscles have been tested under gait evaluation; proximal leg muscles are best tested while observing the patient rise from a chair and with the patient seated or lying down. Walking up stairs, doing a deep knee bend, and rising from kneeling on one knee are excellent tests of proximal muscle strength. With the patient standing, the upper extremity muscles can be readily evaluated. The examination is begun by having the patient stand with feet together, arms extended to 90 degrees in front with palms up. The patient then closes his or her eyes, and the examiner watches the patient's arms for 10 to 15 seconds. In mild hemiparesis the weak arm will pronate and drift downward (pronator drift). Table 1-1 is a simplified chart of muscle testing, with muscle groups, root levels, and peripheral nerves listed. The underlined root is the one principally responsible for the function.

Muscle Bulk and Consistency

The examiner should palpate muscles, particularly any weak muscle in a search for wasting, hypertrophy, or loss of the normal fleshy feeling of the muscle and for muscle tenderness. Muscle bellies should bulge outward. Muscles that are flat or bulge inward indicate wasting of muscles.

Coordination

The performance of a smooth, coordinated movement is a complicated motor task. Successful performance relies on an intact pyramidal system, cerebellum, and basal ganglia and their modulation through proprioceptive and sensory feedback from the lemniscal and vestibular systems. Damage or dysfunction of any portion of the system can produce a defect in coordination. Fortunately, distinctive abnormalities are produced by damage to each structure. During testing, the examiner must carefully compare performance of both sides, making due—but not undue—allowance for the preferred hand. The dominant hand is not necessarily the stronger but clearly is the best coordinated. Box 1-4 outlines a few small tests the patient can do during examination to test coordination.

Spine

The spine is observed for scoliosis. In patients with back pain, the examiner should look for spasm and evaluate mobility. Percussion of spinous processes with a reflex hammer can produce localized or radiating

---

 BOX 1-4

1 *Finger to nose.* The examiner stands with an index finger at arm's length in front of the patient. The patient is asked to touch the examiner's finger with the index finger, then in rapid succession touch his or her nose and return to the examiner's finger. The examiner should look for past-pointing (missing the target consistently to one side), clumsy movement, slowness, tremor (note amplitude, e.g., coarse or fine), and weakness. After several excursions the examiner should move his or her finger and ask the patient to continue the task with a changing target.

2 *Heel/shin (best done with the patient supine).* The patient is asked to place the heel on the opposite knee and then run the heel down the shin. Coarse side-to-side tremor is typical of cerebellar disease.

3 *Finger tapping.* The patient rapidly opposes the index finger to thumb. Speed, clumsiness, maintenance of even rhythm, weakness, and breakdown (taps a few times then is unable to continue because the fingers appear to "stick together") are noted. This further challenges the patient's coordination and can dramatize subtle deficiencies.

4 *Alternating hand movements (diadokokinesia).* The patient is told to rapidly pronate and supinate one hand on the palm of the other. Again, the examiner must look closely for movement breakdown, dysrhythmia, clumsiness, and weakness.

5 *Hand patting and foot tapping.* Note should be made of the rhythm and evenness of the patting.

6 *Circular motion.* The patient is asked to make continuous circular motions with one hand on the back of the other.

TABLE 1-1 Muscle Testing

Action	Muscle(s)
Upper Extremities	
1 Abduct (initial) and external rotation of arm	Supraspinatus, Infraspinatus
2 Abduct arm (hold at 90 degrees against resistance)	Deltoid
3 Flex arm (hand supine)	Biceps
4 Flex arm (hand midway between supine and prone)	Brachioradialis
5 Extend arm	Triceps
6 Extension of wrist	
a Hand abducted (toward thumb)	Extensor carpi radialis longus
b Hand adducted (toward fifth finger)	Extensor carpi ulnaris
7 Flexion of wrist	Flexor carpi radialis
8 Flexion of fingers	Flexor digitorum superficialis (proximal)
	Flexor digitorum profundus (distal)
	a First and second digits
	b Third and fourth digits
9 Palmar abduction of thumb	Abductor pollicis brevis
10 Opposing thumb to base of fifth finger	Opponens pollicis
11 Spreading and adducting fingers	Interossei
Lower Extremities	
1 Flexion of hip	Iliopsoas
2 Extension of hip	Gluteus maximus
3 Adduction of thigh	Adductors
4 Extension of leg (lower)	Quadriceps femoris
5 Flexion of knee	Hamstrings
6 Plantar flexion of foot	Gastrocnemius and Soleus
7 Dorsiflexion of foot	Anterior tibialis
8 Inversion of foot	Posterior tibialis
9 Extension of toes	Extensor digitorum longus and extensor hallucis longus
10 Eversion of foot	Peroneal longus and brevis

Root(s)	Peripheral Nerve
<u>C5</u>,C6	Suprascapular
C5	Axillary
C5,<u>C6</u>	Musculocutaneous
C5,<u>C6</u>	Radial
C7	Radial
C5,<u>C6</u>	Radial
<u>C7</u>,C8	Posterior interosseous
C6,<u>C7</u>	Median
C7,<u>C8</u>,T1	Median
C7,<u>C8</u>	Anterior interosseous
C7,<u>C8</u>	Ulnar
C8,<u>T1</u>*	Median
C8,<u>T1</u>	Median
C8,<u>T1</u>	Ulnar
Lower Extremities	
<u>L1</u>,<u>L2</u>,L3	Direct branches from root
<u>L5</u>,S1	Inferior gluteal
L2,<u>L3</u>,L4	Obturator
L2,<u>L3</u>,<u>L4</u>	Femoral
<u>L5</u>,S1,S2	Sciatic
<u>S1</u>,S2	Tibial
<u>L4</u>,L5	Deep peroneal
L4,<u>L5</u>	Tibial
<u>L5</u>,S1	Deep peroneal
<u>L5</u>,S1	Sciatic

pain in vertebral body disease or root impairment (see Chapter 19).

Skin

The patient's face is observed for butterfly rash, port-wine staining, or adenoma sebaceum; eyelids are examined for heliotrope rash, and elbows and knees are assessed for the erythematous rash of dermato-myositis; the trunk and extremities are checked for café au lait spots or neurofibroma. In addition, the lower spine is examined for a dimple or hair tuft that can indicate spina bifida.

Cranial Nerves

Specific abnormalities in cranial nerve function are demonstrated in many neurologic and systemic medical illnesses. Because of their frequent involvement, all physicians should learn how to examine briefly, yet systematically, the cranial nerves. The examination of the various cranial nerves is outlined, showing the principal function and testing possibilities for these nerves.

First (Olfactory) Nerve

Principal function. Sense of smell (aromatic substances, not strongly irritating ones such as ammonia whose vapor stimulates pain fibers carried by trigeminal nerve). Patients with anosmia also complain of an inability to taste food unless it is highly salted or very sweet.

Testing. The patient closes his or her eyes, occludes one nostril, and then smells some aromatic substance such as cloves, coffee, tobacco, or mild perfume.

Unfortunately, such factors as atrophic or allergic rhinitis, heavy cigarette smoking, or nasal obstruction can interfere with olfaction; therefore the clinical interpretation of anosmia (impaired olfaction) must be made with caution. Olfaction can be abnormal bilaterally in trauma cases. In patients with subfrontal tumors it can be unilaterally or bilaterally abnormal.

Second (Optic) Nerve

Principal function. Vision.

Testing. Several aspects of the second cranial nerve can be assessed:

1   *Visual acuity.* Acuity should be tested in each eye individually and is most practically done at near point (14 cm) with a hand card. Normal vision is 20/15, not 20/20.

2   *Visual fields.* These are most easily tested with the patient facing the examiner; with one eye covered, the patient is asked to focus on the examiner's pupil. A cotton-tipped applicator or hat pin is brought into the periphery of the patient's field until the patient reports first seeing it. The object should be brought in from all quadrants (1:30, 4:30, 7:30, and 10:30 clock positions) to identify partial as well as full-field defects. An alternate method is to simultaneously flash varying numbers of fingers in two fields (e.g., the examiner briefly shows two fingers in the left and right inferior temporal fields) and to ask the patient how many total fingers were seen. If the patient can adequately fix on the examiner's pupil, it is possible to move the object through the entire field of vision and roughly map out the patient's blind spot (the point at which the optic nerve enters the retina) and any scotoma that may be present.

3   *Funduscopy.* With the ophthalmoscope, the heads of the optic nerve, retina, macula, and retinal vessels can all be visualized. Papilledema, usually

secondary to increased intracranial pressure, is the most important sign to search for on funduscopy. The earliest feature of papilledema is the loss of spontaneous pulsations in the veins entering the optic disc. As pressure increases, the veins engorge and become tortuous, disc margins blur, and the optic cup is lost. Finally, the disc elevates, margins are gone, and flame hemorrhages appear in the retina. Visual acuity is relatively spared despite the markedly abnormal appearance of the disc.

A second important disc abnormality to note is optic atrophy. Atrophy is characterized by a small, pale, sharply marginated disc with a decrease in the number of traversing capillaries. In the early stage, temporal pallor may be all that is seen.

4 *Pupillary light reflex.* The afferent limb of this reflex is the second nerve. In optic nerve disease or damage, the light reflex is sluggish or absent. If the light reflex is absent in one eye and the efferent limb via the third nerve is intact, a normal consensual reflex should be present when light is shone into the opposite eye. When the light is swung back to the eye with the damaged second nerve, however, a paradoxic dilation of the pupil occurs (Marcus Gunn phenomenon).

Third (Oculomotor), Fourth (Trochlear), and Sixth (Abducens) Nerves

Principal functions. Ocular rotation, lid elevation (third nerve), and pupillary constriction (third nerve).

Testing.

1 *Ocular rotation.* There are six extraocular muscles, and for many eye movements, groups of muscles work in concert to achieve the desired

degree of ocular rotation. However, the examiner wishes to examine each muscle in isolation to determine which nerve or muscle is dysfunctional. Doing so requires a certain knowledge of the origin and insertion of the muscles and their innervation. The four rectus muscles (medial, superior, inferior innervated by the third nerve, and lateral rectus innervated by the sixth nerve) originate from their corresponding quadrants of the eye and insert in the posterior portion of the orbit at a 23-degree angle nasally from the midline of the globe. The oblique muscles (inferior oblique innervated by the third nerve and the superior oblique innervated by the fourth nerve) originate posteriorly on the globe and pull at a 51-degree angle nasally from the midline (Figures 1-2 and 1-3). To test ocular rotation, the examiner should note any muscle imbalance with the patient looking straight ahead. Next, ocular rotation of each eye separately is tested. First, abduction (pure lateral rectus—sixth nerve) is tested by having the patient follow the examiner's finger laterally. Then, with the patient's eyes in 20-degree to 25-degree lateral gaze, the patient is asked to look up (superior rectus—third), then down (inferior rectus—third), and then adduct the eye (medial rectus—third). Finally, with the eye adducted 50 to 55 degrees, the patient is asked to look up (inferior oblique—third) and then down (superior oblique—fourth).

2 *Lid retraction.* The levator of the upper eyelid is innervated by the third nerve, and a significant lid droop (ptosis) is often caused by a third-nerve paresis. Ptosis can also be seen in lesions of the sympathetic nerves that innervate the superior tarsal muscle.

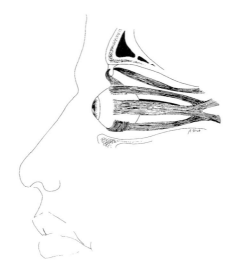

FIGURE 1-2. Attachments of the extraocular muscles. *From Cogan DC:* Neurology of the ocular muscles, *Springfield, Ill, 1948, Charles C Thomas. Copyright 1948 by Charles C Thomas. Adapted by permission.*

3 *Pupils.* First, pupils are observed for regularity and symmetry. The most common cause of unequal pupils (anisocoria) is congenital and clinically insignificant. Next, light reflex, both direct and consensual, is checked by shining a bright light directly into the pupil. The response to light should be brisk; if it is not, a second-nerve (consensual reflex present in eye *without* light reflex) or third-nerve (consensual reflex absent in eye with *absent* light reflex) lesion should be suspected.

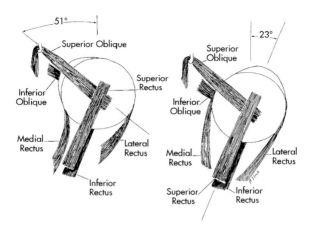

FIGURE 1-3. *Illustration on right*—Right eye. A 23-degree lateral rotation in the horizontal plane, the superior rectus acts as a pure elevator and the inferior rectus as a pure depressor. *Illustration on left*—Right eye. At 51 degrees medial rotation in the horizontal plane, the action of the superior oblique is pure depression and that of the inferior oblique is pure elevation. *From Cogan DC:* Neurology of the ocular muscles, *Springfield, Ill, 1948, Charles C Thomas. Copyright 1948 by Charles C Thomas. Adapted by permission.*

4 *Abnormal spontaneous eye movements.* While testing ocular rotation and observing pupils, the examiner can look for nystagmus or other abnormal spontaneous movements. Nystagmus is described in relation to the rapid phase and position of gaze (e.g., right beating nystagmus on right lateral gaze).

5 *Convergence.* The patient is asked to follow the examiner's finger to the tip of the patient's nose; both convergence and accommodation reflex (pupillary constriction) should be noted.

Fifth (Trigeminal) Nerve

Principal function. Control of the muscles of mastication and sensation of the face, anterior half of the scalp, meninges above the tentorium, and mucous membranes of mouth, nose, and sinuses.

Testing.

1   Muscles of mastication are evaluated by palpation of masseter and temporalis muscles in a relaxed state and with the teeth clenched. The examiner should look for atrophy and poor contraction and ask the patient to open his or her mouth to see if the jaw deviates (with unilateral weakness there is deviation toward the weak side). Finally, strength of lateral jaw motion is checked (weakness of the pterygoids is reflected in an inability to move the jaw to the side opposite the weak muscles).

2   The sensory portion of the fifth nerve has three divisions: ophthalmic (forehead and upper eyelid), maxillary (upper lip and cheek bone), and mandibular (chin and along the jaw line not including the angle). Sensory fibers from the ophthalmic division also supply the cornea.

3   The corneal reflex is tested. The fifth nerve is the afferent limb of this reflex, and the seventh (facial) nerve is the efferent limb. The reflex is tested by touching the cornea with a wisp of cotton in such a way that the patient does not see the stimulus before it touches the cornea. The reflex, integrated in the pons, consists of brisk bilateral eye closure. The bilateral nature of the reflex is important when assessing the integrity of corneal sensation in patients with facial paralysis on the side being tested. In such cases the contralateral blink attests to the adequacy of corneal sensation.

Seventh (Facial) Nerve

Principal function. Control of muscles of facial expression.

Associated function. Running with the seventh nerve are autonomic fibers that control tearing, the tone of the stapedius muscle, taste to the anterior two thirds of the tongue, and secretions of submaxillary and sublingual salivary glands. With peripheral seventh-nerve lesions, these functions can be disturbed.

Testing. Evaluation of facial muscles involves observing the face at rest and in action. The patient is asked to smile, close the eyes, then open the eyes widely and wrinkle the forehead. Any asymmetry should be noted (many patients have mild congenital facial asymmetry, which can suggest unilateral facial weakness). The patient is asked to slightly extend the neck and frown deeply. This causes the seventh nerve–innervated platysma to contract. If the facial asymmetry is due to facial weakness, the platysma will be less prominent on the involved side. Subtle weakness can often be elicited by forcibly trying to open the eyes against effort. If facial weakness is found, the examiner should critically evaluate frontalis muscle strength. In central lesions such as a cortical stroke (supranuclear or upper motor neuron lesion), the forehead moves equally on both sides, whereas with lesions in the nucleus or in the peripheral nerve (infranuclear, lower motor neuron, or peripheral seventh nerve lesion), the frontalis is weak on the side of the lesion. However, partial or recovering peripheral lesions can show good forehead movement and simulate a supranuclear lesion.

Eighth (Acoustic) Nerve

Principal functions. Hearing and vestibular function.

Testing.

1 *Auditory.* The neurologist is most concerned with neural hearing loss, particularly unilateral. A screening examination can be done at the bedside by comparing the patient's hearing with the examiner's (assuming that it is normal). Each ear is tested separately. First, the examiner simply rubs his or her fingers together near the ear; then a tuning fork is used. If differences are found in hearing between patient's ears or between those of the patient and the examiner, bone conduction comparison (again, with patient's and examiner's hearing) is performed to assess sensorineural function. An actively vibrating tuning fork is placed on the bregma (Weber test); with normal hearing, the patient will report equal sound in both ears or on top of the head. Sound that is lateralized to one side indicates either a conductive loss on that side or a neural loss on the opposite side.

The Rinne test (vibrating fork is placed on mastoid process, and, when the patient no longer hears the sound, the vibrating end of the fork is held to the ear) is used to compare bone conduction with air conduction in hearing. Normally air conduction is better, but in patients with a conduction hearing loss (e.g., otosclerosis), bone conduction will be better. If any abnormalities are found, a complete audiometric evaluation should be carried out.

2 *Vestibular.* Vestibular testing is usually only performed if the patient complains of dizziness or unsteady gait. Evaluation of dizziness is discussed at length in Chapter 4.

Ninth (Glossopharyngeal) Nerve

Principal function. Supply of sensation to pharynx, tonsillar fossa, and taste to the posterior one third of the tongue.

Testing. Because of its close anatomic and functional relationship with the tenth nerve, these two nerves are often tested together.

1 The patient's pharynx or tonsil is touched with tongue blade or cotton-tipped applicator.
2 The examiner asks if the patient feels the touch and observes a gag response.
3 Both sides are tested, and any asymmetry of response is noted.

Tenth (Vagus) Nerve

Principal functions.

1 Motor to pharynx, palate, and larynx
2 Parasympathetics to thoracic and abdominal viscera
3 Visceral sensation

Only motor control of pharynx, palate, and larynx is of importance in the clinical neurologic examination.

Testing.

1 The patient's palate is observed for asymmetry or droop.
2 Palate movement is noted with the patient phonating to see if both sides elevate evenly. The uvula will deviate to the normal side.
3 Motor response to stimulation during gag reflex testing is observed.
4 Hoarseness or dysphonia is sought; this can be caused by vocal cord paralysis from a tenth-nerve lesion.
5 The patient is asked to produce a high squeaking sound; this requires very close vocal cord adduction and cord tension and can only be performed

if both recurrent and superior laryngeal branches of the tenth nerve are functioning properly.

6 If there is any suggestion of weakness or inadequacy of the pharynx or palate control, it is advisable to watch the patient swallow some water to see if the swallowing mechanism is smooth and that no regurgitation is present.

Eleventh (Spinal Accessory) Nerve

Principal functions. Turn head (sternocleidomastoids) and assist in shrugging the shoulders (upper trapezius).
Testing.

1 Examiner should place his or her hands on the patient's shoulders and have the patient shrug the shoulders against pressure. The bulk and strength of the upper portion of the trapezius muscles are noted.

2 With the examiner's hand held on the side of the patient's chin, the patient is asked to rotate the head against that hand. Head turning to the right is accomplished by the left sternocleidomastoid and to the left by the right sternocleidomastoid.

Twelfth (Hypoglossal) Nerve

Principal function. Innervation of intrinsic muscles of the tongue.
Testing.

1 With the patient's tongue relaxed in the mouth, atrophy or fasciculations are sought.

2 The patient is asked to protrude the tongue and move it from side to side. The tongue will deviate toward the weak side. The seventh nerve innervates some muscles of the mouth, and some tongue deviation can accompany facial muscle weakness.

3 If weakness is suspected, the patient is asked to press the tongue as hard as possible against the

buccal mucosa while the examiner presses against the cheek. In this fashion it is possible to compare relative strength of the two sides of the tongue. This tests intrinsic tongue muscle strength without interference from facial muscles.

Carotid Arteries

Cerebral vascular disease is a major medical illness, and a high percentage of that disease is found in the extracranial portions of the carotid arteries. Because of this and because surgery of the carotid vessels may control the symptoms of vascular disease, a routine neurologic examination should include an examination of the carotid arteries in all patients.

Initially the examiner gently palpates (one at a time) the common carotids in the neck and compares the strength of the pulse. Then external carotid vessels in the face (temporal, facial, nasal, and infraorbital) are also palpated. In marked internal carotid stenosis or occlusion, the external carotid vessels will often demonstrate exaggerated pulses. Finally, the examiner should auscultate the carotid artery along its course from the angle of the jaw to the base of the neck; in patients with substantial narrowing, a high-pitched bruit can often be heard. The carotid bruit must be differentiated from a referred murmur from the heart or venous hum by auscultating at many points along the course of the vessel.

Reflex Examination

Three principal types of reflexes should be tested.

Muscle Stretch Reflexes

Muscle stretch reflexes, often called deep tendon reflexes, are tested when the examiner rapidly stretches a muscle, usually by striking the tendon with a reflex hammer, and observes the character and intensity of the resultant muscle contraction. The reflex arc is segmental within the spinal cord but is highly influenced by descending inhibitory pathways, particularly the corticospinal tracts. Damage to the upper motor neurons (i.e., cortical motor neurons) or their axons in the brain stem and spinal cord will cause a release of inhibitory influence and thus produce hyperactivity of the muscle stretch reflex. Damage to the lower motor neurons (i.e., the anterior horn cells in the spinal cord) or their axons to the muscle will abolish the activity of the reflex. Because of this effect on reflexes by focal damage in the nervous system, the muscle stretch reflexes are very useful in localization.

A great deal of variation in the activity of reflexes exists in normal people; therefore there is no specific clinical significance to the fact that a patient has hypoactive (0 or 1+) or brisk (3+) reflexes, including brief bursts of repetitive contractions (*un*sustained clonus). The important observations to make in reference to the reflexes are listed here:

- Are they pathologically hyperactive (sustained clonus [4+] present)?
- Is there an asymmetry between the reflexes on the two sides of the body?
- Is there a specific rostral-caudal disparity (e.g., reflexes hyperactive in the legs and less so in the arms, suggesting spinal cord disease) or is there loss of ankle reflexes (often knee reflexes as well) as seen in peripheral neuropathy?
- Is there a loss of a specific reflex such as the ankle jerk on one side, indicating an S1 nerve-root lesion or a sciatic nerve lesion?

In testing the reflex, the examiner should start with a gentle tap and then increase the force with each tap.

In this way, both a threshold for the reflex and the degree of response can be evaluated. Variation in the intensity of response can occur; therefore it is wise therefore, to elicit the reflex several times to appreciate fully its level of activity. If the reflex cannot be obtained, reinforcement is used by having the patient maximally contract other muscles (such as a Jendrassik maneuver in which the patient is asked to flex the arms and tightly interlock the fingers, and then try to pull the two hands apart) while the reflex is being elicited. Reflexes should always be tested in pairs (e.g., right and left biceps, right and left knees) so that ready comparisons can be made.

Jaw jerk (masseter reflex). The jaw jerk is tested by having the patient partially open the mouth. The examiner presses down lightly on the patient's chin with the index finger and gently strikes the finger with a reflex hammer. This stretches the muscles of mastication. The reflex is integrated through the mandibular branch of the trigeminal nerve in the pons. The major importance of this reflex is to decide if a patient with pathologic hyperreflexia in the limbs has a lesion in the upper spinal cord or bilateral lesions in the brain. If the jaw reflex is hyperactive, it favors a brain lesion; but if it is normal, it suggests an upper cord lesion.

Biceps. The patient's arm is bent 60 to 90 degrees. With the patient's arm at rest, the examiner places an index finger on the tendon at its insertion point and strikes the finger to elicit the stretch. The reflex, flexion of the arm, is integrated through the fifth and sixth cervical roots, principally the sixth.

Brachioradialis. With the patient's arm in the same position as with the biceps reflex, the examiner strikes the radius above the wrist and notes arm flexion and finger flexion. The fifth and sixth cervical roots provide innervation via the radial nerve.

Triceps. With the patient's arm flexed, the examiner directly strikes the triceps tendon at its insertion point above the elbow. The response is extension of the arm. The reflex is integrated through the sixth, seventh, and eighth (principally the seventh) cervical roots via the radial nerve.

Finger flexion. The patient rests the fingertips (palms down) on the examiner's fingers. The examiner should strike his or her own fingers and observe the patient's fingers and thumb for flexion. This flexion can also be elicited by holding the patient's middle finger, with wrist dorsiflexed, and flicking the distal phalanx (Hoffmann reflex). This, in effect, stretches the flexor muscles of the fingers. The reflex is integrated through the eighth cervical segment and is considered hyperactive (although not necessarily pathologic) when there is thumb flexion. The Hoffmann reflex is not the upper extremity equivalent of the Babinski sign.

Patellar (knee jerk). The patient is seated with legs dangling freely. The examiner strikes the patellar tendon directly and notes leg extension as the quadriceps muscle contracts. This reflex can be reinforced by having the patient clasp the hands together and then try to pull them apart. The reflex is integrated by second, third, and fourth lumbar segments via the femoral nerve. If the patient cannot sit, a pillow can be placed under the knees with the patient supine so that the legs are slightly bent.

Achilles (ankle jerk). The examiner should passively dorsiflex the patient's foot slightly and then strike the tendon. The response of plantar flexion is due to contraction of gastrocnemius and soleus muscles and is integrated through the first and second (primarily the first) sacral segments via the tibial branch of the sciatic nerve. This reflex can be reinforced by having the patient push the foot lightly down against the examiner's hand. When any stretch reflex, but particularly the Achilles reflex, is pathologically hyperactive (4+), clonus can be elicited. Clonus is an oscillation of contraction between the agonist and antagonist muscles of a joint. For example, in ankle clonus, if the examiner stretches the gastrocnemius muscle by quickly dorsiflexing the foot, that muscle rapidly and forcibly contracts, thus plantar flexing the foot. In doing so, the dorsiflexors of the foot (the anterior tibial muscles) are quickly stretched, and they contract, dorsiflexing the foot again. Because of the hypersensibility of the stretch reflex in these muscles, sustained oscillating contractions (i.e., clonus) are established.

Superficial Reflexes

Superficial reflexes are elicited by lightly stroking the skin and observing contraction of the underlying muscle (innervated by the same spinal segment). The reflex will be absent if there is an upper motor neuron lesion above the level of the segment tested.

Abdominal. The abdominal skin is stroked with a broken applicator stick (or similar sharp object); a swift stroke is used, starting in either the upper (T8-9) or lower (T10-12) outer quadrant and going toward the umbilicus. The reflex quickly fatigues and can be absent in obese persons, the elderly, or women who have had children or patients after abdominal surgery. Deep abdominal reflexes are elicited by pressing down on the muscles and striking the hand with the reflex hammer; these reflexes can be hyperactive when the superficial abdominal skin reflexes are absent.

Cremasteric. The inner aspect of the thigh is stroked and observed for retraction of the testis. Innervation is through the first and second lumbar segments via the ilioinguinal and genitofemoral nerves.

Pathologic or Release Reflexes

Pathologic reflexes are normally found in infants but disappear in the first or second year. With cortical damage in the child or adult, the reflexes return and are useful in diagnosing and localizing central nervous system damage.

Babinski sign or extensor toe sign. The sole of the foot is stroked with a relatively sharp object. This is a nociceptive (pain) reflex; therefore a sharp object is used to stimulate the reflex. The examiner strokes up the lateral side of the foot and then across the ball of the foot to the base of the great toe. A normal response is toe flexion. A pathologic response is extension of the great toe and flaring of the other toes. A positive Babinski sign is always abnormal in patients over age 3 and is the cardinal sign of pyramidal tract disorder.

Thumb adduction (Wartenberg hand sign). The patient and examiner flex distal phalanges, hook their fingers together, and pull against each other's fingertips. Normally the thumb should fix in an abducted position, but in pyramidal tract disease the thumb will adduct across the palm in a simian grasp.

Snout or rooting reflex. The examiner presses or taps on the upper lip. Normally there is no response. An abnormal response consists of pursing and protruding the lips. In marked examples merely touching the cheek or corner of the mouth will elicit the response (rooting).

Grasp reflex. The examiner should rub his or her fingers against the patient's relaxed palm or in the web between the thumb and first finger. An abnormal response consists of the patient's uncontrolled forced grasping of the examiner's finger despite instructions to the contrary. This reflex is usually the last of the so-called frontal release signs to show up; therefore its presence usually indicates significant pathology.

Palmomental reflex. Stroking the thenar entrance with a sharp object will elicit in many patients a twitch of the mentalis muscle of the chin. Unfortunately, this reflex is so commonly seen in the normal population, especially over age 65, that it is usually of little clinical use unless it is asymmetric.

Glabellar reflex. The examiner repeatedly taps the glabellar area lightly with a reflex hammer. The normal patient will blink the eyes several times and then accommodate to the stimulus and stop blinking. Patients with Parkinson's disease or demented persons with diffuse cerebral atrophy tend not to accommodate and will continue blinking as long as the examiner taps.

Sensation

Accurate evaluation of the sensory system requires full patient cooperation and careful instruction by the examiner. The examiner should carefully explain what is going to be done and what the patient should report. The examiner must also have a distinct plan when starting the sensory examination. If the patient has arm pain and the goal of the sensory examination is to determine if the patient has impingement on a nerve root by an extruded cervical disk, the examiner must systematically evaluate the dermatomes in that arm and compare sensation, both in the corresponding dermatomes on the opposite side and with the contiguous dermatomes in the same arm. Testing should be as brief as possible because exhaustive attempts to map out patterns of loss frquently tire and confuse the patient and leave the examiner with an unclear picture.

The sensory examination, like the reflex examination, can provide very useful localizing information:

- Unilateral sensory loss in contralateral central lesions
- Distal loss in extremities in peripheral neuropathies
- Specific dermatomal loss in root lesions
- Specific peripheral patterns in individual peripheral nerve lesions
- Specific level of lesion with spinal cord lesions
- Crossed (ipsilateral face and contralateral body) caused by brain stem lesions

Although many modalities can be tested, there are three main aspects to the sensory system as tested clinically: pinprick sensation, which is pure spinothalamic sensation (temperature is usually not tested routinely because the temperature system parallels pinprick sensation); position and vibration senses, which are almost pure lemniscal sensations (posterior columns); and stereognosis, graphesthesia, and touch localization, which are integrative sensations and are primarily cortical. These cortical sensations are often difficult to assess if primary sensations are impaired. Touch sensation is a complex sensation that is partially lemniscal and partially spinothalamic but can be very useful in localization.

Testing. It is always best to test patients with their eyes closed. The types of sensation tests given are listed in Box 1-5.

Meningeal Irritation

If there is any suggestion of an intracranial hemorrhage or meningeal infection, the patient's nuchal mobility should be tested. The patient lies supine and completely relaxed. The examiner passively flexes the

BOX 1-5

1 *Pin.* The pin is stuck lightly one or two times in each area tested. First the examiner asks if the patient feels the sensation and whether it is sharp. Then the patient is asked to compare the initial stick with a second set of sticks in the opposite side or in a contiguous area. If normal (unaffected) areas are worth 100 cents, the patient is asked to state how much the opposite-side homologous areas are worth. The pin is applied once on each side to avoid a temporal summation effect. If the response is abnormal, the examiner should reverse the order in which the stimulus is applied for confirmation because sometimes in normals the second stimulus is perceived as sharper. Figure 1-4 is a guide to localization of root lesions, and Table 1-2 indicates the most consistent location with least overlap to test for each root or peripheral nerve. There is considerable variation in the distribution of peripheral nerves; thus these are to be used as guides only.

2 *Touch.* Touch can be tested with a cotton swab or light fingertip touch.

3 *Proprioception.* Position is most easily tested using the great toe and distal phalanx of the thumb or other finger. The digit is grasped on the sides and moved through a very short excursion either up or down. Even the slightest movement of a finger should be detected. If the toe or finger is pulled up or pushed down in exaggerated fashion, subtle defects will be missed.

4 *Vibration.* The 128-cps tuning fork is probably the best to use for testing vibration sense. The test is done over bony prominences. This sensation is normally more acute proximally and tends to diminish distally in the elderly.

5 *Stereognosis.* Several small familiar objects are placed in the patient's hand, one at a time. The patient is asked to manipulate the object in the hand, and then identify it. Right side should be compared with left side.

6 *Graphesthesia.* The examiner writes numbers on the patient's palm and asks the patient to identify them.

neck. Any pain or resistance should raise suspicion that the meninges are irritated. When flexing the neck the examiner should observe the patient's legs; in meningitis the patient (particularly a child) will flex

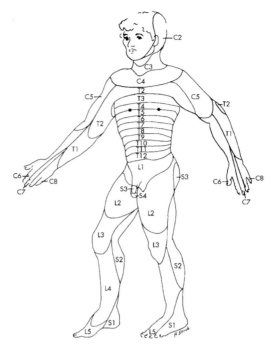

FIGURE 1-4. Sensory distribution.

his or her thighs (Brudzinski sign). Another sign of meningeal irritation is the Kernig sign. In this sign the patient's thigh is flexed on his or her chest, and then the leg is extended; this stretches the meninges, and, if they are inflamed, the patient will report pain and flex his or her neck.

Autonomic Evaluation

In any patient with bowel or bladder symptoms, a rectal examination should be performed. Tone, degree of voluntary contraction of the sphincter, as well as perianal sensation should be noted.

TABLE 1-2 Sensory Localization

Location	Root	Peripheral Nerve
1 Over deltoid muscle	C5*	Axillary*
2 Volar surface distal thumb	C6*	Median
3 Volar surface index finger	C6*	Median*
4 Volar surface middle finger (side toward thumb)	C7*	Median
5 Dorsal surface hand over base of thumb and index finger	C7*	Radial*
6 Volar surface of little finger	C8*	Ulnar*
7 Inner surface of forearm	T1	T1 root
8 Inner surface of upper arm	T2	T2 root
9 Lateral thigh	L2	Lateral femoral cutaneous*
10 Anterior thigh above knee	L3,L4	Femoral*
11 Medial leg (mid-calf level)	L4	Saphenous
12 Dorsal web between great toe	L5*	Deep peroneal* and second toe
13 Lateral foot	S1*	Sural
14 Lateral foot and posterolateral leg	S1,S2	Sciatic
15 Anterolateral leg	L5	Common peroneal

*Indicates that the location tested is almost exclusively innervated by the nerve or root starred.

In patients with syncope, particularly with rapid change in position, blood pressure and pulse should be taken in supine, sitting, and standing positions. Note is made of appearance of symptoms and change in pressure. In dysautonomia, the pressure drops dramatically, yet there is no compensatory tachycardia.

Summary of Examination

At first this examination seems lengthy; with experience the student will learn to perform the many steps rapidly and modify the examination to suit each patient. The complete examination can be performed in 15 to 20 minutes, depending on the patient.

Neurologic Localization

Based on the pattern of the abnormal signs elicited by the examination, the physician must consider if a lesion is localized. The examination findings should indicate if the lesion is unilateral, bilateral, cerebral, spinal, peripheral, or muscular. The clinical sections of this book will discuss the various findings relevant to the different conditions. Box 1-6 is a brief summary of patterns of findings.

Mechanism of Neurologic Disorders

If the onset of symptoms is sudden, vascular or electric disorders (seizures with abnormal cortical discharges) should be considered. Vascular disorders are characterized by loss of function (hemiplegia, hemianesthesia, visual field loss). Seizures are characterized by neuronal hyperactivity (e.g., myoclonic jerks, paresthesias, flashing lights) or impairment of consciousness caused by disturbed reticular formation function. In most patients with vascular disorders, there is rapid stabilization with gradual neurologic improvement. The patient with seizures usually recovers rapidly; however, there can be postictal paralysis (Todd's paralysis).

If the onset of symptoms is less acute, atrophic or mass lesions are suggested. In atrophic disorders there is slow progression over months to years, usually with no plateaus of stabilization. In mass lesions the tempo of progression is more rapid than with atrophic lesions. There is continued worsening, or new symptoms develop. Mass lesions in the brain usually also cause signs of increased intracranial pressure.

▨ SUMMARY

The neurologic history and examination are highly specialized yet not complicated when a systematic

BOX 1-6   **Common Patterns of Abnormal Neurologic Signs**

Cerebral Hemisphere Lesion (e.g., cerebrovascular accident or tumor)

Contralateral weakness, incoordination, sensory loss, increased tone in body and face. Possible visual field loss but no diplopia. Reflexes increased in affected side with positive Babinski and Hoffmann signs. Can have mental status changes, e.g., aphasia, with left hemisphere lesions.

Spinal Cord (e.g., spondylosis with myelopathy)

Cranial nerves normal. Weakness and increased tone and reflexes below the lesion. Babinskis are present, bowel and bladder function can be impaired.

Radiculopathy Secondary to Ruptured Disk

Weakness, decreased sensation, and decreased reflex in the distribution of the nerve root affected.

Mononeuropathy (e.g., carpal tunnel syndrome—median nerve entrapment in the wrist)

Weakness, sensory loss in distribution of that nerve. Reflex will be down if the nerve supplies a muscle involved in one of the major reflex arcs.

Peripheral Neuropathy (e.g., diabetic)

Decreased sensation and decreased reflexes in distal legs. Weakness in distal muscles will occur as the disease progresses.

Myopathy or Myositis

Weakness of proximal muscles of arms and legs without reflex and sensory changes.

---

approach is used. The examination itself usually takes only 15 to 20 minutes, unless full mental status testing is carried out.

Data from the history and examination will usually localize the disease within the nervous system and can often allow the examiner to make a specific clinical diagnosis.

Suggested Readings

Aids to the examination of the peripheral nervous system. Medical Research Council, Memorandum No. 45, London, Her Majesty's Stationery Office.

Alpers BJ, Mancall EL: *Essentials of neurological examination,* ed 2, Philadelphia, 1981, FA Davis.

Cogan DC: *Neurology of the ocular muscles,* Springfield, Ill, 1948, Charles C Thomas.

Dejong RN: *The neurologic examination,* ed. 4, New York, 1979, Harper & Row.

Haymaker W, Woodhall B: *Peripheral nerve injuries,* Philadelphia, 1953, WB Saunders.

Massey EW, Plect AB, Scherokman BJ: *Diagnostic tests in neurology,* Chicago, 1985, Year Book Medical Publishers.

Simpson JF, Magee KR: *Clinical evaluation of the nervous system,* Boston, 1973, Little, Brown.

Strub RL, Black FW: *The mental status examination in neurology,* ed 3, Philadelphia, 1993, FA Davis.

Neurodiagnostic Studies

2

After assessment of patient's symptomatology and neurologic findings, diagnostic studies are performed to confirm clinical impressions. The studies will delineate the presence and location of the neurologic lesion causing the neurologic dysfunction and sometimes delineate the pathologic characteristics of the lesion. To use these studies most effectively, the physician must be aware of methodology, parameters being measured, sensitivity, specificity, indications, contraindications, and risks (Table 2-1).

SKULL AND SPINE ROENTGENOGRAPHY

Skull and spine roentgenograms provide visual representation of intracranial and vertebral distribution of crystallized calcium, and this is displayed on photographic plates. These studies have good spatial resolution with limited contrast resolution. They are ideal for visualizing bone detail. Certain normally calcified structures (e.g., pineal body vertebral bodies) are frequently demonstrated, as are some types of pathological calcification (e.g., neoplasm, angioma). With

TABLE 2-1 Diagnostic Study Use

Study	Parameter Measured
Roentgenogram	Distribution of calcium in head and spine
Electroencephalogram	Surface cortical electrical activity
Cranial ultrasound	Brain acoustical densities
Lumbar puncture	Cellular, chemical, and blood vessel wall morphology of extracranial carotid arteries
Doppler duplex Carotid imaging	Blood flow velocity and blood vessel wall morphology of extracranial carotid arteries
Transcranial doppler ultrasound	Blood flow velocity of major intra-cranial carotid vertebrobasilar arteries
Conventional catheter angiography	Water-soluble iodinated material creates artificial contrast with image extra- and intracranial l blood vessels
Myelography	Iodinated contrast with outline spinal cord and nerve roots—use lumbar puncture
Computed tomography	Distribution of electron densities of brain and spinal cord tissue
Magnetic resonance imaging	Distribution of H^+ ion in brain and spinal cord tissue
Position emission tomography	Distribution of positrons to determine brain blood flow, oxygen, and glucose metabolism
Nerve conduction velocity	Measurement of integrity of myelin sheath
Electromyogram	Electrical characteristics of muscle
Evoked potentials	Summated brain wave after visual, auditory, or sensory stimulation

Clinical Indication	Potential Risk
Trauma Bone lesion	Radiation exposure
Seizure disorder Sleep disorder	None
Pediatric brain disorders in place of CT or MRI as equipment can be brought to bedside	None
Meningitis Subarachnoid hemorrhage Neurosyphilis Multiple sclerosis	Post-LP headache Cerebral herniation
Asymptomatic carotid stenosis TIA Stroke	None
Subarachnoid hemorrhage and vasospasm Stroke	None
TIA Stroke Aneurysm Vascular malformation Venous occlusion Tumor vascularity	Death Stroke Myocardial infarction Puncture hematoma Iodide toxicity
Spinal cord mass	Iodide toxicity
Herniated disc	Meningitis Arachnoiditis
Brain and spinal lesion	Radiation exposure
Brain and spinal lesion More sensitive than CT in epilepsy, MS, ischemic stroke	If patient has cardiac pacemaker or surgical metallic clips or is claustrophobic, cannot be performed
Research technique to measure brain physiology in stroke, epilepsy, dementia, and functional psychiatric disorders	Positrons are generated from cyclotron (limited availability)
Neuropathy	Minimal electrical shock—slightly painful, but not dangerous
Suspected peripheral nerve, anterior horn cell, or muscle disease	Needle inserted in muscle causes discomfort
Optic nerve disease, MS, spinal cord lesion	None

certain modifications in technique, it is possible to visualize one specific thin section of the cranium and blur out intervening structures (geometric or conventional tomography). This enhances the ability to focus on bone detail in one particular region. For example, if an area of calcification appears in the sella region, tomography will demonstrate if this is located within or external (lateral) to sella. Because of the limited contrast resolution, normal intracranial and spinal structures (e.g., brain parenchyma, spinal cord, cerebrospinal fluid [CSF] spaces) are not visualized.

Indications for skull roentgenograms include suspicion of skull fracture in head trauma, suspicion of juxtasellar lesion (endocrine and visual disturbances) to determine sella abnormalities (e.g., enlargement, erosion, calcification), systemic neoplasm with possible occurrence of skull involvement (osteolytic, osteoblastic), and suspicion of intracranial mass lesion to determine position of midline pineal gland, evidence of abnormal calcification, bone change, or sella turcica erosion (Figure 2-1). A complete skull roentgenographic series includes four views (both laterals, anteroposterior, and posteroanterior). Special radiographic projections and tomograms are used to investigate the following: for optic nerve lesions, optic foramen views are necessary; for cerebellopontine angle lesions, internal acoustic canal tomograms are necessary; for lesions of foramen magnum or skull base, craniovertebral junction views are necessary; and for juxtasellar lesions, sella turcica tomography is necessary.

Roentgenograms of the spine are used to visualize bony encasement of the spinal cord in patients with symptoms of spinal root (radiculopathy) or spinal cord (myelopathy) compression. These films are indicated to assess conditions of congenital, degenerative,

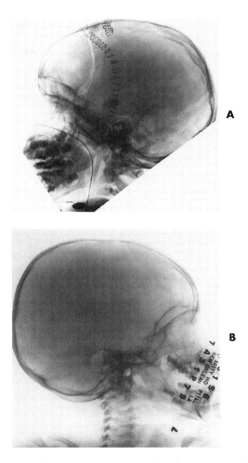

FIGURE 2-1. **A,** Skull roentgenogram showing postoperative defect and surgical clips in a patient with an enlarged sella turcica and suprasellar calcification caused by a craniopharyngioma. **B,** Normal skull roentgenogram with normal-size sella turcica.

neoplastic, traumatic, or infectious etiology. Antero-posterior and lateral views are usually adequate to examine the spine; however, if a herniated disk with neural compression is suspected, oblique projections are necessary to delineate neural foramina through which spinal nerve roots emerge. The major limitation of spine roentgenography is that it does not have sufficient resolution to visualize neural structures, non-calcified soft tissue structures (intervertebral disk, ligaments, spinal cord, spinal nerve roots), or subarachnoid spaces. To define the presence of spinal cord and nerve root abnormalities (e.g., herniated intervertebral disk, spinal cord tumors) myelography, spinal computed tomography (CT), or magnetic resonance imaging (MRI) is necessary. In addition, isotope bone scanning is more sensitive than spine roentgenography to detect certain types of neoplastic or inflammatory bone involvement (e.g., metastases, multiple myeloma, osteomyelitis).

▨ ELECTROENCEPHALOGRAPHY

Multiple electrodes are attached to the patient's scalp. These electrodes sample surface cerebral electrical activity and amplify and record summated potentials of the cerebral cortex. There is a normal pattern for awake and sleep states. Brain lesions can alter the frequency, amplitude, and pattern of brain waves; however, the location of maximal electrical abnormality may not correlate with the precise location of the lesion; for example, temporal neoplasm can cause maximal slow wave discharge in the frontal or parietal region. Electrical activity is sampled in a standard pattern of connections (montages) that represent both hemispheres. Electrical activity generated by the brain varies in frequency and amplitude in different regions. Normally there is a basic symmetrical frequency of

8 to 13 cps. This is maximal in the occipital region and referred to as alpha rhythm. In the frontal region there is a symmetric, more rapid (14 to 30 cps) and lower amplitude beta rhythm. If the patient is aroused by external stimulation (e.g., calling patient's name), there is a change from the alpha rhythm to lower voltage rapid frequency; this is the arousal response. The awake state shows specific electroencephalographic (EEG) findings, and there are characteristic patterns in sleep state (see Chapter 23). Specific responses can also be induced by hyperventilation and photic stimulation and are important to determine in patients with suspected seizure disorders.

Abnormal electrical potentials are recorded as slow waves or spike discharges; these can occur in either a generalized or a focal distribution (Figure 2-2). Superficial cortical lesions are more likely to be detected than deeply located lesions (thalamus or basal ganglia); infratentorial (brain stem or cerebellum) lesions

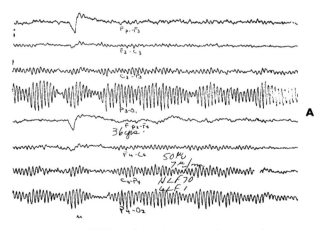

FIGURE 2-2. A, Well-modulated symmetric normal alpha rhythm.

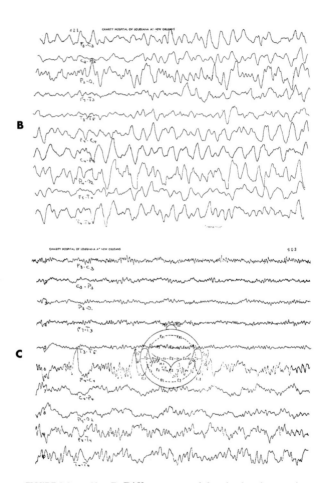

FIGURE 2-2, cont'd.   B, Diffuse severe delta rhythm in a patient with a metabolic encephalopathy. **C,** Right hemisphere (even number of the montages) slow wave focus in a patient with malignant brain neoplasm.

do not usually cause EEG abnormalities. If EEG demonstrates focal abnormality, it may be possible to determine the precise cerebral hemispheric location of a lesion; however, maximal electrical dysfunction does not always correlate with lesion location.

There are two types of abnormal EEG patterns. Spikes are typical of epileptogenic activity. Slow waves can occur in a diffuse distribution as in metabolic conditions (e.g., hepatic encephalopathy) or in focal disturbances as seen with intracranial mass lesions. The slowing can be mild in range of 3 to 7 cps (theta rhythm) or severe with less than 3 cps (delta rhythm). In patients with metabolic disorders, the EEG shows either diffuse slowing or paroxysms of high-voltage bifrontal delta activity. Because of limited EEG response patterns, it is not possible to make specific pathological diagnoses from EEG findings alone. For example, focal slow wave patterns caused by infarct, hemorrhage, neoplasm, or abscess can be identical. In patients with suspected seizure disorder, an EEG is performed to help establish this diagnosis and to be precise in seizure classification. For example, certain seizures appear generalized, but the EEG may show focal abnormality. All patients with epilepsy have abnormal EEGs during seizures; however, if the epileptic EEG discharge occurs intermittently, the EEG can be normal between seizures. Because 10% to 15% of normal persons have nonspecific EEG abnormalities, clinical diagnosis of a seizure disorder cannot be made from the EEG findings alone (see Chapter 11). In patients who have unexplained episodes or "spells" and abnormal nonspecific EEG patterns, combined simultaneous video-EEG monitoring of the patient can differentiate true epilepsy from other conditions such as syncope, breath-holding spells, and pseudoseizures.

CRANIAL ULTRASOUND

A surface probe with an electrically activated piezo-electric crystal transducer is used with an amplifier to record returning echoes. These points of deflection (echoes) represent interfaces between structures of different acoustic densities such as brain ventricles and brain parenchyma. Ultrasonography is of limited value in adults because skull bones cause dispersion of sonar waves before they pass through the intracranial region; however, in the squamous portion of temporal bone located directly above and posterior to the ear, the bone is unilaminar without diploic spaces, and this is adequate for ultrasound propagation.

Ultrasonography is becoming increasingly useful for infants because of the thinness of infant bones. The open fontanelles allow better ultrasound propagation with good spatial and contrast resolution such that the lateral and fourth ventricles can also be visualized. Ultrasound depends more on the skill of the technician performing the study and provides less definition of intracranial anatomy than CT or MRI; however, ultrasound can be performed at the bedside in the nursery and does not require transporting a sick infant to the radiology department. Ultrasonography is an extremely reliable diagnostic technique to image the orbit in patients with visual disturbances and avoids the risk of radiation-induced lens damage.

ISOTOPE BRAIN SCAN

With intravenous injection of radioactive gamma-emitting isotopes (technetium-99m, iodine-131), it is possible to determine the integrity of blood-brain barrier. The complete study includes two parts: one, dynamic image measuring intravascular isotope concentration; and two, static image reflecting brain parenchyma isotope concentration. The flow study is performed immediately following rapid bolus intravenous isotope injection. The isotope count is recorded as it circulates through arterial, capillary, and venous channels. If there is stenosis with reduced flow in one internal carotid artery, the amount of isotope visualized in that vessel is reduced. The static isotope image is obtained 1 to 4 hours later. Because of normal integrity of the blood-brain barrier, there is usually minimal brain parenchyma uptake.

The presence of increased brain uptake implies a breakdown in blood-brain barrier. Certain pathologic processes do not alter this barrier sufficiently or are of such small size to be below resolving capability of the isotope scan (less than 2.67 cm^3 in volume). Other false-negative results are due to image blurring, uptake of isotopes in the overlying temporalis muscle, and the small size of the posterior fossa with large, surrounding venous sinus structures. False-positive results can also occur. For example, a superficial scalplesion with extravasated blood can be incorrectly interpreted as representing a subdural hematoma. With CT and MRI availability, the isotope brain scan is rarely used.

■ ISOTOPE CISTERNOGRAM

In patients with suspected abnormalities of CSF flow, such as hydrocephalus or idiopathic intracranial hypertension, intrathecal injection of gamma-emitting substance demonstrates its distribution in CSF spaces (e.g., basal cisterns, ventricles, convexity sulcal spaces). This valuable study differentiates communicating hydrocephalus from cerebral atrophy (hydrocephalus ex vacuo). It can also be used to demonstrate the location of CSF leaks in patients with rhinorrhea or otorrhea. This is frequently valuable in trauma cases. This study requires a lumbar puncture for the isotope injection. Sequential scans are performed 24, 48, and 72 hours later. Isotope cisternogram is a technically difficult procedure because isotopes can leak out of subarachnoid spaces, and sufficient isotopes do not reach the basal cisterns in 20% of cases.

▇ LUMBAR PUNCTURE

With the insertion of a special spinal needle into the lumbar subarachnoid space, it is possible to measure intracranial pressure and analyze CSF content. For this procedure, the patient is placed in knee-chest position. Under aseptic conditions and with dermal anesthesia, a 19- or 21-gauge needle is inserted below the LA interspace to perforate the dura. After the subarachnoid space is entered, the needle stylet is removed, and the needle is connected to a pressure manometer. For accurate pressure recordings, the patient should be breathing normally and relaxed with legs straightened. If the patient is agitated, performs a Valsalva maneuver (by straining), or shows an increase in intraabdominal pressure (by not being straightened), CSF pressure can by falsely elevated (greater than 22 mm H_2O). If the needle is positioned correctly, fluctuations in pressure occur with respiration and pulse. Hyperventilation causes hypocapnia (low carbon dioxide content), resulting in intracranial vasoconstriction, and this can falsely lower CSF pressure. A spuriously low pressure is recorded if the needle does not freely communicate with subarachnoid spaces. The pressure that is recorded is usually an accurate reflection of intracranial dynamics. In a patient with an intracranial mass who begins to show evidence of a shift of intracranial structures (herniation), CSF pressure can be false low because intracranial and lumbar spaces are no longer in free communication. CSF pressure recorded by lumbar puncture is less reliable than continuous intracranial pressure monitoring with a subdural transducer; however, this requires neurosurgical intervention to insert burr holes. Accurate continuous pressure measurements may be necessary in certain disorders (e.g., Reye's syndrome, head trauma, benign intracranial hypertension).

Lumbar puncture with CSF analysis is necessary to establish the diagnosis of meningitis, subarachnoid hemorrhage, neurosyphilis, and multiple sclerosis. Contraindications for lumbar puncture are relative and not absolute, but usually include suspicion of mass lesion (i.e., altered mentation, focal deficit, papilledema, coagulation disturbance, and local infection at the site of the spinal needle puncture). CT or MRI should be performed initially. If there is lumbosacral infection involving skin, subcutaneous tissue, or bone, a cervical cisternal tap should be performed. The quantity of CSF that is removed does not correlate with the occurrence of postlumbar puncture headache; therefore enough CSF should be removed for all necessary studies. In most cases, 5 ml of CSF is sufficient for cell count, protein content, sugar content, serology, bacterial culture, and Gram stain. It is important to describe the color of CSF (clear, cloudy, bloody, or xanthochromic) and compare this with a tube of water as both the water and CSF are viewed against white background. If CSF appears bloody, the following procedure should be followed: first observe for clot formation to occur because blood-CSF mixture does not clot; next determine if fluid changes to clear appearance after several drops because this is consistent with traumatic spinal tap; and then place bloody CSF in hematocrit tube and centrifuge because in spontaneous subarachnoid hemorrhage, the supernatant appears xanthochromic. Xanthochromic fluid can also occur if the CSF protein content exceeds 1 g/dl. If the tap has been traumatic, white blood cells will also be present in CSF. The correction factor is one white blood cell for every 500 to 1000 red blood cells. In addition, 1000 red cells increase protein content by 1 mg/dl. Complications of lumbar puncture include backache, headache, leg motor or sensory disturbances, bleeding (epidural, subdural, subarachnoid), infection, transient abducens nerve paresis; intraspinal epidermoid tumor other than headache and backache. These other complications are rare. Treatment for headaches include fluid hydration, prone positioning of the patient, caffeine, or, if the headache persists, epidural blood patch.

ULTRASOUND CEREBROVASCULAR IMAGING STUDIES

Noninvasive vascular imaging studies assess the presence of stenotic, occlusive, or ulcerative lesions involving the cerebral circulation and are used most commonly to image the carotid arteries. These tests can be divided into indirect tests (assessing hemodynamic changes in distal carotid blood pressure or abnormal carotid flow velocity) and direct tests (using ultrasonography to image the carotid arterial wall at the carotid bifurcation). In ophthalmodynamometry, ophthalmic artery pressures in both eyes are determined by measurement of central retinal artery systolic pressure. With stenosis or occlusion, distal pressure is reduced compared with the normal side. In oculoplethysmography, central retinal artery pressure is measured by applying negative pressure to the globe with suction cups placed on the cornea. This increases intraocular pressure and obliterates retinal artery pressure. As the pressure is reduced, the pulse reappears. This technique shows reduced pressure and delayed ocular pulse wave arrival with carotid stenosis or occlusion. In thermography, direct measurement of skin temperature is made of the face and orbit area (using an infrared camera) supplied by the internal carotid artery. With severe carotid narrowing this temperature is lowered. In carotid phonoangiography, assessment of turbulent flow is made with a microphone placed over cervical carotid artery. This detects the presence of bruits and determines their amplitude and duration. It is possible to subject the recorded bruit to spectral analysis using a microcomputer to determine the carotid lumen at the region of the carotid artery. With the Doppler technique (based on reflection by moving red blood cells of high frequency sound wave), carotid flow analysis and carotid arterial wall imaging are possible. Stenosis, calcification, and ulcerative changes can be detected in carotid arteries by using Doppler duplex studies and in large basal intracranial arteries by using transcranial Doppler.

▦ DOPPLER DUPLEX ULTRASOUND

With carotid duplex ultrasound it is possible to delineate flow velocity analysis and image the carotid artery bifurcation. This site is a common location for atherosclerotic plaque formation. With increasing severity of carotid stenosis, the flow velocity progressively increases. With high-resolution ultrasound scanners, it is possible to demonstrate morphologic characteristics of the arterial wall. If there is more than 50% carotid stenosis, carotid duplex studies will detect this stenosis 95% of the time. Doppler ultrasound can not differentiate severe stenosis from complete occlusion. This is an important limitation because the patient with occlusion should not undergo endarterectomy.

▨ TRANSCRANIAL DOPPLER STUDY

Using the Doppler principal (signals emanating from an ultrasound probe reflect off red blood cells in the artery such that the frequency of reflected signal is shifted in proportion to velocity of flowing blood), it is possible to perform extracranial (carotid) and transcranial (intracranial) vascular imaging studies. With a pulsed-wave Doppler probe applied at areas of thin skull bone (e.g., temporal bone superior to zygoma between the ears, directly over the orbits, suboccipital region of foramen magnum), intracranial vessels (carotid artery siphon, initial portions of anterior, middle, and posterior cerebral arteries, distal intracranial segments of vertebral arteries and basilar artery) can be insonated. An increased blood flow, as measured by transcranial Doppler technique, indicates arterial lumen narrowing (stenosis, vasospasm). The major limitation is that the study can be technically difficult or even impossible to perform because of an inadequate transcranial temporal ultrasound window.

▨ DIGITAL SUBTRACTION ANGIOGRAPHY

Digital subtraction angiography (DSA) provides a less invasive alternative to conventional arteriography for imaging carotid and vertebral arteries. This test has the advantage of visualizing intracranial circulation compared with other noninvasive tests described earlier. By using intravenous injection of iodinated contrast material with DSA, it is possible to image accurately the carotid artery bifurcation. With selective arterial catheterization and DSA, intracranial small vessel detail can be obtained using much lower contrast volume than with conventional arteriography. DSA uses a radiographic fluoroscope connected to an analog-digital converter and computer. By amplification of signal and subtraction (masking) techniques, it is possible to visualize carotid bifurcation and vertebral arteries following intravenous contrast injection. Intravenous DSA is indicated as a screening procedure for extracranial carotid and vertebral arteries for arteriosclerotic cerebrovascular disease. If adequate visualization of intracranial vessels (aneurysm, arteriovenous malformations, neoplasms, vasculitis) is necessary, arterial DSA is required. This procedure has complications similar to conventional arteriography.

CONVENTIONAL CATHETER ANGIOGRAPHY

Because the intravascular blood pool is slightly more radiodense than CSF and less dense than the brain, water-soluble, iodinated contrast media is necessary to create sufficient artificial contrast to visualize blood vessels. In femoral percutaneous angiography, a flexible, plastic catheter is introduced into this vessel and directed upward through the aortic arch. By using fluoroscopy, it is possible to inject contrast media selectively into carotid and vertebral arteries. Iodinated contrast material is injected into each vessel, and a series of films is rapidly taken to outline arterial, capillary, and venous circulation to visualize anatomical detail of extracranial and intracranial vessels. Tumors are detected because they cause mass effect with distortion and displacement of certain intracranial vessels. On the basis of the direction of major vectors of vascular distortion, the location (e.g., intraaxial versus extraaxial) of the tumor is established; however, this vascular pattern does not define whether the lesion is neoplastic or nonneoplastic (e.g., abscess, intracerebral hematoma). Neoplasms can be associated with new vessel formation (neovascularity). Certain neoplasms (i.e., meningiomas, gliomas) have a characteristic stain pattern. Angiography accurately delineates morphologic detail of abnormal vessels (e.g., aneurysm, vascular malformation). It also shows the degree of stenosis or occlusion of the extracranial vessels and defines the presence of an ulcerated plaque. Since the introduction of CT, angiography has been used to define vascular system abnormalities rather than to demonstrate mass effect (Figure 2-3).

Complications of angiography can result from the technique itself or toxicity of the contrast material. Movement of the catheter can dislodge emboli from intima of the aorta or carotids; in addition, clot formation can occur on the catheter and embolize to the brain. These complications occur more frequently with direct carotid needle puncture than with flexible catheters, which are now routinely used. The organically bound iodide contrast agents can cause systemic (e.g., anaphylactic, cardiovascular) or neurotoxic (e.g., seizures, stroke) reactions. Because the contrast

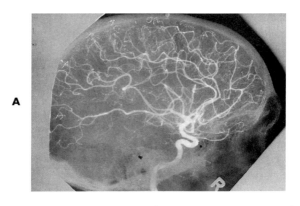

FIGURE 2-3. A, Normal carotid angiogram visualizing the caliber and position of the intracranial vessels.

material is excreted by the kidney, renal dysfunction can preclude angiography.

Using arterial catheterization equipment and fluoro-

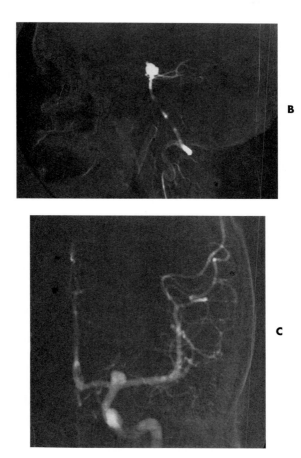

FIGURE 2-3, cont'd. **B,** Giant aneurysm arising from the basilar artery. **C,** Aneurysm arising from the middle cerebral artery.

scopic control, it is possible to reduce regional arterial blood flow (embolization). This is valuable in patients with arterial-venous malformations or in patients with meningioma that has marked neovascularity supplying the tumor. Embolization (with reduction in the blood flow) can be achieved by obliterating abnormal blood vessels with solid materials such as carbon or ferro-magnetic microspheres, detachable balloons, or gelatin sponge. In other patients who have blood vessel occlusion, it is possible to increase blood flow by injecting a thrombolytic agent such as urokinase or streptokinase or to insert and inflate a balloon catheter within stenotic or vasospastic arterial segments. This field of interventional therapeutic neuroradiology is rapidly expanding.

■ MYELOGRAPHY

In myelography the patient is positioned prone on an x-ray table, and 5 to 15 ml of an oil-soluble (e.g., iophendylate [Pantopaque]) or water-soluble (e.g., metrizamide [Amipaque]) substance is injected into lumbar subarachnoid spaces. The dye is maneuvered into lumbar, thoracic, and cervical regions by tilting the x-ray table (e.g., if the lumbar region is to be studied, the patient is erect, and if the thoracic and cervical regions are to be studied, the table is tilted downward). The dye fills the subarachnoid space and outlines the spinal cord and nerve roots. If a herniated disk impinges on a nerve root, myelography shows asymmetry or indentation of the nerve root sheath. If spinal cord compression is present, myelographic findings define distortion and displacement of cord; the position (extradural, intradural, extramedullary, or intramedullary) or mass is defined by findings in laeral or anteroposterior projection. If there is myelo-graphic evidence of a spinal cord block, a cisternal tap is performed to delineate the upper extent of the lesion.

Because iophendylate is oil soluble, it is not spontaneously reabsorbed from subarachnoid spaces and must be removed by the physician. Arachnoiditis is a potential complication of this procedure. An alternative contrast agent is metrizamide, which is water soluble. It is spontaneously removed within 48 hours and does not cause arachnoiditis. However, it is potentially neurotoxic to the central nervous system and can cause seizures or encephalopathy.

▨ COMPUTED TOMOGRAPHY

Computed tomography (CT) is a brain imaging technique that provides direct visual images of intracranial contents (CSF spaces, blood vessels, and gray and white matter) based on radiographic attenuation values (representing tissue density measurements) of these structures. CT scans provide better contrast resolution than other diagnostic procedures, making the brain image essentially equivalent to the findings at autopsy.

The x-ray source is a thinly collimated beam that penetrates the patient's head at multiple angles. Transmitter x-ray attenuation readings are recorded by a series of multiple crystal or gas detectors. These summated x-ray profiles are analyzed by a high-speed computer program. The result reflects radiodensities within specific axial (transverse) tissue sections. These radiodensities are expressed in numerical values; in this scale, water is zero, with bone being +2000, and air being −2000. The value of normal brain constituents represent approximately 120 units (2.5%) of the total scale. These radiodensities are visually displayed on a cathode-ray oscilloscope using a gray scale. The image is displayed on x-ray film; however, the image is a representation of radiodensities. Each brain tissue section is usually 8 to 10 mm in thickness for routine brain CT. Within each section there are multiple rectangular regions (pixels) for which radiodensity values are determined. It is possible to increase the spatial resolution by decreasing the size of each pixel, therefore increasing number of attenuation values obtained.

The characteristic appearance of intracranial content is displayed at multiple levels extending from the base to vertex (Figure 2-4). CT scans are usually displayed in the axial plane, although coronal and sagittal

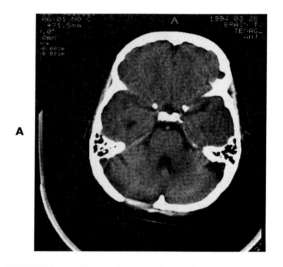

FIGURE 2-4. A, Base of brain shows the triangular-shaped fourth ventricle and directly anterior is the brain stem and surrounding basal cisterns. The dorsum sella is seen and obscures the suprasellar cistern. The anterior clinoids are lateral to the dorsum sella. Anterior to sphenoid bone is frontal lobes. Between sphenoid and petrous bone is temporal lobe. Cerebellar hemispheres are posterior to petrous bone.

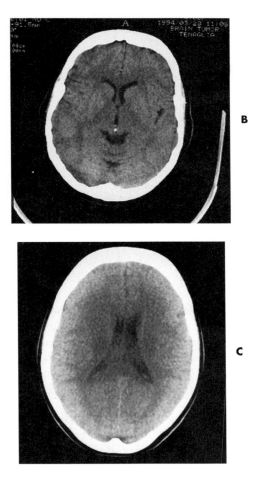

FIGURE 2-4, cont'd. B, Midventricular level shows anterior fontal horns of lateral ventricles, midline third ventricle, calcified pineal gland and quadrigeminal cistern. **C,** High ventricular level shows anterior frontal horns, bodies and occipital horns of lateral ventricles.

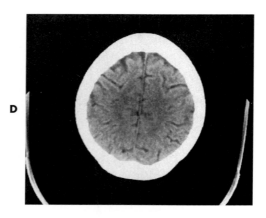

FIGURE 2-4, cont'd.   D, Supraventricular level shows cortical sulcal spaces. The gray matter appears slightly brighter than deep white matter.

sections can be obtained. Pathologic processes cause abnormal radiodensity patterns and can displace normal intracranial structures. Following rapid intravenous infusion of iodinated contrast material (Figure 2-5), it is possible to visualize major intracranial vessels and to detect enhancement patterns caused by impairment in the blood-brain barrier. On the basis of plain and postcontrast appearances, it is sometimes possible to predict underlying pathologic process (Figure 2-6); however, CT findings are not always characteristic enough to make specific diagnoses without surgical biopsy. With improvements in technology, it is possible to image the spinal cord with comparable image quality to myelography, although thick, surrounding vertebral bones and the small size of the spinal cord present significant imaging problems not present with brain CT.

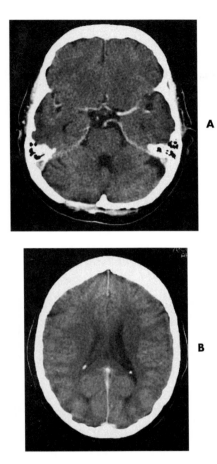

FIGURE 2-5. Postcontrast CT. **A,** Carotid arteries are seen in lateral-anterior aspect of suprasellar cisterns branching into middle cerebral artery extending laterally and anterior cerebral arteries extending medially. The right posterior cerebral artery is seen extending posteriorly from the midline basilar artery. **B,** The round vein of Galen extends to straight sinus and posteriorly into sagittal sinus.

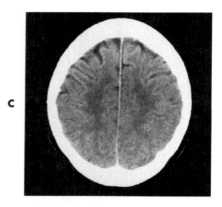

FIGURE 2-5, cont'd. C, The midline falx cerebri appears as linear enhancing band.

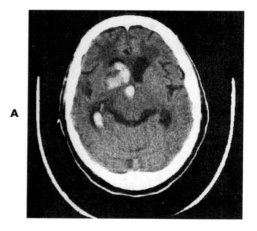

FIGURE 2-6. CT visualized pathological processes. **A,** Blood in the basal ganglia extending into anterior frontal horn, third ventricle, and occipital horn of lateral ventricle.

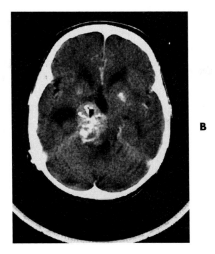

FIGURE 2-6, cont'd. **B,** Enhancing thalamic and posterior third ventricular neoplasm elevating the third ventricle. The large, comma-shaped structure is the dilated temporal horn.

MAGNETIC RESONANCE IMAGING

Magnetic resonance imaging (MRI) uses radiowaves and an externally applied magnetic field to align protons (usually hydrogen ions contained in water molecules) parallel to a magnetic field. When a radiofrequency stimulus is applied, the protons gyrate. As stimulus is turned off, the radioreceiver can detect signals as the protons relax and reorient themselves within the magnetic field. At present, MRI provides brain images based on the distribution of hydrogen ions (Figure 2-7); however, it may be possible to modify the technology to provide images based on sodium ions (this might allow physicians to determine the size of extracellular and intracellular spaces) or phosphate ions (determine amount of high-energy, e.g., adenine triphosphate, brain substances). MRI has the potential to provide quantitative brain biochemistry analysis. Using MRI contrast agents (gadolinium, gadodiamide), the integrity of the blood-brain barrier can be assessed.

The advantages of MRI over CT include no use of ionizing radiation, ease with which multiplanar scanning can be achieved (e.g., axial, coronal, sagittal), and improved contrast resolution such that discrimination of gray and white matter is reliably achieved

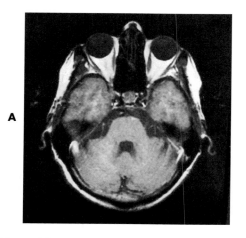

FIGURE 2-7. Normal brain MRI. **A,** T_1 weighted axial MRI shows base of skull, including triangular-shaped fourth ventricles. CSF spaces appear dark, similar to appearance on CT.

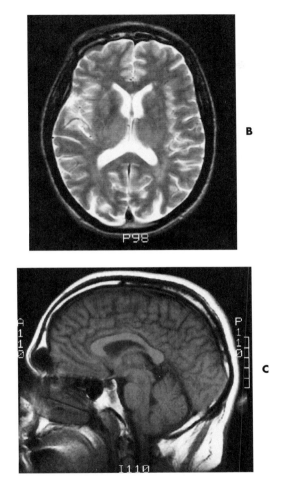

FIGURE 2-7, cont'd. B, T_2 weighted axial MRI shows CSF spaces, including lateral ventricles and spaces appearing white. **C,** T_1 weighted sagittal scan shows cerebral hemispheres, corpus callosum, brain stem, cerebellum, and cervical spinal cord.

(Figure 2-8). Disadvantages are that MRI requires a longer time for data acquisition than CT and that MRI images are susceptible to motion artifacts. MRI cannot be performed on patients who have had prior aneurysm surgery or shunts using cranial metallic clips or who have a cardiac pacemaker. Because of the ease with which multiplanar images can be achieved and because bone does not generate artifacts, MRI provides excellent detail of the posterior fossa and spinal canal.

■ POSITRON EMISSION TOMOGRAPHY

Positron emission tomography (PET) uses positrons (positively charged electrons that are generated using a cyclotron), which are present in normal

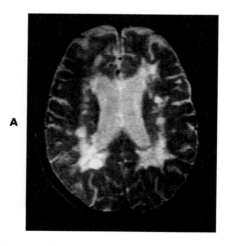

FIGURE 2-8. **A,** High-signal intensity (*white*) periventricular lesions consistent with multiple sclerosis.

brain substances. These include carbon (^{11}C), oxygen (^{15}O), and nitrogen (^{13}N); fluorine (^{18}F) is used to replace hydrogen. The PET technique is similar to that of CT, except that the data collected represents the distribution of photons emitted from isotopes within the brain. With PET, brain physiology and function can be studied in both normal and pathologic states. For example, it is possible to determine brain blood flow and metabolism in aging patients and to compare this with the findings in demented patients. It is possible to determine blood flow and metabolism in the resting state and compare it with changes occurring in specific brain regions after visual or auditory stimulation. Pathologic conditions in which blood flow and tissue metabolism have been studied include ischemic cerebrovascular disease, epilepsy, dementia, and

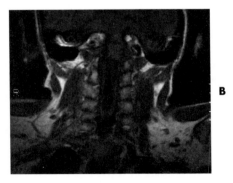

FIGURE 2-8, cont'd.   **B,** Coronal craniospinal study shows large CSF filled (*dark*) space in central spinal cord consistent with syringomyelia.

malignant brain neoplasms. There is also great potential for the use of PET in investigating patients with "functional" psychiatric disorders (e.g., schizophrenia, affective disorders) and to compare these findings in untreated versus treated patients.

▣ SINGLE-PHOTON EMISSION COMPUTED TOMOGRAPHY

For PET, a cyclotron is needed to generate positron-emitting radionuclides. These have a short half-life, which means PET can only be performed in a medical center facility that has a cyclotron. This limits PET; however, with single-photon emission computed tomography (SPECT) the procedure is performed with radionuclides, gamma-emitting isotopes. With SPECT, there is no need for cyclotron, and radionuclides are commercially available; however, spatial resolution of SPECT is lower than that of PET. SPECT uses a routine nuclear medicine camera and is available in most general hospitals; this contrasts with PET, which is available only in specialized centers. SPECT can demonstrate areas of cerebral ischemia as shown by reduced areas of perfusion in patients with Alzheimer's, Parkinson's, and Huntington's diseases can be valuable in showing neurotransmitter (dopamine) abnormalities.

▣ ELECTRICAL DIAGNOSTIC STUDIES

Nerve Conduction Velocity

Conduction velocity of motor nerves is determined by stimulating the nerve at two points (proximally and distally) and recording the action potential over the muscle with surface electrodes. By determining conduction time from distal and proximal stimulation and measuring the distance between these two points, conduction velocity is calculated. The velocities are determined for superficial (median, ulnar, peroneal, and posterior tibial) nerves. More deeply situated nerves are not usually analyzed because their direct stimulation is not technically feasible. Recent technical advances have made possible measurement of sensory conduction velocities.

Nerve conduction velocity depends on the integrity of surrounding myelin sheath. If a pathologic condition has caused peripheral nerve demyelination, generalized slowing of conduction velocity occurs. In other cases, nerve conduction velocity can be slowed in a focal segment; this is characteristic of compression (entrapment) neuropathy. For example, slowing of the median nerve distally (below the wrist) with normal velocities above the wrist occurs in carpal tunnel syndrome.

Electromyography

Electromyography (EMG) is performed by inserting a coaxial needle electrode in the muscle and recording motor unit potentials on a cathode-ray oscilloscope. The muscle potentials are characterized in three phases: resting state, mild muscle contraction, and maximal exertion. At rest, there is normally brief insertional activity and later no spontaneous motor potentials. The presence of prolonged spontaneous discharges is consistent with that of denervating (anterior horn cell or axonal neuropathy) disorder. During mild muscle contraction, muscle potentials are evaluated (e.g., size, amplitude, duration, form). With maximal contraction, there should be sustained electrical activity; this is decreased in myopathic, but not in neuropathic, disorders. On the basis of characteristics of electrical activity, it is possible to define the cause of weakness and usually to differentiate disorders of myopathic or neuropathic origin. If a disorder of neuromuscular junction (e.g., myasthenia gravis) is suspected, repetitive stimulation of a motor nerve should also be performed. The myasthenic syndromes show decremental changes in action potential amplitude with repetitive stimulation.

MUSCLE AND NERVE BIOPSY

In patients with symmetric muscle diseases, EMG is used to define which muscle groups show abnormal electrical response, and a biopsy is performed to define specific pathologic changes in the involved muscles. A biopsy is performed on a muscle that has not been sampled by EMG and is free of needle artifacts. The muscle to be biopsied is determined by clinical, nerve conduction velocity, and EMG findings. It is important to select a muscle that is clinically and electrically in an active phase of involvement. If muscle sampled is not chosen carefully, the biopsy may show no abnormality or only end-stage atrophic changes; therefore it would not be possible to determine if primary pathologic process was myopathic or neuropathic. The biopsy is performed by making an incision in skin and excising a small piece of muscle. This specimen should not be placed in or irrigated with alcohol or saline. The tissue should be divided into three fragments: one fragment is frozen for cryostat sections and histochemistry, the second is fixed for electron microscopic analysis, and the third is used for biochemical (metabolic) analysis.

The sural nerve is a cutaneous sensory nerve that is available for biopsy. Biopsy is indicated in patients in whom the cause of nerve disease cannot be established by other diagnostic modalities. The major limitation is that only sensory nerves can be studied; motor fibers cannot be evaluated. If the pathologic process is multifocal rather than diffuse, the abnormal area can not be included in biopsy specimen. Nerve biopsy is most helpful to delineate these pathologic processes: inflammatory demyelinating neuropathy, amyloid, sarcoid, leprosy, vasculitis, and biochemical disorders affecting peripheral nerve (e.g., metachromatic leukodystrophy).

▪ EVOKED POTENTIALS

The EEG records spontaneous superficial electrical cerebral activity; however, it is not possible to analyze the individual waveforms because of abundant artifacts. The basic signal is buried in background noise or interference. It is possible to amplify the wave by summating and averaging the brain wave recorded after evoked stimulation. The wave can represent an evoked response to sensory stimulation such as a flashing light, auditory sound clicks, and stimulation of peripheral nerve. In usual evoked potentials, an electronic device—average response computer—can summate and average the occipital cortical response to a series of light flashes presented over short intervals (e.g., 256 flashes at 1.5 flashes/sec). Other sensory-evoked potentials assess the auditory system by recording over the primary auditory cortex in the temporal region or somatosensory system by recording over the postcentral parietal region. Each evoked wave has its characteristic latency of response, amplitude, and morphology (form). Sensory-evoked potentials differ from routine EEG in two ways: (1) the response is evoked, and (2) the response is computer averaged to accentuate the response. Evoked potentials (EPs) trace the transmission of sensory nerve impulses through receptor, nerves, spinal cord, and brain stem and to sensory portions of cerebral cortex.

The clinical applications of this technique are rapidly expanding. For example, visual response assesses retinal and optic nerve function. In patients with visual loss, different abnormalities have been reported in patients with demyelinating disease, tumor, or ischemic lesions. In addition, by performing evoked potentials in 50% of the visual field (hemifield), abnormalities or asymmetries of the optic chiasm, optic radiation, or occipital cortex can be assessed. Auditory-evoked potentials are being used to evaluate patients with hearing impairment and vertigo to determine the level of involvement within the auditory system (cochlea, auditory nerve, brain stem, thalamus, auditory cortex). EP can be monitored during surgery to assess the spinal and cerebral pathways, for example.

■ MAGNETOENCEPHALOGRAPHY

Magnetic stimulators have been used to record motor potentials from the motor cortex. This permits assessment of integrity of central motor pathways. Abnormal central motor conduction time is expected in multiple sclerosis, stroke with hemiplegia, or motor neuron disease. Electrical brain stimulation has not been associated with significant untoward effects; however, seizures are a potential, but highly unlikely, complication.

■ SUMMARY

Neurodiagnostic studies are valuable when used appropriately after a careful history and examination have suggested the possible location and type of neuropathological process. With sophisticated neurodiagnostic studies it is not only possible to detect a brain or spinal cord lesion but also to image the effect of the lesion on the surrounding structures. In the future these imaging techniques will provide biochemical and physiological information of brain dysfunction, as well as imaging the brain or spine lesion.

Suggested Readings

Electroencephalography

Kiloh LG, McComas AJ, Osselton JW, et al: *Clinical electroencephalography*, ed 4, London, 1981, Butterworths.

Gumnit RJ: Intensive neurodiagnostic (EEG) monitoring: role in the treatment of seizures, *Neurology* 36:1340, 1986.

Sperling MR: Neuroimaging in epilepsy: recent developments in MR imaging positron emission tomography and single photon emission tomography, *Neurol Clin North Am* 11:883, 1993.

Drury I, Beydoun A: Pitfalls of EEG interpretation in epilepsy, *Neurol Clin North Am* 11:857, 1993.

Daly DD, Pedley TA: *Current practice of clinical electroencephalography*, ed 2, New York, 1990, Raven Press.

Lumbar Puncture and Cerebrospinal Fluid Analysis

Fishman RA: *Cerebrospinal fluid in diseases of the nervous system*, ed 2, Philadelphia, 1992, WB Saunders.

American College of Physicians Policy Committee: The diagnostic spinal tap, *Ann Intern Med* 104:880, 1986.

Hayward RA, Shapiro MF: Laboratory testing on cerebrospinal fluid: a reappraisal, *Lancet* 1:1, 1987.

Marton KI, Geon AD: The spinal tap: a new look at an old test, *Ann Intern Med* 104:840, 1986.

Gower DJ, Baker AL, Bell WO: Contraindications to lumbar puncture as defined by computed cranial tomography, *J Neurol Neurosurg Psychiatry* 50:1071, 1991.

Petito F, Plum F: The lumbar puncture, *N Engl J Med* 290:225, 1974.

Vascular Ultrasound

Lees RS, Kistler JP: Noninvasive diagnosis of extracranial cerebrovascular disease, *Neurol Clin North Am* 2:667, 1984.

Ackerman RH: A perspective on noninvasive diagnosis of carotid disease, *Neurology* 29:615, 1979.

Caplan LR, Brass LM, DeWitt LD: Transcranial Doppler ultrasound, *Neurology* 40:696, 1990.

Petty GW, Wiebers DO, Meissner I: Transcranial Doppler ultrasonography, *Mayo Clin Proc* 65:1350, 1990.

Polak JF, Kalina P, Donaldson MC: Carotid endarterectomy: preoperative evaluation of candidates with combined Doppler sonography and MR angiography, *Radiology* 186:325, 1993.

Masaryk TJ, Obuchowski NA: Noninvasive carotid imaging, *Radiology* 186:325, 1993.

Jacobs NM, Grant EG, Schellinger D: Duplex carotid sonography: criteria for stenosis, accuracy and pitfalls, *Radiology* 154:385, 1985.

Stewart JH, Grubb M: Understanding vascular ultrasonography, *Mayo Clin Proc* 67:1186, 1992.

Conventional Angiography and Magnetic Resonance Imaging Angiography (MRA)

Hesselink JR: Digital subtraction angiography, Neurol Clin North Am 2:823, 1984.

Caplan LR, Wolpert SM: Angiography in patients with occlusive cerebrovascular disease: views of a stroke neurologist and neuroradiologist, *Am J Neuroradiology* 12:593, 1991.

Russell EJ, Berenstein A: Neurologic applications of interventional radiology, *Neurol Clin North Am* 2:873, 1984.

Nakahara I, Pile-Spellman J, Hacein-Bey L: Interventional neuroradiology, *Neurol Chron* 1:1, 1991.

Halbach VV, Higashida RT, Hieshima GB: Interventional neuroradiology, *Am J Radiol* 153:467, 1989.

Computed Tomography and Magnetic Resonance Imaging

Lufkin RB: Magnetic resonance imaging of the central nervous system, *Semin Neurol* 6:1, 1986.

Olendorf WH: The quest for an image of brain: a brief historical and technical review of brain imaging techniques, *Neurology* 28:517, 1978.

Olendorf WH: The quest for an image of brain, New York, 1980, Raven Press.

Edelman RR, Warach S: Magnetic resonance imaging, *New Engl J Med* 328:708, 1993.

Latchaw RE: MR and CT imaging of the head, neck, and spine, ed 2, St. Louis, 1991, Mosby.

Gilman S: Advances in neurology (neuroimaging), *New Engl J Med* 326:1608, 1992.

Positron Emission Tomography and Single Photon Emission Tomography

Lenzi GL, Pantano P: Neurologic applications of positron emission tomography, *Neurol Clin North Am* 2:853, 1984.

Caplan LR: Question driven technology assessment: single photon emission computed tomography, *Neurology* 41:187, 1991.

Baron JC: Positron emission tomography in cerebral ischemia, *Neuroradiology* 27:509, 1985.

Brooks D: Positron emission tomography: its clinical role in neurology, *Neurosurg Psychiatry* 54:1, 1991.

Electromyography and Nerve Conduction Velocity

Kimura J: *Electrodiagnosis in disease of nerve and muscle: principles and practice*, ed 2, Philadelphia, 1989, FA Davis.

Evoked Potentials

Chiappa KH, Ropper AH: Evoked potentials in clinical medicine, *N Engl J Med* 306:1140, 1982.

Greenberg RP, Ducker TP: Evoked potentials in the clinical neurosciences, *J Neurosurg* 56:1, 1982.

Chiappa KH: Transcranial magnetic stimulation of the human motor cortex for evaluation of central motor pathways, *Neurol Chron* 1:1, 1991.

Evaluation of Common Neurologic Signs and Symptoms

Headache and Face Pain

Headache is one of the most common medical symptoms and one that should receive a physician's close attention. Headache can be the first and only symptom of serious intracranial disease such as subarachnoid hemorrhage, meningitis, and brain tumor. Because of the potential seriousness of headache, the physician's first obligation is to rule out these life-threatening conditions.

Fortunately most headaches are benign. The symptoms, however, can be quite disabling, and the physician should carefully characterize the headache and establish a treatment plan to relieve the pain.

▨ HISTORY

The clinical history is very important in diagnosing the cause of a patient's headache. Failure to explore the historical details fully can lead to unfortunate errors. Too many patients with bleeding aneurysms have been sent home from emergency departments with prescriptions for analgesic medication, only to return comatose the following day or week.

The first question in the history should establish whether the patient is experiencing a new or an unusual headache or is seeking help for chronic recurring headache. The patient who has never had headaches and consults the physician for a first-time headache demands careful neurodiagnostic evaluation. Headache of recent onset is much more likely to be the symptom of serious intracranial disease than is chronic (years in duration) recurrent headache.

The second feature of the history that will prove invaluable in establishing the diagnosis is a complete, step-by-step, temporal profile of the headache. Onset, location, and progress of pain all should be meticulously recorded. This temporal profile of the headaches is very important in determining the cause of the pain. Box 3-1 can be used as a guide in history taking.

In patients with chronic recurrent headaches, it is important to obtain a life history of the problem. Some information that should be obtained is listed in Box 3-2.

Because chronic recurrent headaches are frequently caused by emotional stress, it is important to point this out tactfully to the patient and then briefly ask about some aspects of the patient's personal life. Questions can be asked about family relationships, job situations, financial stability, and, if appropriate, sexual relations. Frequently the life stress itself is not unpleasant or emotionally significant but merely the product of a very demanding lifestyle in which many factors must balance perfectly if life is to run smoothly. For example, the single working mother may do well as long as the car works, the children stay well, and she can leave work at 5 P.M. Keeping to such a tight schedule imposes enormous stress by virtue of the ever-present possibility that one element can tip the delicate balance. Finally, it is wise to ask

BOX 3-1

1 Were there any antecedent or associated factors present, such as emotional or physical stress (including such factors as exercise or sexual intercourse); concomitant medical illness (e.g., hypertension); glaucoma; infection of sinuses, ears, or eyes; head trauma; or recent dental work? If the patient is female, is she currently using birth control pills? Does the headache occur most frequently during menstrual periods? Does any food (e.g., monosodium glutamate used in Chinese food, alcohol, cheese, wine) or medication (e.g., vasodilators, drugs containing histamine) precipitate headache?

2 Were any symptoms noticed immediately before to onset of the headache (aura), such as wavy lines in front of the eyes, loss of vision in part of the field, scotoma (holes) in the vision with or without scintillating margins, weakness of one side, numbness, or diplopia?

3 Did the pain come on suddenly or build up gradually? How long did it take to reach maximal intensity? Does the headache awaken the patient from sleep? What time of day does the headache usually occur (e.g., on awakening, late in the day, at work, and so on)?

4 Where was the pain? Unilateral? Occipital? Temporal? Frontal? Generalized?

5 What was the character of the pain? Throbbing? Sharp and stabbing? Tight, steady, and aching? Bandlike?

6 How long did it last?

7 Was the pain associated with nausea, vomiting, or sensitivity to light or sound?

8 Does anything exacerbate the pain, such as coughing, sneezing, leaning over, or exerting physical effort?

9 Did the pain change during the course of the headache?

10 Did the pain suddenly leave, gradually leave, or is it still present?

11 What medication was tried, and how successful was it?

12 Complete review of neurologic and medical symptoms should also be taken. This portion of the history is very important in diagnosing headaches associated with intracranial disease. For example, transient arm weakness at the onset of a unilateral throbbing headache suggests migraine, whereas persistent weakness and prolonged headache is more suggestive of a brain hemorrhage or tumor.

BOX 3-2

1 Age at onset
2 Frequency of the headaches (an important factor in treatment planning)
3 Medications used and their efficacy
4 Periods in life during which headaches were either very frequent or absent (e.g., college, marriage, menopause)
5 Relation to mental state (e.g., depression, stress)
6 Family history of headaches
7 History of motion sickness as a child (a finding in some patients with migraine)

specifically about any feelings or signs of depression (e.g., sadness, sleeping or eating problems, crying spells, and lack of energy) because the patient may not mention these feelings spontaneously.

In addition to the specialized headache history, a complete neurologic examination should be performed. Aspects of the examination that should receive special note are listed in Box 3-3.

The extent of laboratory evaluation will depend on how strongly the physician suspects significant intracranial disease; this evaluation is based on the chronicity of the problem and findings from the history and physical examination.

■ DESCRIPTION OF THE CLINICAL SYNDROMES

The discussions that follow will help the student understand the various diseases that should be considered in the differential diagnosis of headache. The appropriate tests required to establish or rule out each are outlined in each section.

BOX 3-3

---

1 Funduscopic examination: papilledema and subhyaloid hemorrhage (seen in subarachnoid hemorrhage)

2 Level of consciousness: lethargy suggests an intracranial lesion or systemic disease

3 Pupillary asymmetry: aneurysm or herniation from a mass lesion

4 Extraocular muscle weakness: aneurysm or herniation from a mass lesion

5 Reflex asymmetry and lateralizing motor findings: unilateral brain lesion

6 Imbalance and abnormal cerebellar signs: posterior fossa tumors (cerebellum, brain stem)

7 Nuchal rigidity: meningitis and subarachnoid hemorrhage

The most common headache syndromes are discussed in approximately decreasing order of prevalence, not in the order of medical significance. The major features of each are listed in Table 3-1. The boundaries between the principle headache types are quite indistinct, and many patients experience features of both tension and migraine types of headaches concurrently. The pathophysiology of headache is also not as clearly defined as it once was felt to be, but a unifying hypothesis for all headache has been recently proposed (Lance, 1993).[1] The model called the vascular-central-myogenic model proposes a complex interaction between the pain fibers in the muscles and blood vessels with nuclei in the brain stem. The headache process can begin in any of the three structures and then variously affect the other two. Fortunately, this change in the science of headache has led to *improved* treatment rather than therapeutic confusion, an important factor for patient and physician alike.

TABLE 3-1 Headache Profiles

Condition	Character of Pain
Tension headache	Tightness; gradual buildup (occipital, frontal or temporal, or circumferential)
Classic migraine (migraine with aura)	Visual aura then unilateral throbbing pain with nausea and vomiting
Common migraine (migraine without aura)	No aura; unilateral headache at first but then generalized throbbing; can have nausea
Cluster headache	Strong, periorbital, boring, steady or throbbing pain; frequently awakens patient; rapidly reaches maximal intensity
Subarachnoid hemorrhage	Severe generalized headache of sudden onset
Tumor	Dull morning pain that is increased by coughing, sneezing, or exertion
Pseudotumor cerebri	Dull, steady pain frequently with visual complaints
Systemic arterial hypertension	Patient awakens with dull or throbbing pain
Sinus headache	Steady localized pain over sinus
Temporal arteritis	Patients over 60; unilateral head pain
Trigeminal neuralgia	Lancinating face pain
Atypical face pain	Dull, steady, diffuse face pain

Duration	Recurrence	Treatment
1 hour to many days	Tends to fluctuate with life stress	Simple analgesics, amitriptyline, biofeedback, and psychologic support
30 min to several hours	More frequent during or directly after times of stress	Ergotamine preparations, β-blockers, amitriptyline, Bellergal (ergotamine, phenobarbital), calcium channel blockers, methysergide, and analgesics
Hours to days	Similar to classic migraine	Same as classic migraine
15–90 min	Occurs in clusters over a month or two; varying intervals between clusters	Prednisone and ergotamine, methysergide, calcium channel blockers during cluster times
Days	No	Evaluation and often surgical treatment
Weeks to months	No	Surgery
Days to weeks	In some cases	Repeated spinal puncture, corticosteroids, diuretics, and weight reduction
Several hours, lessens during morning	Related to arterial pressure	Antihypertensive medication (see also hypertensive encephalopathy)
Days to weeks	Will recur	Antibiotics and antihistamines
Days to weeks	Can recur	Corticosteroids
Seconds	Recurs throughout life	Carbamazepine, baclofen, phenytoin, or surgery
Hours	Recurs throughout life	Amitriptyline or chlordiazepoxide

Tension-Type Headache (Muscle Contraction Headache or Psychogenic Headache)

Everyone has experienced a tension-type headache (episodic) at some time. Brought on by stress, it is usually promptly relieved by aspirin, rest, and removal of the stress. For some people, however, tension headaches are a severe recurrent problem that does not respond to simple measures; it is usually these patients who seek medical assistance. In many patients the headaches occur almost daily (chronic tension headache with pain more than 180 days per year).

The pain is often caused by steady contraction of the muscles attached to the skull (i.e., frontalis, temporalis, trapezius, and often paraspinous muscles). The sustained muscle contraction causes lactic acid accumulation, and this can trigger vasodilatation so as to induce a vascular component to the headache. It seems that the day-to-day stress of coping with a busy life, often coupled with underlying anxiety, suppressed anger, hostility, and frustration, causes patients to tense these muscles for long periods of time as though they were animals preparing to fight or flee.

The pain itself is most commonly described as a bilateral tightness starting in the occiput, brow, or temples. It often spreads to encircle the head like a tight hatband or vise. The pain starts without warning. It is mild at first but builds over a period of hours. The pain characteristically lasts a few hours or until the patient sleeps or takes adequate analgesic medication. In some patients the pain is very severe, can last for days, and can eventually throb or pulsate as does a vascular headache. When severe throbbing pain occurs, the headache is labeled a tension or vascular headache. In keeping with the new headache model, it is not difficult to see that the active interaction of the cranial musculature, cranial vessels, and central nervous system structures can produce headaches that have overlapping symptoms. With or without medication, the pain recedes gradually as it began. Tension headaches most commonly occur in the afternoon but can be present on arising. Anxiety-producing dreams can also produce nocturnal headaches that can awaken the patient; therefore the belief that nocturnal headaches are always an ominous sign (e.g., brain tumor) is not always correct.

Muscle tension headaches can occur at any age. Women are most commonly afflicted than men, and exacerbations typically occur at stressful times of life. Physical examination demonstrates only tightness or tenderness in the affected muscles.

In a patient with typical tension headaches and a normal neurologic examination, an expensive laboratory evaluation is unjustified. In some patients a screening personality test such as the Minnesota Multiphasic Personality Inventory can be used to delineate depression, somatization tendency, or major psychotic disorder if it appears that a serious emotional disturbance is present.

Treatment is not always simple and above all requires the sympathetic concern of the physician. Therapeutic success rests largely on establishing good physician-patient rapport. Some initial steps that are important and useful are listed in Box 3-4.

Because most tension headaches are caused by the patient's life adjustment, any treatment plan must take this into account. Many patients do not recognize the origin of their problem, and a frank discussion about their life situation is often helpful. Other patients are aware of their emotional difficulty but welcome an opportunity to express their feelings openly. In either case, being able to talk over their

BOX 3-4

1 The physician should acknowledge that real pain is present; too many patients are brushed off or merely handed a prescription and told to live with their problem.

2 Because many patients fear that they may have a brain tumor or other serious disease, it is also advisable to reassure them that no evidence of a serious condition has been found.

3 A realistic goal should be set with the patient. The number and intensity of the headaches can probably be reduced, but not necessarily eliminated completely.

problems with the physician helps many patients gain a new perspective. Obviously, if major psychiatric problems are present, the patient should be referred for a psychiatrist's help.

Other avenues of treatment should also be used. Gentle neck massage and muscle relaxation can be helpful, as can taking a few minutes out of a busy day to lie down. Relaxation can be aided by biofeedback techniques, an approach that has yielded some success. In biofeedback the responsibility for the treatment rests with the patient. This has obvious advantages, but only patients willing to persevere with the program can be helped.

Medications are another approach. Three basic classes of drugs are used: muscle relaxants, psychotropics (antidepressants or tranquilizers), and analgesics. Muscle relaxants such as methocarbamol (Robaxin) (750 mg, 4 to 8 pills daily) help relax tightened muscles in some patients but have certainly not proved to be overwhelmingly effective. Low doses of tricyclic antidepressants (e.g., amitriptyline, doxepin, or nortriptyline, 10 to 50 mg at bedtime) have been very effective in treating chronic headaches. This medication has excellent analgesic properties at these low doses. In patients whose headaches are part of a depression, a full therapeutic dose of antidepressant medication is often very helpful. In anxious or nervous patients, the use of tranquilizers is a serious issue. In patients who have headaches for a week or two twice a year, small amounts of meprobamate or a benzodiazepine medication can often help. These drugs can safely be given as needed or daily during the period of the headache. This, coupled with the judicious use of a mild to moderately strong analgesic medication, can usually carry the patient through a difficult time.

The more significant and all too common problem is the chronic use of medication in patients with almost daily headaches. Stupefying the patient with increasing dosages of medication hardly seems prudent. Most headache experts treat these patients with mild analgesics alone (acetaminophen or aspirin) because the problems of habituation, abuse, and tolerance so frequently develop when stronger medications are used. The side effects (e.g., ulcer, nephropathy, tinnitus) from excessive salicylates must always be considered. Unfortunately, psychotherapy is seldom helpful; therefore intermittent tranquilization and analgesia are used when the headaches are most severe. The use of continuous daily analgesic medication is discouraged; however, daily prophylactic medication can be useful, especially the tricyclic antidepressant.

Patients with chronic headaches tend to "shop" from physician to physician and have tried or are taking a variety of strong medications. Each new pill is effective for a short time, but often the patient requests more and stronger medication. In general, the patient with chronic tension headaches is difficult to treat, and the treatment regimen must be individualized. In some cases the headache has the characteristics of both muscular contraction and vascular types (see next section). If the headaches have a vascular character, some patients will respond to the prophylactic regimen outlined in the next section for chronic frequent migraine headache.

Vascular Headaches

To many persons, any severe headache is called a migraine. This is not always the case, however. Migraine or vascular headaches have rather specific clinical features, and severity is only one. The five basic diagnostic features that strongly suggest migraine are typical visual phenomena, unilateral pounding headache, nausea and vomiting early in a headache before medicine is taken, distinct onset and termination of headache, and a response to ergot preparations. The cause of migraines is uncertain. They are not psychogenic, but emotional stress is certainly known to provoke the attacks. Fatigue, hunger, certain tyramine-containing foods, contraceptive pills, change in hormones during menstruation or menopause, red wine, smoking, monosodium glutamate, smelling certain odors, and a myriad of other factors can also bring on the headache. As in tension headache, there is an increased prevalence in females, but there is also a strong familial tendency to migraine headaches. Onset is usually in the 20s, but an onset in childhood is not uncommon. Frequency of attacks varies but tends to increase during times of stress or major life changes.

The pathophysiology is interesting. The migraine patient has some type of episodic central autonomic imbalance that causes changes in cerebrovascular tone. In the initial stage of a migraine it has been hypothesized that both extracranial and intracranial blood vessels contract. This contraction lasts for 5 to 45 minutes and is rapidly followed by vasodilatation. It is the distention of the extracranial vessels that causes the characteristic throbbing pain. It has been observed that blood levels of serotonin rise during vasoconstriction and fall during vasodilatation. The relationship of the release of this and possible other vasoactive substances (presumably from platelets) to the migraine syndromes is unclear.

Classic Migraine (Migraine with Aura)

In the classic migraine the patient experiences a distinct neurologic warning or aura. This occurs as intracranial vessels constrict. There is considerable controversy whether the neurologic symptoms (particularly the slowly progressing or changing visual phenomena) are caused by a primary vascular phenomena or by a spreading cortical depolarization or depression.

The aura is most often visual (flashing lights, blurring of vision, wavy lines, spreading scotoma with scintillating margins, or hemianopia), although hemiparesis, ophthalmoplegia, hemisensory symptoms, aphasia, and occasionally confusional behavior do occur. When focal neurologic signs appear, such as hemiparesis, the term *complicated migraine* is often applied. The aura typically lasts between 5 and 45 minutes and usually precedes the headache. The headache then rapidly appears. It is unilateral, pounding, and very severe. It is usually associated with an uneasy feeling in the stomach, nausea, vomiting (sick headache), and sensitivity to sound and light. During the headache the neurologic deficits usually fade. The pain lasts from several hours to all day and can recede rapidly or slowly. Attacks occur from once in a lifetime to daily. Each attack starts unilaterally but can spread. Most patients have a usual side for the headache, but it is characteristic that on occasion the headache will begin on the opposite side. If a patient has had all headaches on a single side, the physician must consider the possibility that an underlying focal brain lesion such as a vascular malformation may be present. Headaches that switch sides overwhelmingly suggest the diagnosis of migraine. Vasomotor changes can occur in migraines, which can be responsible for the patient's head feeling warm and hands icy cold. Also, syncope can occur in migraine patients as a result of vasomotor changes, pain, or medication effect.

Common Migraine (Migraine without Aura)

As the name implies, common migraine is the most frequently encountered vascular headache. A distinct aura is not present, but prodromal symptoms such as an uneasy feeling, depression, or malaise can be present for hours or days before the headache. The onset of pain can be somewhat more gradual than in the classic migraine. The pain is severe, usually unilateral at first, but often spreads. Nausea, vomiting, and photophobia are less common. The pain is intermittently pounding and lasts longer than does that of the classic migraine. This type of migraine is sometimes difficult to differentiate from a tension headache, which starts to throb as it increases in intensity. There is, in fact, a significant overlap of chronic recurrent tension and common migraine headaches. Some patients with common migraines can, over the years, develop a chronic daily headache that has features of a background of daily tension-type headache with escalation to migrainelike pain intensity and character on frequent occasions. Such patients tend to overuse analgesics, have depression, have significant life stresses, suffer sleep disturbance, have a greater than expected problem with substance abuse, and often have a family history of a similar disorder.

Cluster Headache

Cluster headache is an unusual but not uncommon headache syndrome that may or may not be related to migraines. These headaches are more common in males; they usually begin between the ages of 20 and 40, but often appear first in middle age. The headaches are characterized by sudden, very severe, steady, boring, or throbbing pain. They often occur at night and awaken the patient from sleep. The pain is exclusively unilateral and usually is located in or around the eye. The pain lasts between 15 and 90 minutes and is often associated with unilateral conjunctival injection, tearing, and nasal stuffiness. The scalp can also feel sore or painful. The pain does not shift sides with attacks as does migraine. The pains occur in clusters over a period of days to months and then disappear for 1 to several years. In some patients, the pain occurs in the lower face (lower half headache) and resembles sphenopalatine neuralgia (Sluder's neuralgia). The pain can be triggered by alcohol consumption or smoking.

There is a variant of the cluster headache in which occurrence is seen equally in males and females; there can be bilateral pain that is more frontotemporal than periorbital; pain is not as severe; autonomic response (e.g., lacrimation) is infrequent; and background vascular headache and jabbing localized head pain are also often experienced. Most cluster headache attacks are episodic with periods of remission; however, some patients experience attacks without remission (chronic cluster). Another variant is the occurrence of short-duration attacks many times each day (chronic paroxysmal hemicrania).

Migraine Equivalents

In some persons episodic aura or prodromata occur without the accompanying headache. Autonomic disturbances such as tachycardia, nausea, or visceral pain can be experienced as well as neurologic signs. Classic visual aura with spreading scotoma are occasionally experienced initially in middle or old age without headaches. Most of these patients do not have any demonstrable cerebral vascular disease to explain them. The reason for the appearance of the migraine equivalents at this age is unclear. (Fisher, 1986)[2] These isolated migraine equivalents are at times reported by migraine patients but are also experienced by people who have never had an associated headache.

Laboratory Evaluation

If the patient has had only a few headaches and they are all on one side or if the patient has either abnormalities on the neurologic examination or suspicious factors in the history, full evaluation is advisable. In addition, if the headache precedes the neurologic aura or if the patient is seen during the first ever attack, neurodiagnostic studies are warranted. In patients with a typical history of chronic recurring vascular headaches, an extensive evaluation seems unnecessary. Electroencephalograms will often show focal abnormalities that are not significant clinically and only serve to worry both the patient and the physician. Routine CT or MRI scanning seems unjustified in most headache patients.

Treatment

Treatment of vascular headaches is usually much more rewarding than the treatment of tension headaches. Significant improvement is expected in the majority of patients. The choice of medication depends both on the character of the headache and on its frequency. In patients with occasional headaches with a distinct aura or prodrome, ergot preparations or sumatriptan should be used at the onset of symptoms (Table 3-2). These drugs maintain mild vascular constriction and prevent the painful vasodilatory phase. They are quite safe and can be used even in complicated migraines. If nausea prevents oral intake, suppositories can be used. Dihydroergotamine (DHE) may soon be available in a nasal spray. Hopefully, this will prove to be a good alternative to suppositories. Ergot must be started early in the course of the attack because it is rarely effective once the severe headache has started. If the patient has no warning of the headache's onset or it awakens him or her at night, ergot derivatives are usually ineffective, and the only effective treatment is sumatriptan injections. Oral ergot is much cheaper than the sumatriptan and is the initial drug of choice. Sumatriptan is available in a self-injecting form that can be given at any time during the headache; it is highly effective with minimal significant side effects. In a minority of patients the headache can rebound, and a second shot needs to be given. If the shot is not effective, strong analgesic medications plus medication for nausea must be used. Parenteral use of dihydroergotamine (1 mg) preceded by metoclopramide (Reglan, 10 mg) may also abort the migraine attack, but this preparation is not available in an autoinjectable form.

TABLE 3-2 Drugs Commonly Used to Abort Acute Migraine

Drug	Dose
Imitrex (sumatriptan)	Injection 6 mg
Cafergot (ergotamine, 1 mg and caffeine)	Two tablets at first sign of migraine, then one tablet every 30 minutes; maximum six tablets in 24 hours
Gynergen (ergotamine, 1 mg)	Same
Midrin (acetaminophen plus a sympathomimetic and mild sedative)	Same
Wigraine (ergotamine, 1 mg, belladonna, caffeine, and phenacetin)	Same

In patients with daily or severe weekly headaches, a daily prophylactic medication seems justified. The medications in Table 3-3 have been shown to be effective and are listed roughly in descending order of effectiveness. In episodic cluster inhalation of oxygen administered via a mask can abort the attack. Chronic paroxysmal hemicrania may respond to indomethacin (Indocin) in a dose of 25 mg three times daily. Patients using contraceptive pills are often helped by switching to an alternate form of birth control; in some cases switching to a low estrogen preparation can reduce migraine frequency.

The length of therapy depends on the patient and the type of headache. Cluster headaches typically last only a few weeks or months; thus medication can be tapered after headaches have abated. In the classic or common migraine, it is suggested that patients remain on medication for 6 to 12 months and then taper off

---

Side Effects and Precautions

Burning at injection site, tightness in chest or throat, tingling or
burning sensation

Numbness and coolness of extremities
Chest pain and tachycardia
Nausea and vomiting. Do not use in patients with cardiovascular or
peripheral vascular disease. Never use in pregnant women.

Gynergen (ergotamine, 1 mg)

Midrin (acetaminophen plus a
sympathomimetic and mild sedative)

Wigraine (ergotamine, 1 mg, belladonna,
caffeine, and phenacetin)

---

the medication until headaches recur. Breakthroughs
from prophylactic therapy do occur and are treated as
a regular migraine.

The prognosis of migraine is similar to that of tension
headaches. Most patients have more frequent headaches
around the times of major stresses and life changes.

Headaches Associated with Hypertension

A significant number of hypertensive patients complain of headache. Interestingly, headache is much
more common in patients who are aware that they
have hypertension. This suggests that knowing about
hypertension and its possible sequelae, such as brain
hemorrhage, promotes headaches. The hypertensive
headache itself is not particularly distinctive. It is
often, although not always, throbbing. It is frequently
localized in either the occipital or the frontal area and
can be lateralized to one side. It is present in the

TABLE 3-3 Prophylactic Medications

Trade Name (Generic Name)	Dose
Migraine	
Beta Blockers	
Inderal (propranolol) or Corgard (nadolol)	Start with Inderal 60 mg LA or Corgard 20 mg; increase to 240 mg maximum.
Tricyclic Antidepressants	
Elavil (amitriptyline), Sinequan (doxepin), Pamelor (nortriptyline)	10 to 25 mg at bedtime; can increase as needed
Calcium Channel Blockers	
Verapamil	180 to 240 mg sustained
Sansert (methysergide)	2 mg twice daily up to four times a day
Nonsteroidal analgesics	
Bellergal-S (phenobarbital, ergotamine, belladonna)	Two to four tablets daily
Periactin (cyproheptadine)	4 mg, two to four tablets daily
Anticonvulsants	
Tegretol	Must titrate
Depakote	Must titrate
Cluster headache	
Calcium channel blocker	As above
Prednisone plus ergotamine	10 mg four times a day for 7 days then taper off to four tablets daily for 7 days, then taper off
Sansert	As above
Periactin	As above
Lithium (chronic cluster)	300 mg tid
Cluster variant	
Indomethacin	25 mg three times a day
Aspirin	Eight 5-grain tablets daily

Because of β-blocking properties, it is not safe in patients with asthma or heart failure. Can slow heart rate.

Nervousness, drowsiness, dry mouth, and other anticholinergic side effects. Seizures in very high doses.

Can cause cardiovascular effects such as hypotension and arrhythmias, including heart block. Do not use with β-blockers.

Retroperitoneal, pulmonary, and cardiac valve fibrosis. This can almost always be prevented by not giving the drug longer than 6 months without a month drug holiday. Never give more than 8 mg daily.

May cause stomach problems. Anaprox (naproxen) is particularly useful in catemenial (menstrual) migraine when used before and throughout the menstrual period.

Drowsiness plus other side effects of ergot and belladonna

Drowsiness and antihistamine effects

Can reinstitute full treatment regimen if headaches break through while tapering medications

Watch blood level

Confusion, tremor, polyuria, nausea, diarrhea, weakness

Monitor complete blood count

Gastric distress

mornings in about half of the patients, particularly those with throbbing pain, and scattered throughout the day in the others. In some the pattern is migrainous, whereas in others it is not. Treatment of the hypertension helps many patients; thus it seems that the increased arterial pressure in the vessels is in some way related to the headaches in some patients. In hypertensive encephalopathy the headache is more persistent and is the direct result of cerebral edema and increased intracranial pressure.

Sinus Headache

Inflammation of mucosa of the nose and ostia of the perinasal sinuses can give rise to localized pain in the head and face. When a sinus is actually blocked, an intense pain can be caused by the vacuum created by absorption of trapped air. The pain is steady, dull, and aching. It is localized over the area of the affected sinus. Table 3-4 shows the location of pain based on the sinus infected.

The pain is aggravated by coughing, sneezing, bending over, or straining. Tearing is often seen, and there is usually evidence of nasal inflammation. The bone over the sinus is often tender to firm pressure. In acute sinusitis the pain is quite severe, whereas in chronic sinusitis the pain is less intense and less often associated with nasal symptoms. Sinus headache is often diagnosed in patients with simple tension headaches, and sinus disease has become the scapegoat for many psychologic headaches. Allergic rhinitis can be associated with sinus headache on occasion, but again tension headache is much more common in the allergy sufferer than is true sinusitis.

The diagnosis of sinusitis and sinus headache is usually made on history, examination of the nose, and

TABLE 3-4	
Sinus infected	*Location of pain*
Frontal	Forehead above eyebrows
Ethmoidal	Bridge of nose
Maxillary	Below eye and in upper teeth
Sphenoidal	Behind eye and at vertex

sinus roentgenograms. Treatment consists of decongestants, antibiotics, and analgesics.

Chronic Pain from Cervical Spine Disease

Degeneration of intervertebral disks in the cervical region (cervical spondylosis, see Chapter 19) can be the source of occipital headache. The syndrome is principally seen in laboring middle-aged males and after whiplash types of injuries. Pain can be caused by local degenerative changes or pressure on cervical nerve roots. The pain is steady, often exacerbated by neck motion, and can spread into the shoulder or arms, particularly with root impingement.

Examination usually reveals only minor spasm of the upper trapezius, but a careful neurologic examination for signs of nerve root and spinal cord compression should be carried out. Cervical spine roentgenograms are important in establishing the diagnosis.

Treatment in the absence of neurologic deficit is conservative: heat to the area, simple analgesics, occasional muscle relaxants, cervical traction, and intermittent use of a soft collar are the most helpful.

Posttraumatic Headaches

Posttraumatic headaches can be chronic and recurrent. These headaches usually occur immediately after the head injury and are seen after mild as well as severe injuries. Three patterns of headache have been described: one, constant, bandlike, generalized headache; two, superficial tenderness at the local injury site; and three, episodic, throbbing, unilateral headache. The headaches can be intermittent or constant, worsened by head movement or emotional stress, and associated with dizziness and difficulty concentrating. It is imperative to perform a careful neurologic examination to exclude a structural trauma-related lesion. If the findings of this examination are normal, computed tomography (CT) is not usually necessary. The majority of posttraumatic headaches resolve within several weeks or months after head injury; however, some are quite prolonged and intractable. Treatment depends on the headache pattern and if the symptoms suggest a predominantly vascular or muscle contraction component. When the headaches begin to increase in severity 2 to 4 weeks after the trauma, it is wise to obtain a CT scan to rule out a slowly developing subdural hematoma.

Headache Associated with Brain Tumor and Other Lesions Causing Increased Intracranial Pressure

Mass Lesions

The brain itself does not have pain fibers; the pain from tumors and other mass lesions comes from the distortions and traction on such pain-sensitive structures as the dura, dural sinuses, and the great vessels at the base of the brain.

This type of headache has several very important clinical features. There is seldom a long history. The pain is a dull, steady, aching feeling that is usually much less intense than migraine. The pain is usually worse in the morning and is acutely exacerbated by rapid assumption of the upright position. Coughing, sneezing, and straining will also cause acute worsening of the pain. The pain is often localized to the area of the mass. In subtentorial tumors, headache is very common and is principally in the occipital region. The supratentorial tumors in the temporal lobe are most likely to create pain.

A history of headache developing gradually over several months is a possible indication of a mass lesion. If the history is associated with any other neurologic symptoms such as seizure, decreased level of awareness, vomiting, and language difficulty, the likelihood of tumor increases dramatically.

If a mass is suspected, it is imperative that a full neurodiagnostic evaluation be undertaken. *A spinal puncture should never be performed when an intracranial mass lesion is suspected.* Treatment is usually neurosurgical. Corticosteroids can decrease pressure, but it is prudent to discuss the case with a neurosurgeon first (dexamethasone, 12 mg intravenously stat, with 4 mg intravenously every six hours is usually used).

Hydrocephalus

Hydrocephalus (expansion of the cerebral ventricles because of obstruction of flow) results in dull frontal and occipital pain. This can be very severe if there is acute obstruction as occurs in posterior fossa and midline third ventricular tumors. CT scanning, magnetic resonance imaging (MRI), and shunting of cerebrospinal fluid (CSF) are the mainstays of evaluation and treatment.

Benign Intracranial Hypertension (Pseudotumor Cerebri)

Benign intracranial hypertension is an unusual, yet by no means rare, condition that occurs primarily in young (20 to 35), overweight females who have menstrual irregularities. The symptoms are primarily diffuse headache and occasionally intermittent blurred vision (obscuration) and diplopia. The headache is a nondescript intermittent, generalized pain that is worse in the morning and exacerbated by coughing or sneezing. On examination the patients are alert, have papilledema, and occasionally show lateral rectus weakness, reduced visual acuity, and enlarged blind spots.

Evaluation should include first a CT and MRI scan to rule out a mass or hydrocephalus and then lumbar puncture. CSF pressure is usually more than 300 mm H_2O but with normal CSF content (no cells, normal protein, or sugar). With the tap, the pressure should be brought down to 50% of the opening pressure.

The treatment varies. If the cause is known (e.g., anemia), correction of the basic problem will reverse the condition. When no cause is known, often the initial lumbar puncture with a decrease in pressure can be curative. When unsuccessful, repeated therapeutic taps (every other day) have been used although without a theoretic basis. Corticosteroids (prednisone, 80 mg daily) and (acetazolamide [Diamox], 1 to 3 g daily) have also been used with some success. In rare cases in which these measures have failed and vision is in jeopardy, an optic nerve sheath decompression or a lumbar peritoneal shunt may be necessary.

Most cases resolve without permanent visual loss, but some cases (less than 10%) become recurrent or chronic and present a severe management problem.

Subarachnoid Hemorrhage

When blood suddenly invades the subarachnoid space, it stretches and distorts and irritates the pain-sensitive vessels and meninges. This produces an acute and very severe headache. The patient can usually report the exact time of the onset of a pain and will frequently exclaim that it was the "worst headache I have ever had." Such a history should immediately alert the physician to the possibility of a serious intracranial disaster, very probably a subarachnoid hemorrhage. The headache usually strikes without warning. It is severe, steady, and generalized. There can be an immediate alteration in the level of consciousness, and some patients become comatose within seconds. The alert patient usually complainsof neck stiffness, photophobia, dizziness, and nausea. With more serious hemorrhages focal neurologic signs can be present. On examination nuchal rigidity is usually present. Subhyaloid hemorrhages in the retina, oculomotor nerve paralysis, and other neurologic signs can be present.

Evaluation should begin with a CT scan; this will show hematoma formation as well as subarachnoid blood in most cases. If no clot or subarachnoid blood is demonstrated, a spinal puncture should be performed. At this point a neurologist or neurosurgeon should be consulted. If blood is present, a four-vessel arteriogram should be planned and specific treatment dictated by the findings therein.

Meningitis

Although not common, meningitis is a serious but treatable disease that is frequently heralded by headaches. The pain originates in the inflamed meninges. The headache is usually occipital but can be present in other locations. Stiff neck and fever are almost always present and certainly point to the diagnosis.

Other neurologic signs can be present, including an altered level of consciousness, cranial nerve palsies, and major motor abnormalities. Diagnosis is made by spinal puncture. Viral, fungal, cryptococcal, tubercular, and bacterial organisms can all produce the classic symptoms. Treatment and prognosis are related to the organism isolated (see Chapter 18).

One note of caution concerning occipital headache and nuchal rigidity: these disorders can be caused by herniation of the cerebellar tonsils in posterior fossa masses. A careful search should be made for lower cranial nerve abnormalities and nystagmus before attempting lumbar puncture. If the patient is afebrile and any question about the diagnosis exists, a CT or MRI scan should be obtained before lumbar puncture.

Temporal Arteritis

Temporal arteritis is a variety of diffuse granulomatous arteritis in which the majority of the patients (60%) experience headache. The disease most commonly affects the ophthalmic artery and branches of the external carotid artery (superficial temporal, occipital, facial, and maxillary). The condition is rare in persons under the age of 50 and in most cases (85% to 90%) patients are over the age of 60. Headache is the most common feature. Classically the pain is steady, localized, and strong, with intermittent sharp, stabbing pains. This is not always the case, however, and because of this the diagnosis is often delayed.

Unilateral or bilateral rapid (12 to 48 hours) *irreversible* visual loss can occur. Jaw claudication (pain with chewing) from involvement of the maxillary artery is also common. A variety of signs of generalized illness can be seen (e.g., malaise, fever, depression, anorexia), and the condition is often associated with polymyalgia rheumatica (aching pains in the joints and muscles without objective signs of arthritis). On examination the temporal artery can be tender or at times pulseless and hard secondary to thrombosis. The scalp skin is often tender. The most specific laboratory test is the erythrocyte sedimentation rate, which is elevated in more than 90% of cases, often to very high levels. A temporal artery biopsy can also be performed to establish the diagnosis pathologically.

Treatment should be started immediately to preserve vision; prednisone, 60 to 80 mg, is given daily for 4 to 6 weeks and then gradually tapered to 5 to 10 mg. Treatment at low doses should be continued for at least 1 year. Periodic erythrocyte sedimentation rates will document treatment effectiveness.

Pain from Structures in the Head

When taking the history and examining the headache patient, it must be remembered that many structures in the head can be responsible for pain. Ocular pathology (particularly glaucoma), severe refraction errors, and masses or inflammation either within or behind the orbit are also sources of pain. Unless there is a marked refractive error or the eye appears clinically involved (e.g., red or swollen), the eye is not the source of the headache. Abscessed teeth, middle ear infections, and mastoid infections can also cause headaches.

A final fairly common source of headaches is the temporomandibular joint dysfunction. When there is malocclusion of the teeth, unbalanced force is transmitted to this point. This results in pain that can run up into the temple, occiput, face, teeth, or neck. The joint itself is often painful to palpation, a sign that will confirm the diagnosis. This condition, often called Costen's syndrome, frequently occurs after dental work. When the diagnosis is made, referral to a dentist should be made. Indomethacin, 25 mg three times a day, is often useful in treatment.

Headache Associated with Other Systemic Diseases

Headache is often an accompanying symptom of systemic disease such as infection, endocrine disorders, and allergic and immunologic disorders and, of course, can be a prominent secondary symptom in anyone with chronic illness. The headache itself is a nonspecific tensionlike headache and is best handled by promptly treating the underlying disease.

Face Pains

Trigeminal Neuralgia

There are several important syndromes of severe face pain. The most common is tic douloureux, or trigeminal neuralgia. Age at onset is usually 50, and the disorder is twice as common in females. The cardinal symptom is a lightninglike (lancinating), excruciating, unilateral face pain that shoots down one or a combination of the fifth (trigeminal) nerve branches. The syndrome has also been described in ninth (glossopharyngeal) and tenth (vagus) nerves. Some patients may describe a similar type of pain that occurs in the back of the throat and can radiate to the ear. These are stabbing or electric-like pains that can be precipitated by swallowing or yawning. This pain is characteristic of glossopharyngeal neuralgia. The pains frequently come in bursts over a few seconds to a few minutes and leave the region with a soreness after the pain. Pain can often be triggered by touching the face, eating or drinking hot or cold substances, talking, or jarring the head in any way. The pain is most frequently experienced in the distribution of both mandibular and maxillary divisions (36%); mandibular pain alone occurs in 19% of the cases; all divisions, 15%; maxillary alone, 14%; maxillary and ophthalmic, 11%; and ophthalmic alone, only 3%. Initially these pains occur in bouts over a few days and then remit for months; in time, however, the bouts lengthen and the remission shortens. In chronic trigeminal neuralgia the pains can last many minutes.

On examination there should be little or no abnormality in the appreciation of sensation over the affected areas. The presence of significant facial hypalgesia or other cranial nerve abnormality (e.g., loss of corneal reflex or weakness) usually indicates a structural lesion either in the nerve, such as a neurofibroma, or in the posterior fossa, such as a multiple sclerosis plaque, cerebellar tumor, or acoustic neuroma.

In the absence of any positive neurologic findings, the only advisable laboratory test would be dental roentgenograms to rule out an apical abscess or other similar conditions.

The pathophysiology of the pain is not known; however, the two main theories are pressure from a blood vessel lying on the nerve as it exits from the brain stem and chronic infection with herpes simplex virus.

Treatment can be either medical or surgical. It is usually advisable to try medication initially. The drugs prevent the pains by stabilizing the nerve membranes. The most effective are carbamazepine (Tegretol, 200 mg bid, then increasing by 200 mg daily every 3 to 4 days until either the pain stops or the patient is taking 1600 mg daily), phenytoin (Dilantin, 300 to 400 mg daily), and baclofen (Lioresal, 20 to 60 mg daily). If medication fails, alcohol injection into the nerve or percutaneous radiofrequency trigeminal gangliolysis is effective but can produce anesthesia and residual hyperpathic pain. Retromastoid craniectomy with dissection of the vessels off the nerve is also a successful procedure.

Atypical Face Pain

The second important face pain syndrome is atypical facial pain. This condition is seen in young as well as older adults and is characterized by rather diffuse, nondescript pain. The pain aches or burns rather than stabs. It is often quite widespread and can involve half or occasionally all of the head and spread to the neck. The pain is quite persistent and can last for years.

Many pathologic conditions such as sinus tumor, tooth abscess, and temporomandibular joint abnormalities can be present with face pain and must be ruled out. If no specific lesion is found, a diagnosis of idiopathic or atypical facial pain is made. The cause is not known, but psychotropic medications, particularly antidepressants or minor tranquilizers, have been the most successful treatment.

▨ SUMMARY

There is a spectrum of headache from classic migraine at one end to simple tension headache at the other. The history of the clinical characteristics of the headache will place the headache on the appropriate location in that spectrum. Specific medications can then be prescribed basis on the of the character of the headache and its frequency.

References

1. Lance JW, editor: Advances in biology and pharmacology of headache, *Neurology* 43(suppl 3):S1, 1993.
2. Fisher CM: Late-life migraine accompaniments—further experience, *Stroke* 17:1033, 1986.

Suggested Readings

Evaluation

Day JW, Raskin NH: Thunderclap headache: symptom of unruptured cerebral aneurysm, *Lancet* 2:1247, 1986.

Edmeads J: Emergency management of headache, *Headache* 28:675, 1988.

Edmeads J: The worst headache ever, *Postgrad Med* 86:93, 1989.

Headache Classification Committee of the International Headache Society: Classification and diagnostic criteria for headache disorders, cranial neuralgias and face pain, *Cephalgia* 7(suppl 8):1, 1988.

Mathew NT, editor: Headache, *Neurol Clin* 8:781, 1990.

Pearce JMS: Headache, *Neurol Neurosurg Psych* 57:134, 1994.

Raskin NH: *Headache*, ed 2, New York, 1988, Churchill Livingston.

Migraine Headache

Appenzeller O, Feldman RG, Friedman AP: Migraine, headache, and related conditions—panel 7, *Arch Neurol* 36:784, 1979.

Sumatriptan International Study Group: Treatment of migraine with sumatriptan, *N Engl J Med* 325:316, 1991.

Welch KMA: Drug therapy of migraine, *N Engl J Med* 329:1476, 1993.

Cluster Headache

Kudrow L: Cluster headache, *Neurol Clin North Am* 1:369, 1982.

Kudrow L: Diagnosis and management of cluster headache. Med Clin North Am 75:579, 1991.

Medina JL, Diamond S: Cluster headache variant, *Arch Neurol* 38:705, 1981.

Intracranial Mass Lesions

Forsyth PA, Posner JB: Headaches in patients with brain tumors, *Neurology* 43:1678, 1993.

Benign Intracranial Hypertension

Wall M, George D: Idiopathic intracranial hypertension, *Brain* 114:155, 1991.

Weisberg LA: Benign intracranial hypertension, *Medicine* 54:197, 1975.

Muscle Contraction Headache

Edmeads, J: The cervical spine and headache, *Neurology* 38:1874, 1988.

Riley TL: Muscle-contraction headache, *Neurol Clin North Am* 1:489, 1983.

Facial Pain

Penman J: Trigeminal neuralgia. In Vinken PJ, Bruyn AW, editors: *Handbook of Clinical Neurology,* vol 5, 296–322, Amsterdam, 1968, Elsevier North Holland Publishing Co.

Solomon S, Lipton RB: Atypical facial pain, *Semin Neurol* 8:322, 1988.

Temporal Arteritis

Buchbinder R, Detsky AS: Management of suspected giant cell arteritis, *J Rheum* 19:1120, 1992.

Goodman BW: Temporal arteritis, *Am J Med* 67:839, 1972.

Dizziness

4

Dizziness is a common, multifaceted, yet often elusive symptom. In its broadest sense, it is a feeling of uncertainty about one's physical orientation in space. The feeling is unphysiologic because the patient is not actually having his or her environment moved but is receiving false or conflicting information about his or her position or motion relative to the environment. For example, when getting off a merry-go-round, a person feels as if he or she is still moving when, in fact, this is not the case. Patients describe many abnormal sensations as dizziness; the first task of the physician, therefore, is to elucidate exactly what the patient means when reporting dizziness.

▦ TERMINOLOGY

The general symptom can be separated into five major categories, each with its own diagnostic significance. The physician must inquire specifically about each to firmly establish the type of dizziness the patient is experiencing (Box 4-1).

BOX 4-1

1 *Vertigo.* This is a spontaneous feeling or illusion of movement. This is usually a rotational sensation in which either the patient or the environment is moving. Vertigo represents an illusion of movement. True vertigo is usually due to dysfunction of the vestibular system—peripheral labyrinth, vestibular nuclei in the pons, and the flocculus of the cerebellum.

2 *Syncopal sensation or presyncope.* This is the sudden feeling of faintness that occurs when circulation to the brain is inadequate. This is due to diffuse cerebral ischemia with inadequate oxygenation of the brain secondary to hypotension, cardiac arrhythmia, stenosis of cerebral vessels, or other circulatory factors. Syncopal sensations can also be caused by hyperventilation with a reduction of carbon dioxide blood levels and constriction of cerebral blood vessels.

3 *Dysequilibrium.* An imbalance can occur when the patient is standing or walking; this feeling of being off-balance is often called dizziness by the patient. Imbalance or dysequilibrium can be caused by numerous motor and sensory disorders, such as mild hemiparesis, Parkinson's disease, hydrocephalus, spasticity from myelopathy, sensory loss in the legs from neuropathy, cerebellar disorders, and others.

4 *Visual-induced dizziness.* A change in visual acuity caused by ocular pathology or a recently modified eyeglass prescription can cause dizziness as a result of an altered vestibulo-ocular reflex system. This dizziness and feeling of spatial disorientation can be accompanied by occipital or base-of-skull headache of the muscle contraction type.

5 *Lightheadedness or giddiness.* This is an all-inclusive category for other vague or nondescript sensations of uneasiness in the head. Patients can also complain of a floating or spinning sensation inside the head. It is important to recognize that this symptom is not true vertigo and therefore not necessarily of vestibular origin. This type of complaint is often attributed to emotional causes, but many patients probably have subtle vestibular dysfunction, circulatory problems, sensory disturbances, or visual disturbances.

In general, dizziness is of a benign etiology but at times can signal significant neurologic or otologic disease.

▨ PATHOPHYSIOLOGY

To understand the various clinical syndromes associated with *dizziness,* it is useful to have some basic understanding of the symptom pathophysiology. Dizziness arises when orientation in space is disturbed. Knowing where the body is in relation to the environment and being able to move efficiently throughout that environment without feeling dizzy requires the integration of a set of delicate sensing devices (i.e., proprioceptive, visual, and vestibular) that feed information about the environment and a motor system that responds to the sensory information to maintain equilibrium. Whenever any portion of the system is damaged or gives false information, the system becomes unbalanced and there is a mismatch between the actual orientation of the body in space and what the patient perceives. This mismatch produces a false sense of motion that results in the patient's feeling of dizziness or vertigo.

Of the various sensors, the eyes are the most important because vision is the basic orienting sense. Even though primary visual disorders infrequently cause dizziness, unless the patient has developed diplopia, a person has only to close one eye and passively move the open eye by applying gentle pressure to the side of the eyeball to appreciate what can happen when the visual information received from the eye is not what the brain expects. How visual input affects balance and orientation is complex and involves integration of vision and eye movement. If such integration does not take place, every eye movement is interpreted by the brain as a sudden movement of the environment. Most eye movement is initiated in the cortex and then relayed to the vestibular nuclei and lateral gaze center in the pons. From this point, eye movements are integrated by the medial longitudinal fasciculus to the nuclei of the extraocular muscles. Simultaneous with the corticovestibular discharge is what has been called a corollary discharge to the visual cortex to prepare it for the imminent movement. This prevents the potential disorienting effect of the change in visual information.

The second critical sensor of body orientation is the labyrinth. Two types of sensors are present in each labyrinth: the saccule and utricle, which are static receptors to relay information in reference to gravity, and the cristae in the semicircular canals, which are kinetic receptors that sense angular or rotational movement. The labyrinths are in a tonic balance, and dysfunction in one or both will distort information about balance and body movement. This imbalance in labyrinthine input produces a sensation of movement when none is present (i.e., vertigo).

Nerve impulses from the labyrinth are carried by the vestibular portion of the eighth cranial nerve and terminate in the vestibular nuclei and flocculus of the cerebellum. From the vestibular nuclei there are four efferents: to the medial longitudinal fasciculus to integrate eye movements; to the cerebellum for balance and limb control; to reticular formation to maintain or stir arousal to prepare for the movement; and to the spinal cord via the vestibulospinal tract to control muscle tone for balance maintenance. Some vestibular efferents project to the cortex in the deep posterior temporal lobe. The major clinical significance of these temporal lobe projections is that when they are stimulated by an epileptic discharge, vertigo will result.

The third major sensor is the proprioceptive system. This system brings in information concerning position and movement of the joints. Particularly rich in proprioceptive receptors are the zygapophyseal joints of the upper cervical spine; these provide all-important information about head position and movement. Touch, pressure, and auditory input also are involved in the overall concept of spatial orientation, but much less so than the three principal sensors. In conjunction with this complex sensory system, a responsive motor system is also needed to make the necessary postural adjustments to maintain balance. An impaired motor system will produce imbalance but alone should not produce true vertigo.

◾ CLINICAL EVALUATION

The neurologic history and examination must be expanded to assess the complaint of dizziness properly.

History

The physician must review the primary complaint several times to establish what the patient is actually experiencing when complaining of dizziness. A series of specific questions should be asked about the symptom. Box 4-2 lists such questions.

Once the full character of the patient's complaint has been delineated, other pertinent medical history can be explored (Box 4-3).

Examination

Standard physical and neurologic examinations should be performed; particular attention should be paid to cerebellar testing and the cranial nerve examination. Look for nystagmus: rotatory, vertical, and horizontal. Check finger to nose to examiner's finger;

BOX 4-2

1 Is the problem acute or chronic?

2 Was the onset sudden or gradual?

3 Are the symptoms constant or intermittent? If they are intermittent, what will precipitate an exacerbation?

4 Do nausea and vomiting accompany the dizziness?

5 Are the symptoms exacerbated by motion?

6 Are the symptoms exclusively related to the position change or to the assumption of a specific position?

7 Is hearing impaired during the attack?

8 Is tinnitus present?

9 Is there an accompanying sensation of fullness in one or both ears?

10 Do any other neurologic symptoms accompany the dizziness, such as diplopia, weakness, perioral numbness, dysphagia, dysarthria, ataxia, or headache?

11 Does the patient feel off-balance? Is there a tendency to fall to one side?

12 Are symptoms worse with the eyes opened or closed?

 BOX 4-3

1 Is there cardiac disease or other chronic medical illness?

2 Does the patient have a decrease in vision, hearing, or peripheral sensation in legs or arms?

3 Has there been any recent viral illness?

4 Does the patient have an ear or sinus infection?

5 Has there been recent head trauma? If so, is it related to the symptoms?

6 Has there been neck trauma, or does the patient have neck pain or stiffness?

7 Has the patient been exposed to any toxic substance (e.g., pesticides, hydrocarbon vapors)?

8 Is the patient on any medications?

9 Does the patient use alcohol? What effect does its use have on the symptoms?

10 Are there psychiatric or emotional problems?

patients with vestibular disease will past-point *toward* the affected side because the healthy vestibular apparatus is tonic and forces the response to the weak side in the same way in which the eyes are forced to that side (i.e., the slow phase of the nystagmus). The patient can also turn to one side if asked to close eyes and take 50 steps in place. After performing the routine examination, the physician should carry out a series of maneuvers in an attempt to reproduce the patient's symptoms. After each maneuver, the patient is asked if it mimics the patient's complaint. The patient is assessed for nystagmus, past pointing, and imbalance while symptomatic. The testing procedure was developed by Drachman and is called a Dizziness Simulation Battery. The different maneuvers are carried out to attempt to reproduce exactly what the patient means by dizziness.

Dizziness Simulation Battery Maneuvers

Box 4-4 details the seven maneuvers carried out in Drachman's Dizziness Simulation Battery tests.

▆ DIAGNOSTIC ASSESSMENT

Based on the clinical features, it is possible to characterize the type of disorder causing the complaint of dizziness and to determine the diagnostic studies that are most useful. If dizziness is associated with an illusion of motion, this is most likely due to a primary vestibular disorder. If there is tinnitus and autonomic dysfunction (e.g., perspiration, nausea) without hearing loss or neurologic dysfunction, this indicates a peripheral vestibular or a labyrinthine disorder. If symptoms caused by a peripheral vestibular disorder do not resolve rapidly, referral to an otologist is warranted. Further testing, including hearing tests with

BOX 4-4

1 Blood pressure and pulse rate change from supine to erect posture. Pressure is checked with initial rise and again in 3 minutes to see if the patient compensates for the normal initial drop. Observe for orthostatic hypotension.

2 Hyperventilation for 3 minutes. This normally causes lightheadedness.

3 Valsalva maneuver. The patient squats 30 seconds, then strains 15 seconds. This will usually simulate syncopal sensation.

4 Carotid sinus stimulation. Gentle unilateral noncompressive stimulation is provided for 10 seconds with careful pulse monitoring. This can induce bradycardia and a syncopal sensation.

5 Rapid turns when walking and rapid passive head movements by the examiner (flexion and extension as well as rotation) are performed. If vertigo is elicited only when the neck is twisted and not with a change in body position with the neck immobile (e.g., lying down or full body turn), the problem is not due to labyrinth disease, but either cervical spine disease or vascular compression of the carotid or vertebral arteries.

6 Nylen-Bárány or Hallpike maneuver. Seat the patient on the examining table or hospital bed, hold the patient's head in both hands and then gently, but rapidly lower the patient backward until the head is 45 degrees below the edge of the table or bed. While lowering the patient back, the examiner simultaneously turns the patient's head to the side. This maneuver will test for positional vertigo.

7 Spinning. The patient is seated in a swivel chair that is rapidly spun around (10 times in 20 seconds). This will produce true vertigo in most patients.

pure tone audiography (impaired with cochlear disorders) and speech discrimination (impaired with retrocochlear disorders), is indicated. If vertigo is associated with cochlear hearing loss pattern, Ménière's disease is suggested. If vertigo is not associated with hearing loss or tinnitus, the patient may have a drug-induced or toxic disorder.

If vertigo is not associated with tinnitus and the neurologic examination is normal, it is important to perform hearing tests and caloric testing. Based on results of auditory or vestibular function tests, it should be possible to differentiate labyrinthine and cochlear disorders from retrolabyrinthine and retrocochlear (lesions affecting eighth nerve, brain stem, cerebellum) conditions. Electronystagmography demonstrates nystagmus by recording eye movement deflections by a patient and can detect nystagmus too subtle to be visualized by observation alone. Electronystagmography can also help diagnose dysfunction of the vestibular system and determine if the lesion is in the peripheral or central portion of the system.

Retrolabyrinthine disorders include mass lesions affecting the eighth nerve and cerebellopontine angle, brain stem (including multiple sclerosis) and cerebellar lesions, vascular lesions (aneurysm, angiomas, ectatic vessels) of vertebrobasilar arterial system, and petrous bone apex and tentorial lesions. If an eighth nerve or a cerebellopontine angle lesion is suspected, MRI or contrasted CT scan should be performed. MRI scanning also delineates the brain stem, cerebellum, and petrous apex. If a retrolabyrinthine or retrocochlear lesion is suspected and the imaging procedures are negative, brain stem (auditory) evoked potentials can be helpful in delineating the location of the lesion and can help differentiate cochlear from retrocochlear hearing loss.

If a patient's complaint of dizziness is not associated with an illusion of motion but is more of a vague lightheadedness, this is frequently *not* a vestibular dysfunction, and in such cases vestibular and auditory tests are not needed. If the symptoms seem secondary to anxiety, the dizziness can often be reproduced by hyperventilation. If there are associated cardiac symptoms, a medical-cardiac evaluation may be required. If symptoms are precipitated by standing, postural hypotension is suggested. In the elderly patient there can be multiple factors, including sensory loss, hearing decrease, visual decrease, medical problems, and also the effects of medications.

▨ CLINICAL SYNDROMES

Labyrinthine or Peripheral Vestibular Disorders

In general, labyrinthine or peripheral vestibular disorders are characterized by intense vertigo. The vertigo is dramatically exacerbated by movement. The onset is occasionally so sudden and severe that the patient falls to the floor. Nausea and vomiting are common. Nystagmus is usually present and is rotational or horizontal but never vertical. Ocular fixation can suppress both the vertigo and the nystagmus. Because of the tonic effect of the labyrinth, the slow phase of the nystagmus is toward the side of the damaged labyrinth. Nystagmus decreases with gaze toward the impaired side and increases with gaze toward the intact side. On finger-to-finger testing, the patient will past-point toward the damaged side and will fall to that side on tandem walking. Symptoms are worse when laying with the involved side down. Caloric testing shows a decreased response on the affected side. The condition can be episodic; in fact, any patient with episodic vertigo most likely has a peripheral rather than central (i.e., brain stem or cerebellar) disorder.

Acute Peripheral Vestibulopathy (Acute Vestibular Neuronitis, Acute Labyrinthitis)

Acute peripheral vestibulopathy occurs most commonly in young adults. The onset is acute in 75% of the cases. Vertigo, nausea, oscillopsia (experience of objects moving in the environment caused by marked coarse nystagmus), imbalance, and motion sensitivity are present. Nystagmus caused by peripheral labyrinthine or vestibular disorder can be horizontal or rotatory but never vertical (this indicates brain stem disease). The patient frequently is sweaty and has skin pallor. Tinnitus and a sensation of fullness in the ear are experienced by some patients. Posterior headache and fatigue can also be present in the recovery period. The cause is uncertain, but approximately 50% of the patients report a recent upper respiratory tract infection. The severe symptoms last from a few days to about a week, and a mild, gradually diminishing uneasiness typically continues for 2 to 6 weeks. Rapid movement, strenuous exercise, emotional stress, and alcohol consumption can exacerbate the symptoms. Treatment is symptomatic, with bed rest and anticholinergic medication every 4 to 6 hours affording some relief (scopolamine, 0.6 mg; promethazine [Phenergan], 25 to 50 mg; meclizine or cyclizine [Antivert, Bonine], 25 to 50 mg; diphenhydramine [Benadryl] 25 to 50 mg; or dimenhydrinate [Dramamine], 50 mg). Side effects include sedation of dryness of mucous membranes. In intractable cases diazepam (Valium), lorazepam (Ativan), and methylphenidate (Ritalin) have been used. In some cases symptoms will recur 6 weeks after the initial bout.

Benign Recurrent Vertigo

Benign recurrent vertigo is an uncommon condition that occurs both in children (ages 3 to 7) and adults. In children, it is characterized by abrupt onset and short duration (often less than 1 minute). The child looks pale during the attack and can vomit. The attacks recur from daily to semiannually, with an average of 8 to 12 per year. Caloric testing is usually abnormal. Spontaneous remission occurs. In adults the condition tends to be familial. The attacks last hours rather than seconds, the condition tends to be chronic, and caloric testing is normal.

Infection

The labyrinth can be affected by either systemic illness (particularly viral disease such as mumps, measles, rubella, and herpes zoster) or as an extension of otitis and mastoiditis. In chronic suppurative otitis (an increasingly rare disease) labyrinthine fistulas can develop. When this occurs, any abrupt rise in middle ear pressure from a sneeze or cough will trigger a sudden severe attack of vertigo. In syphilitic labyrinthitis progressive impairment of vestibular and auditory function causes vertigo and deafness.

Benign Positional Vertigo

Some patients experience vertigo only when they place their heads in a specific position. Most commonly, symptoms occur when the patient lies down or turns over in bed. Symptoms begin after a 2- to 10-second latency period and usually last about 20 seconds. The symptoms can be reproduced with the Nylen-Bárány maneuver (see p. 126), and during the period of vertigo nystagmus is present. The response will fatigue with repeated testing and subsequently remains resistant to further change for many hours. For some patients repeated self-produced attacks with the resultant immune period become a satisfactory method of treatment. Most cases are idiopathic, but predisposing factors include head trauma, advancing age, inactivity, and other ear disease. Age of onset is usually in the late 50s. The cause is uncertain but probably is due to a loose otolith or loose calcified

particles in the ampullae of the semicircular canals—
so-called cupulolithiasis.

Ménière's Disease

Ménière's disease is relatively common and is characterized by an excess of endolymph with resultant distention of the membranous labyrinth. Onset is usually
in the 40s. The classic syndrome consists of recurrent
attacks of acute vertigo, tinnitus, decreased hearing,
and full feeling in the affected ear. In the initial attacks
the vertigo can be the only symptom. The frequency
of attacks varies and long periods of quiescence are
not uncommon (e.g., 2 to 3 years). The caloric response is decreased on the side of the disease.

The hearing loss is sensorineural with cochlear
features. This cochlear pattern of hearing loss is characterized by low-frequency hearing loss with preserved speech (word) discrimination. The hearing
impairment is usually unilateral but can be bilateral.
When bilateral, the hearing loss can be asymmetric.
This cochlear pattern is contrasted with the findings
in retrocochlear lesions such as cerebellopontine
angle tumors. In these cases there is unilateral high-
frequency hearing loss and impaired speech discrimination. If there is any question, the differentiation
between a cochlear and retrocochlear lesion can be
made by brain stem (auditory) evoked potentials and
other hearing tests.

Tinnitus can persist between attacks, and in some
cases the hearing loss precedes the vertiginous attacks.
With repeated attacks hearing is gradually lost; low-
frequency tones are the first to be lost. The labyrinth
can eventually be destroyed, and at that point clinical
symptoms disappear. The disease has a familial tendency and is bilateral in 10% to 20% of the cases.

Diagnosis is usually made by history; however, documentation of a fluctuating low-frequency hearing loss is diagnostic. Medical treatment with anticholinergics, diazepam, and diuretics has not been very rewarding, and many patients are treated with surgical procedures that destroy the labyrinth or cut the vestibular portion of the eighth nerve. Abstaining from smoking, drinking, and stressful situations is helpful.

Ototoxic Substances and Metabolic Etiologies

Aminoglycoside antibiotics (kanamycin, streptomycin, and gentamicin), phenytoin, phenobarbital, quinidine, diazepam, aspirin, and alcohol are all known to have vestibular toxicity. Usually prompt withdrawal will reverse the problem, but unfortunately this is not effective in every case. In some alcoholic patients with or without Wernicke-Korsakoff syndrome, dizziness can be a prominent symptom. Hypothyroidism can also cause vestibular dysfunction.

Vertigo Caused by Migraine

Some patients with basilar migraines will experience vertigo as an aura or concurrent symptoms with their migraine headaches. At times, vertigo can be the *only* symptoms of the migraine attack—the so-called migraine equivalent or migraine accompaniment.

Disease of the Eighth (Acoustic) Nerve

Acoustic neuromas (neurinomas, schwannomas) or granulomatous disease such as sarcoid will occasionally affect the eighth nerve. Vertigo, when present, is persistent yet much less severe than in labyrinthine disease. Because of its close association with the auditory nerve, hearing is usually impaired. The eighth nerve is joined by the seventh nerve along its course through the petrous bone, so facial weakness may be observed. Tinnitus is usually present, but fullness in the ear is not. Motion sensitivity is not common but can be present.

Tumors in the Cerebellopontine Angle

The eighth nerve is often involved in mass lesions in this area, but vertigo is seldom a symptom. Hearing loss and decreased facial sensation and motility are often present. Cerebellar signs and eventually fifth, sixth, ninth, and tenth nerve dysfunction occur in larger lesions.

Central Lesions

Lesions involving the flocculonodular lobe of the cerebellum or the vestibular nuclei in the pons will produce vertigo. Ischemia, with or without infarction or hemorrhage in these areas, frequently produces acute and severe vertigo. Multiple sclerosis plaques and mass lesions also produce vertigo, but they present a more subacute course. Vertigo can actually be the initial symptom in some patients with multiple sclerosis; however, the patient usually has other associated neurologic signs on examination. Several clinical features differentiate central lesions. Most important is the presence of other signs and symptoms of brain stem or cerebellar damage (Horner's syndrome, diplopia, weakness with upper motor neuron signs, sensory signs, and cerebellar findings). Nystagmus is vertical or horizontal and not usually rotatory. Ocular fixation will not suppress the vertigo or the nystagmus. On the Nylen-Bárány maneuver, nystagmus appears as soon as the head is positioned and, unlike labyrinthine-induced nystagmus, is prolonged and nonfatiguing. Positional exacerbation can occur but is not as dramatic. With a structural lesion such as a brain stem infarct, symptoms usually last several months, but they can be present as long as a year. The best symptomatic treatment of central lesions is with diazepam (Valium). Anticholinergics may help, but their efficacy is marginal. MRI scanning is the preferred imaging study when a central lesion is suspected. CT scans do not usually adequately image the brainstem and cerebellum and are also very insensitive in diagnosing multiple sclerosis.

Dizziness as a symptom of cerebrovascular disease has been misunderstood and greatly overdiagnosed. This is particularly true of transient ischemic attack (TIA). Fisher's statistics are useful in helping place the symptom in its proper perspective. First, documented vertigo in ischemia or completed stroke from carotid or middle cerebral lesions is very rare. In posterior cerebral artery occlusion there is a 25% incidence of vertigo, but the symptom is usually not severe. Basilar artery occlusion renders 75% of its victims dizzy, and in 25% dizziness is the first symptom. Finally, 80% of the patients with vertebral artery occlusion experienced dizziness, along with the other symptoms and signs of Wallenberg's syndrome. As a general rule, dizziness is only found in vertebrobasilar vascular disease, *not* in carotid disease, and is always accompanied by other brain stem or cerebellar signs. Dizziness alone, particularly if it is recurrent and has been present for months or even years, should *not* be attributed to vertebrobasilar insufficiency.

One final comment on dizziness in vascular disease: potentially treatable cerebellar hemorrhage often appears as vertigo. For this reason, any older patient, especially the hypertensive person who is seen for the sudden onset of vertigo, should be examined very carefully for cerebellar signs and undergo computed tomography as soon as possible.

Epileptic Dizziness

Some seizure patients will experience true vertigo as an initial symptom of their seizure or as the sole manifestation of their epilepsy. Epileptic dizzy spells usually begin suddenly and only last for a few seconds. There is no exacerbation with position change. Nausea is common. In most cases an epileptic focus is demonstrated in the posterior temporal region on the electroencephalogram. Most patients have other manifestations of a partial complex seizure disorder and not vertigo as the sole manifestation of their epileptic disorder.

Medical Illness

Dizziness, at times vertiginous, is known to occur in diabetes mellitus, thyroid disease, and other endocrine diseases. Hypotension (often secondary to medications) and a host of cardiac diseases are also causes of the presyncopal variety of dizziness.

Sensory of Multisensory Disorder

Because spatial orientation is directly related to the information received through the sensors, any imbalance, disruption, or distortion of input can lead to a feeling of spatial disorientation, dysequilibrium, or dizziness. Severe proprioceptive loss such as that seen in tabes dorsalis or severe peripheral neuropathy will often cause dysequilibrium but rarely vertigo unless the patient is in the dark.

The elderly often suffer with multisensory deficit—decreasing vision, hearing, and proprioception. These factors coupled with slower righting reflexes produce a cautious, uncertain gait (presbystasis).

Minor missteps or rapid movement can trigger imbalance, lightheadedness, and vertigo. Treatment for this condition basically falls on the patient, who must learn to be cautious, not to move quickly, and to carefully focus the eyes in the proper direction before starting off. Some patients benefit by dragging a long cane along so they always feel and hear where the ground is located. The elderly often take medications that affect blood pressure or have heart conditions that allow variations in cardiac output; therefore the combined effect of many factors leads to dizziness in these persons.

Cervical Spine Disease

Experimental studies have shown that stimulation of the proprioceptive fibers in the zygapophyseal joints of the upper cervical spine can produce vertigo. The extrapolation from these studies is the hypothesis that cervical spondylosis and arthritis of the facet joints can cause irritation of the receptors for proprioception and thus induce clinical vertigo. If cervical vertigo is suspected, antiinflammatory medications are often useful in treating the condition.

Psychogenic Dizziness

Many patients with emotional problems experience dizziness; this can be lightheadedness, giddiness, or true vertigo. This type of problem is most commonly seen in anxiety states, but it is also present in depression, hysteria, and schizophrenia. The symptoms are often vague. In some patients hyperventilation is a major factor in their lightheadedness sensation.

The vestibular system in the brain stem has rich interconnections with the reticular formation, so it is not surprising from an anatomic point of view to find the heightened arousal state of anxiety associated with vertigo and lightheadedness. In anxiety eye and head movements tend to be furtive, thus producing rapidly changing visual input that further taxes the integrative capacity of orientation mechanisms. These and probably other physiologic and chemical changes are responsible for complaint of dizziness in anxious or depressed patients.

Other Disorders

There are always patients who cannot be neatly classified or diagnosed. Some patients can have partial syndromes or a combination of many factors. The examiner must also realize that there is much variation in the sensitivity of the vestibular apparatus in the normal population. Some patients are sick after one turn of a merry-go-round, whereas others can fly into space or barrel-roll high-speed aircraft all day without the slightest degree of disorientation.

■ SUMMARY

Dizziness is a common yet complicated complaint to evaluate. Exact characterization of the complaint will separate the principal types of dizziness: vertigo, presyncope, imbalance, and nonspecific light-headedness. True vertigo is usually caused by a disturbance in the labyrinthine system either peripherally or centrally. Separating central from peripheral lesions is very important because the peripheral diseases tend to be benign, whereas the central lesions are often destructive, for example, tumor, stroke, or demyelinating plaque.

Suggested Readings

Evaluation of Dizzy Patient

Baloh RW, Honrubia V: *Clinical neurophysiology of the vestibular system,* Philadelphia, 1979, FA Davis Co.

Drachman DA, Hart CW: An approach to the dizzy patient, *Neurology* 22:323, 1972.

Drachman DA, Posner J: *Doctor I'm dizzy,* Tape B3, American Academy of Neurology, 1981.

Kroenke K: Causes of persistent dizziness, *Ann Intern Med* 117:898, 1992.

Kumar A, Valvassori G: Neurological diagnosis of intracranial lesions: an algorithm for neurologic disorders, *Neurol Clin North Am* 2:779, 1984.

Lerner SA, Matz GJ: Aminoglycoside ototoxicity, *Am J Otolaryngol* 1:169, 1980.

Wolfson RJ, editor: Symposium on vertigo, *Otolaryngol Clin North Am* 6:1, 1973.

Positional Vertigo

Baloh RW, Honrubia V: Benign positional vertigo, *Neurology* 37:371, 1987.

Harrison MS, Ozsahinoglu C: Positional vertigo, *Arch Otolaryngol* 101:675, 1975.

Koenigsberger MR, Chutorian AM, Gold AP, et al: Benign paroxysmal vertigo of childhood, *Neurology* 20:1108, 1970.

Schuknecht HF: Cupulolithiasis, *Arch Otolaryngol* 90:765, 1969.

Slater R: Benign recurrent vertigo, *J Neurol Neurosurg Psychiatry* 42:363, 1979.

Vertigo Due to Neurological Disease

Fischer CM: Vertigo in cerebrovascular disease, *Arch Otolaryngol* 85:529, 1967.

Grad A, Baloh RW: Vertigo of vascular origin. *Arch Neurol* 46:281, 1989.

Korgeorgos J, Scott DF, Swash M: Epileptic dizziness, *Br Med J* 282:687, 1981.

Kumar A, Torok N: Neurological diagnosis of intracranial lesions, *Otorhinolaryngology* 30:138, 1982.

Treatment of Dizziness

Hain TC: Treatment of vertigo, *The Neurologist* 1:125, 1995.

Tinnitus

Marion MS, Cevette MJ: Tinnitus, *Mayo Clin Proc* 66:614, 1991.

Meniere Disease

Shea JJ: Classification of Meniere disease, *Am J Otolaryngol* 14:224, 1993.

CHAPTER

Weakness and Gait Disturbances

5

▢ WEAKNESS

Normal voluntary muscle contraction can be described as an integrated sequential neuromuscular function. Impulses originate in the large upper motor neurons, primarily in the Betz cells, and travel through the corticospinal tracts to the lower motor neurons in the anterior horns of the spinal cord and motor nuclei of the brain stem. The impulses from these lower motor neurons travel through the peripheral and cranial nerves to reach the nerve terminals, where acetylcholine that has been synthesized and stored in vesicles is released to reach the acetylcholine receptors on the postsynaptic muscle membrane. When acetylcholine reaches the acetylcholine receptors, there is a transient increase of permeability to sodium and potassium resulting in electrical depolarization of the muscle membrane, which initiates the sequence of events that leads to voluntary muscle contraction. Lesions at any site along these pathways can cause weakness. Clinical manifestations differ according to the lesion level. The clinician should be able to determine if the weakness is due to a lesion in the corticospinal tract, anterior horn cells, peripheral nerves, neuromuscular junction, or muscles. Observations that help the clinician are listed in Box 5-1.

In Table 5-1 lesions at any level of the corticospinal tract (upper motor neurons) can produce paralysis or weakness (paresis) of large groups of muscles, an increase in muscle tone (spasticity), hyperactive stretch reflexes, and pathologic reflexes, including extensor-plantar response (Babinski sign).

 BOX 5-1

1 *Location of the weakness:* Is the weakness distal or proximal, symmetrical or asymmetrical? If asymmetrical, does it involve a group of muscles innervated by one nerve, several nerves, or a plexus? Does it involve ocular or bulbar muscles? Does it involve breathing muscles?

2 *Muscle atrophy:* Is wasting of muscles present? In what distribution: a nerve, root or plexus distribution? Is it distal, proximal, or generalized? Is it an early or late event in the disease? Are fasciculations present? If there is hypertrophy, is it localized to certain muscles such as the calf, or is it generalized?

3 *Stretch reflexes:* Are the reflexes normal, hyperactive, or hypoactive? Are they symmetrical? Are pathologic reflexes present, such as a Babinski sign?

4 *Sensory alterations:* Are there unilateral or bilateral sensory deficits, dermatomal or stocking-and-glove losses of sensation?

5 *Muscle tone:* Is it normal, increased (rigidity, spasticity), or decreased (hypotonia)?

6 *Myotonia:* When the muscles are contracted or percussed, can the muscle relax easily and fast, or do they relax slowly but without pain as in myotonia? Or do the muscles relax slowly and painfully as in muscle cramps? Are the cramps spontaneous, or are they induced by exercise or ischemia?

▨　**TABLE 5-1　Neuromuscular Diseases**

	Level of Lesion	Site of Weakness
	Corticospinal tract	Large group of muscles; one extremity (monoplegia) or two (diplegia); if the arm and leg are paralyzed on the same side, this is hemiplegia; if both legs are paralyzed, this is paraplegia
	Anterior horn cell	Variable, proximal, and/or distal; small group of muscles
	Peripheral nerve	Distal extremities (feet, hands) are initially involved, and this can extend proximally
	Neuromuscular junction	Fatigability, ocular, bulbar, or generalized
	Muscle	Proximal involvement

All of these findings usually appear 1 to 3 weeks after the acute onset of a destructive lesion, as in an infarct, or evolve slowly, as in infiltrative or degenerative lesions. Anterior horn cell lesions (lower motor neurons) tend to cause severe weakness and early atrophy of individual muscles or muscle groups, fasciculation, flaccidity, and loss of stretch reflexes but no pathologic reflexes. Lesions in peripheral motor nerves cause weakness in the muscles supplied by the nerve. In polyneuropathies the weakness usually begins distally in the extremities (hands and feet), can "ascend," and can be associated with atrophy, flaccid-

Muscle Atrophy	Stretch Reflexes	Sensation	Tone
Mild, disuse can develop	Hyperactive	Normal	Spastic
Severe, early, fasciculations muscles	Hypoactive or absent	Normal	Flaccid
Mild to severe, early	Hypoactive or absent	Abnormal in sensory or mixed neuro-pathies	Flaccid
Minimal, late	Normal	Normal	Normal
Late, skeletal abnormalities	Normal early, absent late	Normal	Normal or myotonia

ity, and loss of stretch reflexes. Pathologic reflexes are not part of the syndrome. Sensory deficits can be present if sensory nerves are also affected (sensory neuropathy or mixed sensorimotor neuropathies). Diseases that affect the neuromuscular junction are manifested by fatigability or weariness during exertion, variability of weakness that worsens during the day and improves with rest, minimal or no atrophy, no change in muscle tone or reflexes, and no sensory deficit. Primary diseases of muscle (myopathies) usually cause proximal muscle weakness with late atrophy, no changes of stretch reflexes except very late in the disease (areflexia caused by muscle atrophy or joint contractures), and no change in sensory functions. Myotonia or painless delay in relaxation of muscles after contraction occurs in some myopathies. Myotonia is frequently associated with weakness and atrophy of muscles in myotonic dystrophy and with hypertrophy in myotonia congenita.

When a patient complains of weakness, a detailed inquiry into the symptoms should be made. By definition weakness is a diminution of strength. Some patients complain of weakness when they are experiencing easy fatigability, numbness, or problems of balance or coordination. It is important to inquire about the onset of weakness, its progression or regression, its distribution, and any associated symptoms, such as cramps. A differentiation should be made between weakness as defined here and fatigability as defined by weariness during exercise. Objective ("pathologic") fatigability is seen in diseases that affect the neuromuscular junction. The fatigue should diminish with rest. Fatigue is also seen with other disorders that affect the motor system, for example, anterior horn cell disease, peripheral nerve disease, muscle disease, and upper motor nerve disease. The fatigue is most prominent after activity. If the patient reports fatigue upon awakening or immediately after initiating activity, this suggests a psychogenic cause of the fatigue (neurasthenia). On describing the symptoms the patient frequently localizes the site of the weakness. Patients with *hip weakness* complain of difficulty getting up from a sitting (chair) or squatting position; they also complain of having difficulty going up stairs and mention that they have to pull themselves up by pulling with their hands on nearby objects or pushing on their knees. *Weakness at the ankles* frequently affects dorsiflexion and produces footdrop. Patients complain of stubbing their toes, tripping, and twisting their ankles. *Weakness of the shoulder muscles* is described by patients as difficulty in combing their hair or difficulty with any activity that requires raising the arms above the head. Shoulder girdle weakness produces forward and lateral displacement of the scapulae with compensatory pronation of the arms (palms facing backward) when the arms are down. Patients with *weakness of the hand muscles* have difficulty turning door knobs, unscrewing caps of jars of bottles, or holding objects in their hands. Eating or writing becomes quite laborious. Weak *finger muscles* produce difficulty pinching, buttoning and unbuttoning, and using zippers. In *neck muscle weakness* the patients have difficulty lifting their heads when in a supine position, indicating involvement of the neck flexors. Rarely are the neck extensors primarily affected. Patients with *weakness of the facial muscles* have difficulty drinking through a straw, whistling, or blowing. Difficulty in chewing or closing the mouth indicates weakness of the masseter and temporalis muscles. Difficulty in articulating or in removing food particles from between and around the teeth with the tongue can suggest weakness of tongue muscles. Diplopia can indicate weakness of extraocular muscles. Blurred vision can be caused by double vision, and this should be clarified during the interview. *Respiratory insufficiency* caused by intercostal or diaphragmatic muscle weakness is a late and usually terminal event in neuromuscular diseases, is manifested by abdominal breathing, and should be differentiated from the different breathing patterns seen in central nervous system lesions. Respiratory insufficiency can be the first manifestation of some myopathies such as adult Pompe's disease (glycogenosis type II).

GAIT DISTURBANCES

Careful observation of the patient's gait as he or she walks into the examining room frequently can reveal what muscles are affected and where the lesion is even before any questions are asked. Although impairment of gait can be caused by mechanical factors, such as diseases of bones, tendons, joints, or muscles, lesions at different levels of the nervous system are very important causes of gait abnormalities. Patients should be observed as they walk and then be asked to walk with their eyes closed, backward, around objects, on their toes, on their heels, and in tandem fashion (placing one heel directly in front of the other foot). Different patterns of gait develop when different muscles are affected, indicating different levels of lesions that can be considered from distal to central involvement.

Steppage or Equine Gait

Steppage or equine gait results from weakness of the peroneal and anterior tibial muscles and is characterized by a slapping quality produced when the knee and hip have to be flexed and lifted to compensate for lack of foot dorsiflexion (foot drop). The slapping noise is produced when the anterior end of the foot has to be thrown upward to avoid tripping or twisting the ankle. This type of gait is seen in patients with ankle weakness that produces dropfeet, such as in the distal peripheral neuropathy of lower extremities, lesions involving the L4-5 root, anterior horn cell disease of the lower extremities, pressure or stretch injuries of peroneal nerves, and more rarely in distal dystrophic processes. Patients with this type of weakness are unable to walk on their heels when asked.

"Back-Kneeing"

Weakness of the thigh muscles can result in poor stabilization of the knee with resultant hyperextension of that joint (so-called back-kneeing) causing a peculiar gait. This gait is seen with some of the femoral neuropathies and with any other cause of quadriceps muscle weakness.

Waddling Gait

Waddling gait is a result of hip girdle muscle weakness. The lack of fixation of the hip by the weak gluteal muscles on taking a step makes the opposite side of the pelvis drop, producing compensatory lateral movement of the pelvis. Very frequently the hip and back extensors are concomitantly affected, which explains the marked lumbar lordosis with protrusion of the abdomen seen while the patient stands or walks. This type of gait is seen in all myopathies that affect the hip girdle musculature, such as in patients with most dystrophic myopathies (limb-girdle, Duchenne, Becker, and so forth), in the intermediate form of spinal muscular atrophy (Kugelberg-Welander type), in inflammatory neuropathies (dermatomyositis, polymyositis), and in hip dislocation.

Sensory Ataxic Gait

Sensory ataxic gait is a result of lesions in the posterior column of the spinal cord, posterior nerve roots, dorsal root ganglion, or peripheral nerves and is associated with loss of sensation in a variable distribution according to where the lesion is. The muscle strength is normal, and, if there is some weakness, it is out of proportion to the sensory deficit. In predominantly dorsal spinal cord disease there is loss of position and vibratory sense in the lower extremities and a positive

Romberg sign (the patient falls or sways when standing with feet together and eyes closed, but not with eyes open). The inability to sense the positions of the joints in space and in relationship to themselves makes the patients produce an unsteady broad-based gait to correct the instability and causes the hard slapping character of the steps. The patient has to use his or her sight to maintain these spatial relationships and consequently has more difficulty walking in the dark or with the eyes closed. This type of gait is seen in patients with tabes dorsalis, subacute combined degeneration, Friedreich's ataxia, and some types of spinocerebellar ataxias (SCA1 and SCA2). In sensory neuronopathies there is distal loss of all modalities of sensation and severe distal limb ataxia and truncal ataxia.

Cerebellar Ataxic Gait

Cerebellar ataxic gait is produced by cerebellar lesions, either focal, as in midline (vermal) lesions of chronic alcoholism, multiple sclerosis, and neoplasms, or diffuse, as in the various types of diffuse cerebellar atrophy, such as paraneoplastic immune disorders, degenerative diseases, and intoxications (mercury). In truncal ataxia, as seen in midline cerebellar neoplasms, and in chronic alcoholics with anterior (dorsal) vermal degeneration, the patient walks in a broad-based unsteady gait with short but somewhat regular steps and forward inclination of the trunk. In these patients, the limb movements are generally well coordinated, and the speech is not affected. Pancerebellar (involving both the midline vermis and lateral cerebellar hemispheres) disease and multiple sclerosis produce a very unsteady gait with irregular short or large steps, lateral or vertical truncal swaying, and severe incoordination of extremities frequently associated with slurred speech. Standing with feet close together results in marked instability, even with the eyes open. Patients are unable to walk tandem gait (heel-toe in a straight line).

Dyskinetic Gait

In dyskinesias, which are diseases that affect the extrapyramidal system such as the choreas and dystonias, the gait exacerbates the abnormal involuntary movements and can result in jerky movements of one or several extremities or grotesque writhing movements of all four extremities, face, neck, and pelvis. The dystonic gait is slow and deliberate because of inversion of the feet or pelvic distortion (see Chapter 20).

Parkinsonian (Festinating) Gait

Parkinsonian gait is produced by nigrostriatal lesions as seen typically in Parkinson's disease and is characterized by slowness in initiating movement and a shuffling character with a tendency to accelerate (festination). The steps are short and irregular (*marche à petits pas*). The patients have a characteristic forward displacement of their trunks and have difficulty stopping suddenly. Any change in the direction of the gait is difficult and laborious.

"Senile" Gait

Gait impairment and falls are frequent in the elderly population, worsen with age, and are more frequent in females than males. There is a significant correlation between hypodensity of the white matter on brain CT scans and both gait disturbance and balance disorders in the elderly. However, there is more likely a multifactorial cause, including vision and hearing deficits, decreased neuromuscular function caused by peripheral nerve and central nervous system deficits, and arthritis. The gait is characterized by a truncal and head forward flexion, diminished arm swing, and increased flexion of both knees and elbows. There is a decreased walking speed and stride length.

Spastic Gait

Spastic gait is due to lesions of the corticospinal tracts and can be a unilateral hemiplegic spastic gait or a bilateral paraplegic spastic gait. Spastic hemiparesis is frequently the result of a cerebrovascular accident or trauma affecting one corticospinal tract. The leg is overextended at the hip and knee, and the foot is plantar flexed. The patient's inability to flex the hips and knees forces the leg to circumduct with each step (i.e., the leg is dragged in a semicircular movement external to the pelvis). The upper extremity is immobile, held in a posture characterized by flexion of the shoulder, elbow, wrist, and fingers with adduction at the shoulder. In spastic paraparesis both legs are affected. The leg features described in the hemiparetic gait are similar. There can be shortening of the Achilles tendon and lumbar lordosis. The gait is slow, staggering, stiff, and shuffling with short steps, producing a scissoring quality to the gait.

Abnormal Gait in Frontal Lobe Disorders

Abnormal gait in frontal lobe disorders, such as normal pressure hydrocephalus or frontal lobe infarcts, is quite elaborate, very laborious, severely imbalanced, and frequently difficult to predict and describe. It has a magnetic quality as if the feet were glued to the ground. The legs move easily and rapidly if the patient is lying in bed with the feet off the ground. There is no associated weakness of the legs.

Hysterical Gait

Hysterical gait, associated with no lesion of the neuromuscular system, has bizarre, nondescript qualities with an unpredictable changing character. At times normal movements can be detected along with abnormal ones. Patients may be able to run or walk backward or to the side without difficulty or may be unable either to stand or walk (astasia-abasia).

▉ EXAMINATION

After observing the patient's ordinary routine gait, observing the performance of simple daily necessary activities will also help localize the area of weakness. Patients with hip-girdle weakness will have difficulty arising from a sitting position and will need to use their hands to push themselves up. These patients will place their hands on their knees or thighs to push themselves, push with their hands on the sides of a chair, or actually pull themselves with their hands by grabbing a static object. When back extensor muscles are also weak, the patient will get up from a chair and remain with the trunk flexed over the hips. He or she then has to get into an erect truncal position by using both hands to "climb up his or her thighs" as described by Gowers. Such patients will prefer to use a high stool at home so that arising from the sitting position is easier. Arising from the floor is a very elaborate and slow maneuver for patients with proximal hip-girdle weakness, and observing a patient during this procedure will provide information that can obviate complicated muscle strength testing, which can be particularly difficult in children. Such patients tend to break the movement into parts by first extending the knees in a sitting position, then rotating the trunk to place their hands on the floor, then flexing the knees and rising to an erect position by pushing themselves with their hands in an alternating displacement of the hands from leg to knee to thigh (Gowers' sign). This complicated maneuver can be modified according to the patient's degree of weakness. Observing a patient going up stairs or stepping onto a stool will demonstrate mild hip weakness if the patient uses his or her hands on the knees or lower thighs to push himself or herself up. The patient may need to use handrails to pull himself or herself upstairs.

Manual muscle testing: Because of normal variations from person to person and differences in age, all muscle testing and grading are subjective. We prefer to describe the patient's ability to perform tasks, such as the ability to dress oneself, to eat, to brush one's teeth, to groom oneself, and so on. When using a grading system, we prefer the one recommended by the British Medical Research Council (see Box 5-2).

After or during the observation of gait, the observation of a few simple tasks, and manual muscle testing, the examination of the neuromuscular system should include simple *inspection* of the muscle bulk. In neuromuscular diseases the muscles can be wasted or atrophic, or they can be enlarged because of true hypertrophy or pseudohypertrophy (hypertrophy of

---

 BOX 5-2

1+ Flicker or trace of contraction
2+ Active movement with gravity eliminated
3+ Active movement against gravity
4+ Active movement against gravity and resistance
5+ Normal power

some muscle fiber with infiltration of muscle by fat and fibrous tissue). During inspection, look for fasciculations, which are easily seen in thin persons but can be masked by subcutaneous fatty tissue in infants and obese patients. An accessible site to find fasciculation is the tongue. The tongue should be in a resting position within the mouth to avoid confusion with tremor. The irregular jumping of isolated muscles frequently associated with atrophy should be differentiated from the rhythmical generalized movements seen in tongue tremor. Facial inspection will detect ptosis, which is frequently compensated for by corrugating the forehead or tilting the head backward. Atrophy of the temporalis and masseter muscles causes a cadaveric appearance of the face that frequently is associated with prominent puckered lips and tapiroid mouth caused by facial muscle weakness. Inability to close the eyelids and upward deviation of the eyeballs when trying to close the eyelids (Bell's phenomenon) indicate nuclear or infranuclear (peripheral) seventh nerve palsy if associated with flattening of the nasolabial fold and lack of facial expression. Sparing the eyelids and forehead in facial weakness indicates supranuclear (central) seventh-nerve palsy, except in some myopathic processes (facioscapulohumeral dystrophy). Shoulder muscle atrophy makes the bony prominence more prominent and causes winging of the scapulae. The scapula deviates laterally, upward, and backward when the patient pushes his or her hand against the wall or when the arms are stretched in front of the chest. Shoulder weakness also will produce internal rotation of the arm in such a way that the dorsal side of the hand faces forward. Atrophy of the intrinsic hand muscles will cause a guttering appearance between the metatarsal bones. A "knife edge" configuration of the tibia indicates atrophy of the peroneal innervated anterior tibial muscles. An exaggerated variation of leg muscle atrophy with sparing of the thigh muscles results in the "stork leg" appearance or "inverted champagne bottle" sign.

Palpation of the muscles can aid in determining whether the muscles are of normal consistency or whether they are rubbery as is usually seen in the pseudohypertrophic calves of patients with Duchenne's muscular dystrophy. Muscle nodules can be palpable in some cases of myositis. Subcutaneous calcifications can be palpable in the infantile form of dermatomyositis. Palpation of muscles can be painful in myositis, polyarteritis nodosa, poliomyelitis, and polyneuritis.

Percussion of muscles can help the examiner detect myotonia and myoedema. Percussion of normal muscles produces a sudden, brief contraction followed by a quick relaxation of the muscle. In myoedema the muscle contracts and produces a localized but electrically silent bulge. In myotonia the entire muscle contracts in a sustained involuntary fashion, then slowly relaxes and has electrical changes.

Skeletal abnormalities are frequently associated with hereditary, degenerative neuromuscular problems and include lumbar lordosis, kyphoscoliosis, pes cavus, and pectus excavatum.

◼ SUMMARY

Gait can be impaired by nonneurologic disorders such as orthopedic, rheumatologic, vascular, or neurologic disorders (weakness of upper or lower motor neuron type, cerebellar, proprioceptive, vestibular, or basal ganglia disorders, normal pressure hydrocephalus, frontal lobe lesions). By examining the patient the location of the neurological disturbance causing the gait impairment can be ascertained. This includes assessing base and station and the ability to arise from a chair; tandem walk; balance on either leg for 10 seconds with feet close together, stand with eyes open, and then, with eyes closed, walk on heels and toes; and walk forward and backward and around a chair. When the gait disorder is due to weakness, the pattern of weakness and any accompanying motor, reflex, or sensory disturbances can determine the level of abnormality in the neuro-axis. This includes the corticospinal tract, anterior horn cell, spinal nerve root, peripheral nerve, neuromuscular junction, and muscle. By clinically determining the cause of the gait disorder or weakness the most cost-effective evaluation for each patient can be determined.

Suggested Readings

Weakness

Brooke MH: *A clinician's view of neuromuscular diseases,* Baltimore, 1986, Williams & Wilkins.

Dubowitz V: Muscle disorders in childhood. In *Major problems in clinical pediatrics series,* vol 16, London, 1978, WB Saunders.

Engel AG, Franzini-Armstrong C: *Myology: basic and clinical,* ed 2, New York, 1994, McGraw-Hill.

Haerer AF: *DeJong's the neurologic examination,* ed 5, Philadelphia, 1992, JB Lippincott.

Kennedy HG: Fatigue and fatigability, *Lancet* 1:1145, 1987.

McHardy KC: Clinical algorithms; weakness, *Br Med J* 1:1591, 1984.

Shafran SD: The chronic fatigue syndrome, *Am J Med* 90:730, 1991.

Gait Disorders

Grim RJ: Disorderly walks, *Neurol Clin* 2:615, 1984.

Keane JR: Hysterical gait disorders, *Neurology* 39:586, 1989.

Nutt JG, Marsden CD, Thompson PD: Human walking and higher level gait disorders particularly in the elderly, *Neurology* 43:268, 1993.

Wolfson L: Falls and gait. In Katzman R Rowe JW, editors: *Principles of geriatric neurology,* Philadelphia, 1992, FA Davis.

Sensory Disorders (Including Selected Pain Syndromes)

6

DEFINITIONS

Following lesions of the central or peripheral nervous system, sensory disturbances can be characterized by positive features such as too much sensation, spontaneous sensations such as pins and needles, or negative sensory deficit such as too little sensation or numbness. For describing sensory deficit, use these terms: one, hypesthesia (partial impairment of sensory perception) and anesthesia (total loss of sensory perception); two, hypalgesia (partial loss of pain sensation) and analgesia (total loss of pain sensation). Some patients report that normal nonpainful superficial sensory stimulus (pin, light touch) causes severe discomfort (hyperalgesia or hyperesthesia). Hyperpathia refers to an uncomfortable sensation elicited by normally nociceptive stimulus such as pin, and there is a lowered pain-eliciting threshold for the stimulus. Neuralgia refers to tingling, electrical, or shock sensations in specific nerve (cranial nerve dysfunction, as in patients with facial pain due to trigeminal neuralgia, or peripheral nerve impairment, as in patients with leg pain due to sciatic nerve dysfunction [sciatica]) or nerve root (e.g., cervical, thoracic, lumbar) distribution. Causalgia describes intense burning pain usually associated with hyperesthesia-hyperalgesia; this is usually due to partial nerve injury. Paresthesias are abnormal sensations of pins and needles or tingling caused by normally nonnoxious events, for example, when socks or bed sheets are applied to the feet of a patient with peripheral neuropathy. Dysesthesias are uncomfortable painful abnormal sensations that occur with or without any external stimulus being applied. When local anesthetic is given for dental procedures, an area of the mouth is initially "dead or numb" (analgesia), and while sensation in the "blocked" nerve returns, paresthesias are reported.

■ SYMPTOMS

Sensory abnormalities are characterized by loss of sensation, pain, or paresthesias. These subjective symptomatic disturbances can precede or occur without objective neurologic findings. Because sensory symptoms can be very subjective, physicians must attempt to determine these characteristic features, which are listed in Box 6-1.

Sensory symptoms can occur in nonneurologic conditions such as vascular insufficiency or arthritis; therefore the examination should be directed toward detecting objective neurological findings, for example, areas of abnormal sensation, decreased reflexes, motor weakness, muscle wasting, trophic skin, or joint changes.

Paresthesias can be characterized as "pins and needles," "limbs falling asleep," or simply as "tingling"; however, if paresthesias are unusually intense, they can be perceived as painful (dysesthesias). Paresthesias can

BOX 6-1

1 What is the patient actually experiencing, and what are specific descriptive terms used by patient?

2 What is the location of the sensations (e.g., localized or diffuse, superficial or deep)?

3 What is the pattern of onset (e.g., maximal at onset or progressively intensifying, worsen with activity, awaken patient from sleep)?

4 Are symptoms constant or episodic (intermittent)?

5 Is there radiation or spread?

6 What factors exacerbate or relieve sensory disturbances (e.g., position, rest, movement, or sleep)?

occur in the absence of involved body parts, such as phantom limb phenomenon after an amputation. Paresthesias occur in distribution of isolated sensory nerve (mononeuropathy) or spinal root (radiculopathy), in distal extremities (e.g., peripheral polyneuropathy), over the entire body and limbs below the level of spinal cord lesion, on one side of the face and on contralateral extremities and trunk (crossed hemianesthesia) in brain stem lesions, or on one side of the body (hemianesthesia) contralateral to thalamic or cerebral hemispheric (cortical or subcortical) lesion.

In simple, partial (focal) somatosensory seizures caused by lesions involving the parietal sensory region, paresthesias are episodic and paroxysmal. They usually spread proximally from fingers to arms, shoulders, hips, legs, feet, and then to the face. Paresthesias caused by peripheral neuropathies can be provoked by minimal tactile stimulation (e.g., bed coverings placed on top of bare legs). Neuropathic pain is worse at night. Limb movement or neck flexion can cause electrical paresthesias that extend down the back to thighs and legs (Lhermitte sign) in patients with multiple sclerosis or cervical myelopathy. This is believed caused by irritation of demyelinated posterior columns of the cervical spinal cord. It is clear that paresthesias can be caused by disturbances at any level of neuraxis from peripheral nerve to parietal cortex.

Numbness is the word commonly used by patients to describe the sensation of deadness, heaviness, or coldness in the affected body part. In certain neuropathies and spinal cord lesions (e.g., syringomyelia), patients are not aware of any sensory impairment and will report no subjective sensory symptoms; however, they may burn, injure, or mutilate themselves because of the profound sensory loss that can be demonstrated on neurological examination.

▨ EXAMINATION FINDINGS

Sensory examination depends on the patient's subjective interpretation of the applied stimulus. Thoroughness of examination is determined by the patient's symptomatology and neurologic findings (reflex changes, Babinski sign, motor weakness, muscle wasting, trophic skin, joint changes). These findings suggest the possible level of involvement in the central or peripheral nervous system. The patient's response to pinprick, vibration, light touch, and position-sense testing is carefully assessed (see Chapter 1). In assessing the significance of sensory disturbances, two general rules should be considered: one, sensory symptoms can occur in the absence of objective sensory findings such as paresthesias in a radicular pattern caused by a herniated disk; and two, objective sensory findings rarely occur in the absence of sensory complaints such as an anesthetic limb that feels different to the patient than does a normal limb; if anesthetic limb does not feel different, consider functional conversion reaction (see pp. 167–168).

CLINICAL SYNDROMES

Polyneuropathy

Neuropathic disorders include symmetrical polyneuropathies and asymmetric mononeuropathies (single or multiple). There is symmetric loss of sensory perception that initially involves the longest and largest diameter nerve fibers. Sensory impairment is most severe distally, that is, the feet and hands; there is less deficit proximally, that is, the thighs and shoulders, with the trunk usually being spared. This causes a stocking-and-glove pattern of sensory impairment. The sensory deficit of polyneuropathy does not correspond to any specific peripheral nerve or root and is usually quite symmetric. Sensory symptoms begin on bottom (soles) of feet and later involves the top (dorsum) of the foot. It would be most unusual for polyneuropathy symptoms to begin in hands rather than feet (consider an alternative diagnosis such as carpal tunnel syndrome), and if initial sensory symptoms are on the dorsum of feet or appear asymmetrical, consider a diagnosis of radiculopathy. The anesthetic zone gradually merges into a zone of less diminished sensation (hypoesthesia); this subsequently blends into a region of normal sensory perception in sensory disturbance caused by objective sensory neurological disturbance. Sensory loss usually involves all modalities, but in some cases proprioception and vibration sense seem to be involved earlier and more severely than are pinprick, light touch, and temperature sensation. This indicates that faster-conducting, thickly myelinated fibers (mediating vibration and position sensibility) are usually damaged before slower-conducting, thinly myelinated and unmyelinated fibers (mediating pain, temperature, light touch). Large-fiber nerve dysfunction is characteristic of diabetic neuropathy, whereas early thin-fiber nerve involvement is more common with amyloid neuropathy. Other findings in patients with sensorimotor polyneuropathy include one, decreased or absent deep tendon reflexes especially at ankles; two, distal extremity weakness and muscle wasting; and three, trophic skin and joint changes. Loss of deep tendon reflexes in neuropathy is usually due to sensory afferent portion of reflex arc such as large sensory fibers rather than being caused by efferent motor portion of reflex. Polyneuropathies usually include both sensory and motor abnormalities; in rare cases pure sensory neuropathy caused by amyloid or remote effect of carcinoma occurs. These predominantly sensory neuropathies show dorsal column sensory loss such as impaired proprioception and vibration sense with less severely involved pain perception. Sensory ataxia can develop in certain neuropathies. These patients have broad-based unsteady gaits with clumsy, awkward finger manipulations of objects and utensils. There can be involuntary finger movements that simulate athetosis (pseudoathetosis), and these result from severe proprioception impairment. Pseudoathetoid movements are seen in other conditions such as tabes dorsalis, multiple sclerosis, and parietal lobe lesions.

Mononeuropathy

Mononeuropathies involve single nerve trunks. The majority result from trauma; others have vascular or toxic causes. Mononeuropathy of vascular etiology can involve single or multiple (mononeuritis multiplex) nerve(s). Entrapment (compressive) neuropathy is due to pathologic disturbances (demyelination) in

isolated nerve segments. Sensory symptoms are frequently the initial complaint in mononeuropathies.
Numbness and tingling in the hand (especially first
three fingers) are initial symptoms of median nerve
compression (carpal tunnel syndrome). Clinical findings such as sensory, motor, and trophic abnormalities are localized to the known distribution of the specific involved nerve. The anesthetic zone can be
smaller than the nerve's anatomic cutaneous distribution because of overlap of the contiguous sensory
nerves. The diagnosis of neuropathy is confirmed by
nerve conduction velocity measurement and electromyographic findings (see Chapter 16).

Plexus (Brachial and Lumbosacral) Syndromes

Sensory symptoms depend on the specific nerve
trunks damaged. Brachial plexus dysfunction can be
caused by trauma (stab injuries or gunshot wounds),
infection (following immunization, viral, or bacterial
illness), or neoplasm (lung or breast). If there is
involvement of the upper portion (C5, C6), sensory
impairment occurs in the shoulder, lateral forearm,
and arm; there is motor weakness and wasting of
intrinsic hand muscles with sensory loss along the
medial (ulnar) region of the forearm and hand. In
most brachial plexus disorders, the predominant sensory symptoms is anesthesia; however, in certain conditions (e.g., brachial plexitis, neoplastic infiltration)
there can be pain. Certain traumatic injuries can
result in causalgia (burning pain).

The lumbosacral plexus is less frequently damaged. Causes include vertebral or hip disorders
(pelvic and retroperitoneal neoplasms, osteomyelitis,
pelvic surgery or fractures, psoas abscess) and inad-
vertent injury into the nerve(s) of the plexus from

local injections. The patient usually describes pain and paresthesias located in the gluteal region or thigh; this can radiate down the back of the calf and lateral portion of the leg to the ankle region. This local pain can be constant, dull, and aching, and the radiating component pain can be intermittent and lancinating. Pain is worsened when the sciatic nerve is stretched or palpated. Lumbosacral plexus involvement can be confused with disk disease, but the lack of back pain is an important differentiating feature.

Radicular Syndromes

Subjective symptoms and objective sensory findings of dorsal spinal roots are referred to segmental dermatomal distribution. Because of the overlap between several dorsal roots, objective delineation on sensory examination of sensory impairment can be less reliable than the patient's description of sensory radiation. Pain and paresthesias of radicular involvement usually are lancinating, radiate along nerve root distribution, intermittent, increased by activities that increase intraspinal pressure (coughing, straining) or stretch the nerve root, and respond to treatment by inactivity (e.g., bed rest and traction). Reflex changes can be present if the dorsal (sensory) root is involved. If the ventral root is involved, weakness and muscle wasting can be prominent. Radicular syndromes can be caused by lesions compressing spinal nerve roots (intervertebral disk, extradural or intradural extramedullary tumors). Less common causes include herpes zoster infection and diabetes mellitus. Herpes zoster can invade the dorsal root ganglia. This can cause severe burning trunk (girdle) pain localized to a specific thoracic segmental pattern. Herpes zoster neuralgia is usually accompanied by cutaneous vesicular eruption. Vesicles may resolve, but neuralgia can persist within an anesthetic zone (post-herpetic neuralgia). This pain can be treated with capsaicin (derived from Hungarian red pepper) that is applied topically. This drug blocks the release of the chemical pain mediator substance P. Other drugs used to block substance P include opiates, tricyclic antidepressants, clonidine, and carbamazepine.

Certain patients with diabetes mellitus complain of severe and constant pain in the upper back, rib, thoracic, or abdominal region. This has either radicular or girdlelike distribution. Clinical findings include decreased sensation in the thoracic region, weakness of abdominal muscles, and weakness of iliopsoas or quadriceps muscles. There is frequently minimal evidence of generalized peripheral neuropathy, although the patient can experience significant weight loss. The presence of pain and weight loss can lead to extensive evaluation for thoracic, abdominal, or pelvic lesions or pathological conditions originating from the spine. The diagnosis of diabetic thoracoabdominal radiculopathy is established by electromyography findings.

Spinal Cord Syndromes

Central Gray Matter Commissural Syndrome

Sensory fibers subserving pain and temperature travel in the lateral spinothalamic tract and decussate centrally in anterior commissure. If these are damaged, sensory loss is usually symmetrical and segmental; less frequently it is asymmetrical. Because certain sensory modalities such as light touch, vibratory sensation, and proprioception do not decussate in this region, they are initially spared. This sensory dissociation (loss of pain sensation with sparing of touch vibration and position sense) and shawl-like sensory loss that extends for several levels (segments) is characteristic of intramedullary lesions (e.g., syringomyelia). If a lesion involves the fourth through sixth cervical fibers, sensory loss has a shawl-like distribution involving the anterior neck, shoulder, and upper arm. Because sensory fibers involving the sacral region are located peripherally in the spinothalamic tract, the buttock (saddle region) is not affected by central spinal cord lesions located above the thoracic region. Ventral extension of the syringomyelic cavity into the anterior horn of cervical region can cause accompanying weakness, fasciculations, muscle wasting, and hypoactive reflexes in upper extremities.

Posterior Spinal Cord Syndromes

If a spinal lesion, for example, cervical spondylosis, neoplasm, or abscess, causes compression and distortion of the posterior spinal cord, there is loss of proprioception and vibration sensation below the level of the lesion. With proprioceptive impairment in cervical region, searching, writhing movements (pseudo-athetoid) of outstretched hands and fingers can occur. With flexion of the neck, electrical shocklike sensation is felt in the back and down the legs (Lhermitte sign).

Hemisection (Brown-Séquard) Syndrome

If lesions are restricted to one side of the spinal cord, hemiparesis often with impaired position and vibration sense occurs ipsilateral to the lesion, and impaired pain and temperature perception are present in extremities and trunk contralateral to the lesion (usually beginning two spinal segments below the lesion level). This pattern results from extradural or intradural extramedullary lesions such as meningioma, neurofibroma, and cervical spondylosis.

Complete Spinal Cord Transection Syndrome

Complete transection syndrome is characterized by the complete loss of all sensory modalities below the level of the lesion with associated paralysis and loss of spincter function. The deficit develops rapidly in trauma or demyelinating disorders (acute transverse myelitis); it evolves more gradually when caused by spinal cord neoplasm or abscess. Spinothalamic tract fibers have a laminar pattern, sacral fibers are lateral, and cervical fibers are medial. If the spinal cord is damaged from extrinsic compression (extradural or intradural extramedullary tumor), the sensory level gradually can ascend to a higher level. Initially, a lesion acts to compress externally located sacral fibers; later, internally located (medial) fibers—which represent lumbar, thoracic, and cervical regions—are compressed. It is important to consider the evolution of the pattern of sensory involvement caused by spinal cord lesions; this differs depending on the location of the spinal cord lesion, for example, intramedullary lesions initially spare the sacral region, and extramedullary lesions cause early sacral involvement with prominent autonomic (bowel and bladder) impairment.

Anterior Spinal Cord Syndrome

This is most commonly caused by ischemic spinal artery disease. Initial symptoms of spinal stroke caused by infarction within anterior spinal artery territory can be diffuse back pain or radicular dysesthetic pain. Pain is followed by the rapid onset of weakness in arms and legs (occlusion of cervical portion) or legs only (occlusion of thoracic region), usually with incontinence. Initially, the limb tone is flaccid; reflexes can be diminished, and bilateral

Babinski signs are present. There is absent pain and temperature sensation below the lesion level. Proprioception and vibration sensation are *intact* because posterior columns are supplied by posterior spinal artery. This pattern of dissociated sensory loss is differentiated from that seen with mass lesions including hematomyelia (hemorrhage into substance of spinal cord), in which there can be complete transection syndrome in which there is involvement of *all* sensory modalities.

Tabes Dorsalis

Tabes dorsalis is usually due to neurosyphilis but can be caused by diabetes. There is damage to proprioceptive fibers of dorsal roots. This damage initially involves lumbosacral roots but can extend to the thoracic and cervical regions. Clinical symptoms include lightning or lancinating pains. Findings include hypotonia, areflexia, and loss of proprioception and vibration sensations.

Brain Stem Syndromes

With lesions in the medulla and those extending to midpontine level, there is crossed anesthesia; loss of pain and temperature sensation on the face is on the same side as the lesion (because fibers traveling in the trigeminothalamic tract initially descend in the brain stem on same side before their synapse) and on trunk and extremities contralateral to lesion (caused by the immediate crossing of the ascending lateral spinothalamic tract within the spinal cord). If the lesion is located above the nucleus of spinal tract of the trigeminal nerve, all sensory loss is located contralateral to lesion. There is impairment of sensation of sensory modalities supplied by the lateral spinothalamic tract (pain and temperature) and medial lemniscus (position sense and vibration) because at this level of neuraxis these sensory tracts are parallel and contiguous.

Thalamic Sensory Syndromes

Patients with thalamic sensory syndromes invariably demonstrate contralateral hemianesthesia for superficial and deep sensations as well as having astereognosia (inability to recognize objects placed in hand). There can sometimes be accompanying hemiparesis, hemiataxia, or hemichorea. Sensory abnormalities include all modalities involving the face, arm, trunk, and leg contralateral to the lesion. This is usually caused by infarction that is due to the occlusion of thalamogeniculate branches of the posterior cerebral artery or hemorrhage involving the thalamus; it can also be due to parietal white matter subcortical lesions. Several days to weeks after the onset of the vascular episode, painful sensations develop in the region of sensory impairment (Dejerine-Roussy syndrome). These sensations have a burning and unpleasant causalgic quality. Tactile stimulation of the involved region or emotional disturbances can evoke dysesthesias in anesthetic regions (anesthesia dolorosa). Pain can be spontaneous or evoked by touching the limb. This "thalamic pain" is usually unresponsive to any analgesic medication. It may respond to tricyclic antidepressants or anticonvulsants, agents effective in treating neuropathic pain.

Cortical Sensory Syndromes

Sensory information is modulated and interpreted in the neocortex (parietal lobe). In parietal lobe lesions there can be inattention or neglect of sensory stimulation on contralateral limbs and trunk. These are most common with nondominant lesions but can also occur with dominant cerebral hemispheric lesions. These cortical sensory parameters are mentioned in Box 6-2.

In simple partial seizures originating in parietal (somatosensory) cortex, the patient may describe paresthesias, dysesthesias, or the sensation and the motionless limb feels as if it is moving; these sensations occur contralateral to the side of the parietal lesion.

Functional Sensory Loss

Patients with conversion symptoms and hysteria frequently have sensory disturbances. The possibility of functional sensory dysfunction is considered when there is discrepancy between the patient's symptoms with neuroanatomical and neurophysiologic realities. For example, the patient may report stocking-and-glove anesthesia; however, this pattern is characterized

---

 BOX 6-2

1 Stereognosis, or the ability to recognize objects placed in hand (impairment is astereognosia)

2 Graphesthesia, or the ability to recognize numbers traced on skin of hand (impairment is agraphesthesia)

3 Recognition of shape, weight, or texture of objects placed in hand

4 Two-point discrimination, or the ability to recognize two points as separate when applied simultaneously 3 mm apart on fingertips

5 Double simultaneous stimulation, or the ability to recognize two independently applied or presented sensory stimuli (e.g., tactile and visual) on symmetrical body regions

6 Position and vibration sense; impairment involving sensory modalities is valid only if primary sensory modalities (e.g., pain, temperature, and light touch) are intact

by an abrupt or precise change from abnormal to normal without an intervening area of partial anesthesia as is consistent with polyneuropathy. In other cases the functional sensory pattern does not conform to that seen in peripheral nerve or spinal root lesions. In patients with functional hemianesthesia other special systems can be involved (hearing, vision, and olfaction), and functional loss has sharply defined borders between areas of absent and normal sensibility without an intervening zone of mildly impaired sensation. In functional sensory disorders impairment of position sense is equally impaired in distal and proximal joints (equal numbers of errors when toes and knees are tested), whereas there is most severe impairment in distal joints in true proprioception abnormalities. Despite a profound loss of position sensation, the patient does not fall and does not appear unsteady. In functional hemianesthesia there is an abrupt change in the patient's ability to perceive vibration in the central region of the face and sternum. Because this sensation is transmitted through one bone, the patient should perceive vibration equally on both sides of this bone except if the sensory loss if functional. Also, in functional sensory anesthesia, the patient does not report that the limb feels different than the normal limb.

▨ SELECTED PAIN SYNDROMES

Pain Related to Peripheral Nerve Lesions

Neuralgia literally means "nerve pain" and is used to describe paroxysms of electrical or shocklike sensation caused by spontaneous discharges within demyelinated areas of the nerve. This can result from compression or stretching of nerves. Following nerve trauma, this neuropathic pain is due to abnormal discharges involving thinly myelinated or unmyelinated fibers. The pain is usually intermittent as is the characteristic of short-lived, but frequent paroxysms of trigeminal neuralgia, but can be more continuous as reported in postherpetic neuralgia. With partial nerve injuries, the painful limb usually shows other characteristics (Box 6-3).

In patients with partial nerve injuries there is reduced function of large, thickly myelinated fibers serving vibration sensibility, proprioception, and two-point discrimination. These large-fibers are believed to initiate a mechanism within the dorsal horn of the spinal cord (substantia gelatinosa) that should normally inhibit conduction of painful impulses to CNS. When this mechanism is impaired, CNS is flooded with painful impulses, and the patient reports limb pain. By using transcutaneous electrical stimulation to activate afferent sensory fibers or by applying a sympathetic nerve block used to terminate abnormal electrical impulses, neuropathic pain can be reduced.

Phantom-Limb Pain

Amputation of a limb can be followed by awareness of deafferented (amputated) body part. This experience can range from a vague diffuse tingling in the

 BOX 6-3

1 Painful discomfort to testing with normally nonnoxious stimulus such as pin, cotton, or temperature (cold or warm)

2 Delayed appreciation of sensory stimulus

3 Continued pain after stimulation with the pin has stopped

region of the amputated limb to reporting the exact experience that previously emanated from the amputated limb. Less commonly, the patient experiences painful sensations in the region of the missing limb or at the remaining amputation stump. This pain can have these characteristics: stabbing, throbbing, deep ache. The pain is exacerbated by emotional stress, autonomic (sympathetic) reflex activity, or touching the stump; this pain can be relieved by rest or massage of the stump. Pain usually disappears within 1 year of amputation. The mechanism of phantom-limb pain is not established but may relate to persistence of sensory reflex signals transmitted to spinal cord and brain following amputation of the painful limb.

Peripheral Neuropathy

Certain patients with neuropathies report severe uncomfortable paresthesias and limb pain; this can be deep aching in limbs or superficial burning pain. It would seem logical that painful neuropathies would have selective large fiber loss; however, there are other painful neuropathies (amyloid) in which there is selective small-fiber type loss. This indicates that the mechanism for pain in neuropathy is not established.

Reflex Sympathetic Dystrophy

The cardinal features are the following: one, burning pain (causalgia); two, sympathetic dysfunction (edema, increased sweating pattern, cold limb temperature, thin shiny skin, cracked brittle nails, reduced extremity hair pattern, osteoporosis); three, pain evoked by usually painless stimulus (allodynia) and hyperesthesia. When this pattern occurs after peripheral nerve injury, it is referred to as "causalgia," and when there is no evidence of nerve injury, the term reflex sympathetic dystrophy (RSD) is used. The pain is usually located distally (hand, foot) and is exacerbated by limb movement; therefore the involved limb is held motionless, usually in a guarded position. This disuse of the limb can lead to joint fibrosis, muscle atrophy, contractures, and osteoporosis. The diagnosis of RSD can be confirmed by thermography (reduced limb temperature caused by reduced blood flow), limb radiogram (demineralization, osteoporosis), and bone scan abnormalities (impaired blood flow, abnormal soft tissue and bone uptake of radionuclide isotope); however, symptom relief by nerve block is essential to establish the diagnosis. Nerve block can abolish symptoms for several weeks; however, symptoms can recur. Some patients' symptoms respond to physical therapy and transcutaneous nerve stimulation; however, in persistent cases where there has been response to nerve block but the effect wears off after several weeks, sympathectomy may be necessary. It is important to establish the diagnosis of RSD in the early stages when the condition responds to nerve block and sympathectomy. In later stages of RSD the disorder may no longer respond to these treatments and patients may require neurosurgical pain-relieving procedures including dorsal column stimulation, morphine pump, or oral narcotics to control pain. RSD is an important consideration in any patient who reports unexplained limb pain.

▣ SUMMARY

Sensory disturbances can be reported as symptoms by the patient even when there are no objective neurological findings. These symptoms can include numbness, paresthesias, or pain. Based upon the history, it is crucial to ascertain if those symptoms are of neurological or nonneurological (vascular, rheumatological) origin. If these symptoms are of possible neurological origin, ascertain the sensory symptom characteristics (pattern, duration) and the exact distribution of the sensory abnormalities. This permits localization of the lesion causing sensory disturbance within the peripheral or central nervous system. It is important to recognize that sensory symptoms can be caused by neurological processes, for example, numbness or paresthesias in the arm or hand caused by cervical nerve root compression or compression of the median nerve at the wrist, even if the neurological examination is normal. Careful history and examination are crucial to determine the exact nature of the reported sensory symptoms, which can be caused by neurological, medical-systemic, or psychiatric disturbances.

Suggested Readings

Pain Syndromes

Dawson DM, Katz N: Reflex sympathetic dystrophy, *Neurol Chron* 2:1, 1992.

Levine DZ: Burning pain in an extremity, *Postgrad Med* 90:175, 1991.

Schwartzman RJ, McLellan, TL: Reflex sympathetic dystrophy, *Arch Neurol* 44:555, 1987.

Pain—General

Critchley M: *Disorders of tactile function in the parietal lobes,* New York, 1966, Hafner Press.

Cross SA: Pathophysiology of pain, *Mayo Clin Proc* 69: 375, 1994.

Melzack R, Wall PD: Pain mechanisms: a new theory, *Science* 150:971, 1965.

Melzack R: *The puzzle of pain,* New York, 1973, Basic Books.

Shephard DI: Sensory disturbances, *Br Med J* 288:1147, 1984.

Sensory System Evaluation

Chad DA: The evaluation and diagnosis of peripheral neuropathy, *Neurol Chron* 4:1, 1994.

Evans BA, Stevens JC, Dyck PJ: Lumbosacral plexus neuropathy, *Neurology* 31:1327, 1981.

Sun SF, Streib EW: Diabetic thoraco-abdominal neuropathy: clinical and electrodiagnostic features, *Ann Neurol* 9:75, 1981.

Tsairis P, Dyck PJ, Mulder DW: Natural history of brachial plexus neuropathy, *Arch Neurol* 27:109, 1972.

Visual System Disorders

7

DIAGNOSTIC ASSESSMENT

The patient's complaints are usually caused by two types of abnormalities: defective visual perceptions (sensory visual disorders) and abnormal ocular movements (ocular motor disorders). To analyze these visual disturbances attention must be directed toward seven important points (Box 7-1).

With these findings, it is usually possible to localize the lesion within the visual system.

SIGNS AND SYMPT0OMS OF DISEASE IN THE AFFERENT VISUAL SYSTEM

Symptoms

Patients are frequently aware of bilateral visual acuity impairment, but if acuity loss is unilateral it may not be detected early and only when patients close the nonaffected eye. Patients may complain of visual blurring or visual dimming. Ask the patient, "What did you initially notice was wrong with your vision?" Determine the temporal pattern of visual

177

BOX 7-1

1 Precise delineation of visual symptoms including accompanying facial, orbital, and cephalic sensory (pain) symptoms or other neurological complaints

2 Measurement of best corrected visual acuity

3 Visual field examination

4 Analysis of pupillary size and reactivity

5 Examination of optic fundus

6 Eye movement analysis

7 Detection of associated neurologic findings

complaints (evolution or resolution) by asking, "When did you first notice visual symptoms?" and "Has there been subsequent improvement or deterioration in your vision?" Determine exacerbating factors: one, exercise (Uhthoff's phenomenon in which visual dysfunction is worsened by exercise in patients with optic nerve demyelination) and elevated body temperature, which also worsens vision in multiple sclerosis patients; and two, medication administration as it relates to visual symptoms (digitalis or ethambutol can cause visual disturbances) in drug effects.

Sudden unilateral visual loss is caused by retinal or optic nerve lesions. These include vascular conditions (retinal artery occlusion, temporal arteritis with optic nerve head infarction), demyelinating disorders (optic neuritis), or primary ophthalmologic disorders (detached retina). Amaurosis fugax is temporary unilateral loss of vision caused by a microembolism originating from the carotid artery. This can be accompanied by other signs of transient ischemia caused by ipsilateral cerebral hemisphere, for example, contralateral weakness, sensory disturbance, aphasia. Amaurosis fugax can be a harbinger of carotid artery disease (high-grade stenosis, occlusion). Other causes of sudden unilateral visual loss include central retinal artery occlusion (CRAO) and anterior ischemic optic neuropathy (AION). In CRAO, unilateral visual loss occurs rapidly. Findings include the pupil not reacting to light and funduscopy showing ischemic retina appearing pale (white) with normal red-colored choroid reflecting through fovea (cherry-red spot); and optic atrophy develops later. In some cases a retinal embolus that is occluding the retinal artery can be visualized by funduscopic examination as it is observed moving from one vessel region to another, usually migrating to a more distal segment. In AION, sudden painless visual loss occurs; this is usually an altitudinal defect (described as if a curtain is pulled over one eye). Signs of AION include: unilateral altitudinal visual field defects or total blindness; impaired pupillary response to light; and funduscopy showing narrowed retinal arteries, hyperemic (swollen) pale disc, flame-shaped hemorrhages, and later optic atrophy.

Lesions responsible for sudden bilateral visual loss include pituitary apoplexy, cortical blindness caused by bilateral occipital lobe infarcts, and hysteria. Bilateral visual loss is due to bilateral retinal, optic nerves, optic chiasm, optic tracts, optic radiations, or occipital lesions. Bilateral cortical (occipital) blindness is usually due to bilateral posterior cerebral or basilar artery occlusion. Visual disturbances include bilateral homonymous hemianopsia; however, the patient may not be cognizant of blindness (Anton's syndrome).

Transient monocular visual loss that resolves rapidly within seconds or minutes indicates amaurosis fugax caused by carotid diseases or papilledema caused by intracranial hypertension, although the latter condition more commonly causes bilateral episodic visual obscurations (Box 7-2). Sudden monocular visual loss that stabilizes and improves during a period of several days or weeks is consistent with demyelinating disease (optic neuritis). Visual loss can also develop insidiously. This indicates a compressive optic nerve lesion if unilateral or metabolic

---

BOX 7-2   Mechanisms of Acute Visual Loss

Transient

Unilateral	Amaurosis fugax
	Retinal migraine
Bilateral	Systemic hypotension
	Systemic arterial hypertension
	Retinal dysfunction
	Intracranial hypertension
	Systemic hyperviscosity syndromes
	Uhthoff's syndrome

Persistent

Unilateral

Painless	Central retinal artery occlusion
	Anterior ischemic optic neuropathy
	Macular or vitreous hemorrhage
	Retinal detachment
Painful	Glaucoma
	Temporal arteritis
	Optic neuritis
	Iridocyclitis
	Vitreous hemorrhage

Bilateral

Painless	Bilateral occipital infarction
	Eclampsia
	Hysteria-conversion reaction
Painful	Pituitary apoplexy

and a toxic or degenerative optic nerve lesion if bilateral. These patients may report sensations that a film is developing over one eye or the patient can have difficulty focusing when reading. Other visual symptoms of optic nerve dysfunction include dimming of color or light brightness under different sources of illumination (e.g., sunlight, twilight, watching color television).

Abnormal visual sensations can be initial migraine symptoms. These include flashing lights (scintillation), bright zigzag or picket fence lines (fortification spectrum), or flickering colored lights moving across the visual field. These symptoms can be accompanied by central areas of impaired vision (scotoma); this may be initially noted in center of visual field and extend peripherally within a 10 to 30 minute interval. Perception of unformed flashing lights moving rapidly across the visual field within seconds or minutes is characteristic of occipital epilepsy.

In patients with sensory visual symptoms reporting cephalic or orbital pain, consider acute glaucoma, temporal arteritis, retrobulbar neuritis, migraine, or cluster headache; however, orbital pain can indicate a local ophthalmological disorder. In patients with diplopia and ocular motility disorders reporting cephalic or orbital pain, consider a ruptured carotid aneurysm or ischemic extraocular nerve lesion. Other causes of painful ophthalmoplegia include superior orbital fissure or cavernous sinus conditions of neoplastic, inflammatory, or vascular origin.

Examination

Determine the patient's best corrected visual acuity at 20 feet; however, this is usually tested with a pocket-sized eye chart held 12 to 18 inches from the patient.

It may be possible to improve acuity by having the patient view this card through a pinhole if reduced vision is due to refractive changes. Observe the patient manipulate the card; patients with hemianopic defects may ignore part of the visual acuity chart extending into affected visual field. Visual acuity loss not correctable with lenses (refraction) or not attributed to retinal disease, strabismic amblyopia (lazy eye with loss of acuity caused by failure of visual potential to develop because of wandering or crossed eye), lens disease, corneal disease or other primary ophthalmological disease is presumed caused by optic nerve or chiasmal dysfunction. Test color vision using Ishihara color plates. Acquired color vision defects (color desaturation) is early sign of optic nerve dysfunction.

Examination of visual fields is best initially performed using confrontation techniques (Chapter 1). Visual field defects can be delineated by tangent screen examination, Goldmann kinetic perimetry, or automated static threshold perimetry, but these require specialized equipment. Confrontation technique is quite accurate if certain rules are considered. Box 7-3 lists these rules. Characteristic visual field defects are shown in Figure 7-1.

Pupillary size, shape, and light reactivity must be assessed. Have the patient fixate on distant object; maximal pupillary size is then measured. Twenty to 30% of normal subjects have clinically observable differences in pupil size; however, light reactivity should be symmetrical in both eyes, and there should be no difference in the degree of anisocoria in different illumination states, such as sunlight versus a dark room. To test pupillary reactivity bright light is directed to one eye and rapidly moved to the opposite eye. Rapidity and degree of change in pupillary size

BOX 7-3

1 Lesions of the optic chiasm and postchiasmal region cause defects that change abruptly as an object is moved across the vertical meridian from the nasal to temporal sectors.

2 Superior and inferior quadrants are separately tested because quadrantanopic defects have more localizing value than hemianopic defects.

3 Monocular visual field defects are due to retinal or optic nerve lesions.

4 Binocular visual field defects developing at the same time are caused by chiasmal and postchiasmal lesions. Bilateral scotomas caused by bilateral optic neuritis can develop at separate times, but it is unlikely that these will develop at exactly the same time.

5 The hallmark of postchiasmal visual lesions is homonymous hemianopsia; chiasmal lesions cause bitemporal hemianopsia.

is determined in both the eye directly illuminated and the opposite eye (consensual reaction). Response should be equal in both eyes because the Edinger-Westphal nucleus located in midbrain summates the total light received and sends an identical pupil diameter message to both eyes.

If the afferent (optic nerve) portion of a light reflex is defective, the response of defective eye is diminished when light is directly applied and normal when the light is applied to the opposite eye (consensual reaction). Unilateral optic nerve lesions can be detected by rapidly moving a light from one eye to the other eye (swinging flashlight test). Abnormal response consists of less brisk pupillary constriction or dilatation (pupillary escape) when a light is rapidly moved from a normal to a defective pupil (Marcus Gunn phenomenon). This test is helpful in unilateral—but not bilateral—optic nerve lesions. Despite

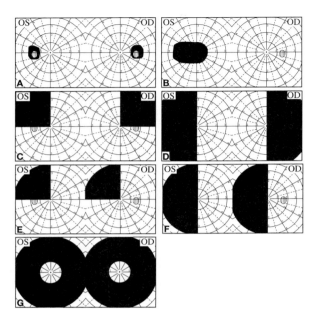

FIGURE 7-1. A, Bilateral enlarged blind spots caused by papilledema. **B,** Left centrocecal scotoma caused by dysfunction of the left optic nerve in a patient with unilateral optic neuritis. **C,** Bitemporal quadrantanopia caused by compression of the undersurface of the optic chiasm by a pituitary adenoma. **D,** Bitemporal hemianopia caused by optic chiasmal compression, which is due to pituitary tumor. **E,** Left superior homonymous quandrantanopia, which may be caused by a lesion involving the temporal lobe. **F,** Left homonymous hemianopia, which may be due to a right-sided cerebral lesion. **G,** Concentric constriction (tubular visual fields) is cylindrical and measures the same size irrespective of the distance of the patient from the visual chart or the size of the test object. This can be seen in hysteria.

abnormal response to light stimulation in unilateral optic nerve lesions, the pupils are equal in size in the resting state. If the efferent portion of the light reflex (oculomotor nerve) is defective, pupils are unequal in size, with the abnormal pupil dilated and poorly reactive to both direct and consensual stimulation.

In patients with optic nerve dysfunction, there is reduced visual acuity, central scotoma (blind or black spot within field of vision), and afferent pupillary defect. Another important feature of optic nerve dysfunction is defective color perception (dyschromatopsia) and decreased appreciation of color or light brightness. Impairment of color vision can be tested by having the patient look at colored objects (such as the Ishihara color plates) with each eye independently. In assessing the presence of impaired color vision, remember that 10% of men have congenital color blindness. The eye in which color is less rich and less bright is the affected eye. Patients rarely complain of this symptom, and this is demonstrated by visual testing only.

Examination of the retina and optic disc (papilla) is performed at bedside by the neurologist using hand-held ophthalmoscope. The ophthalmologist uses an indirect light-source ophthalmoscope; this has much brighter light source and pupil if fully dilated and prevented from constricting by locally instilled dilating agent. This allows better visualization of a larger portion of the retina (including periphery) by the ophthalmologist. Optic disc edema appears as optic nerve swelling. If this is due to increased intracranial pressure, it is referred to as papilledema. When caused by intracranial hypertension, papilledema is present bilaterally; papilledema can be asymptomatic or cause transient visual obscurations. Headaches are usually prominent in intracranial hypertension. If papilledema is unilateral, this indicates local vascular inflammatory or neoplastic orbital lesions; *unilateral* papilledema is rarely due to increased intracranial pressure. The diagnosis of papilledema is established by funduscopic findings (Figure 7-2). Box 7-4 outlines the diagnostic features of papilledema.

Spontaneous venous pulsations are present in 80% of normal people. Their visualization usually excludes diagnosis of increased intracranial pressure; however, absence of spontaneous venous pulsations is not helpful as 20% of normal people have no evidence of pulsations despite normal cerebrospinal fluid (CSF) pressure. It may not be possible to differentiate ophthalmoscopic signs of optic disc edema from pseudopapilledema such as optic disc drusen. Fluorescein angiography, three-dimensional fundus photographs, and serial ophthalmoscopic examinations can improve diagnostic accuracy. The presence of intracranial hypertension can only be *definitively* established by the finding of elevated opening pressure when lumbar puncture is performed with the patient in a

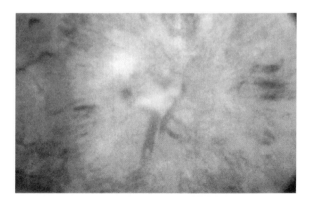

FIGURE 7-2. Optic disc blurring of disc margins with loss of central cup; consistent with papilledema.

BOX 7-4

1 Absence of spontaneous venous pulsations
2 Presence of hemorrhages and exudates located contigious to optic disc region
3 Inability to focus on vessels at center and periphery of disc without changing diopter settings; this is due to central disc elevation
4 Blurring of nasal disc margins and later extending to temporal margins
5 Loss of central physiologic optic cup; this is usually a late finding
6 Blurring of the retinal nerve fiber layer as seen with green light on the ophthalmoscope
7 Engorged veins and increased disc redness (disc hyperemia)

---

lateral recumbent position. Optic disc edema can occur in the absence of elevated intracranial pressure without any neurological signs, and in this case ophthalmologic evaluation for possible vascular or inflammatory causes is warranted.

Funduscopic findings of optic atrophy reflect the loss of nerve fibers with a decrease in the number of small blood vessels crossing the optic disc with accompanying gliotic reaction (Figure 7-3). Funduscopic criteria for optic atrophy include the following: white coloration of the optic disc representing glial changes, a decrease in the number (usually 8 to 12) of arterioles seen extending across the disc margin, and thinning of the retinal nerve fiber layer, best appreciated by looking at very small caliber branches of retinal arterioles. In ischemic optic atrophy, such as temporal arteritis, retinal arteries can be markedly narrowed; in glaucomatous atrophy the disc

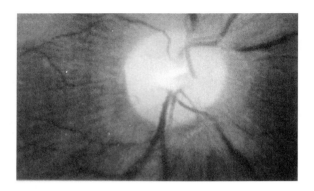

FIGURE 7-3. Pale gliotic-appearing optic disc with loss of nerve fibers consistent with optic atrophy.

is enlarged and deeply cupped. In patients with optic atrophy there is decreased visual acuity in the involved eye with afferent pupillary defect (minimal pupillary constriction with direct light stimulation but brisk response of involved eye when light is applied to the normal eye).

Patients with retrochiasmal lesions have homonymous visual field defects. Certain patients can be unaware of this deficit (visual inattention), whereas others initially complain of difficulty reading or problems bumping into objects in affected visual field. In patients with retrochiasmal hemispheric (temporal, parietal, occipital) lesions and during certain drug intoxications, unusual visual disturbances can be present, including these:

- Prosopagnosia—the inability to recognize faces
- Palinopsia—the persistent visualization of an image after stimulus has been removed
- Metamorphopsia—the distortion of the shape or form of objects

- Micropsia or macropsia—the abnormal perception of size—or teleopsia—the distance of an object from the patient
- Phosphenes—the flashing of bright lights or colors
- Chromatopsia—the perception that the environment is tinted in single color
- Visual hallucinations

With occipital lesion such as neoplasm or hemorrhage, perceived visual sensations are unformed and consist of flashing lights or spots, whereas parietal-temporal lesions cause complex hallucinations and illusions, including entire pictures or scenes. It is important not to falsely identify the cause of these bizarre and unusual visual phenomena as hysteric in origin or caused by psychotic disorders without careful assessment of visual system.

◼ SIGNS AND SYMPTOMS OF DISEASES IN THE EFFERENT VISUAL SYSTEM

Symptoms

Patients with ocular motility abnormalities may have no symptoms; more commonly they complain of double vision (diplopia) or movement of objects in the environment (oscillopsia). In patients with congenital strabismus (misalignment or lack of parallelism of visual axes of eyes) there may be no diplopia because the visual image from the deviated eye is suppressed. If ocular misalignment is observed, it is called tropia (turning), for example, exo- or esotropia, hypo- or hypertropia; however, there can be phoria, which is misalignment brought out by cover-uncover testing of each eye. Observe whether the eyes appear in parallel alignment and whether they move conjugately. Specific characteristics of diplopia must be determined. Box 7-5 lists four questions specific to the characteristics of diplopia.

BOX 7-5

1 Are images horizontal side by side (this indicates dysfunction of lateral or medial recti), or located vertically one above the other (this indicates superior or inferior recti or oblique muscles)?

2 Is diplopia more prominent on near gaze as a result of superior oblique or medial recti paresis or on far gaze as a result of lateral rectus paresis?

3 With closure of one eye, does diplopia disappear or persist (monocular diplopia is usually caused by ocular disease, e.g., lens opacities, dislocated lens, psychogenic origin, or occipital-parietal lesions causing metamorphopsia)?

4 Has double vision subsequently improved (vascular), become more severe and persistent (tumor), or does it fluctuate during the day (myasthenia gravis)?

Examination

Evaluation of eye movements includes observation of eyelids, orbits, and facial movements. The presence of proptosis (protrusion of globe) is evaluated by standing behind the seated patient and looking directly down at the orbits. To measure proptosis objectively a small and inexpensive exophthalmometer is necessary. The upper limit of normal forward eye protuberance is 22 mm; there should be no more than a 3-mm intereye difference. When observing eyelids, note any degree of eyelid asymmetry. Ptosis caused by levator palpebrae weakness is initially detected on upward gaze. The finding of ptosis does not necessarily imply neurologic abnormality. Compare the patient's present appearance with old photographs to differentiate congenital from recently developing ptosis. Ptosis can be caused by myopathic conditions such as myasthenia gravis, by neurogenic conditions such as third nerve or sympathetic disorders, or by the loss of tension (laxity) in levator tendons (dehiscence); the latter is of nonneurological origin. Ptosis can cause visual impairment if the pupil is covered. The diagnosis is based on these general facts:

- Ptosis of myopathic origin is usually bilateral, and the pupil is spared.
- Ptosis caused by third nerve disorders is unilateral and produces paresis of medial and superior gaze; the pupil is dilated and unreactive.
- Ptosis caused by oculosympathetic paresis (Horner's syndrome) is unilateral, the pupil is miotic, reduced sweating occurs on the involved side of face, and no motility abnormality occurs.

If the third nerve is compressed by an extrinsic mass lesion (aneurysm or neoplasm), the pupil is dilated and unreactive to light stimulation, whereas the pupil is usually normal in diabetic ophthalmoplegia caused by vascular ischemia. This results because pupillary fibers are located peripherally and are initially affected by compressive lesions, yet are spared in ischemic lesions as blood vessels initially traverse the external nerve surface and are less vulnerable to vascular ischemia.

Pupils that respond poorly to light should be tested for reactivity (constriction) on near fixation. Miotic pupils having normal near reflex (pupilloconstriction, convergence, lens accommodation) but reacting poorly to light are indicative of neurosyphilis (Argyll Robertson pupil). Tonic (Adie's) pupil shows absent constriction to light with slowed and tonic constriction to near target (accommodation). The pupil can show slowed writhing movements when viewed with a slit lamp. This condition can be unilateral or bilateral, is most common in young women, and can be associated with decreased or absent deep tendon reflexes. Tonic pupil is a benign condition; however, certain patients report visual blurring especially when shifting from far to near objects. The diagnosis of tonic pupil is confirmed by pharmacologic testing. There is rapid and complete pupillary constriction using 0.125% pilocarpine; this indicates denervation cholinergic sensitivity. Tonic response to accommodation and pharmacologic testing differentiates Adie's pupil from Argyll Robertson pupil (Box 7-6).

The effect of drugs on pupillary size and reactivity must be considered; pupillary dilatation can be secondary to anticholinergic drugs; constriction can result from heroin abuse. In comatose patients, pupillary size or reactivity is quite important, and four general rules should be remembered (Box 7-7).

BOX 7-6   Features of Pupillary Syndromes

Argyll-Robertson Syndrome
Visual function intact
Intact accommodation response
Abnormal pupillary light response
Irregular shaped miotic and asymmetric pupils
Iris atrophy
Usually caused by neurosyphilis
Adie's Tonic Pupil Syndrome
Dilated pupils
Absent reaction to light stimulation
Slow pupillary reaction to near response
Slow (tonic) dilation after near response
Iris sphincter sector paresis
Impaired accommodation
Pupils constricts to 0.125% pilocarpine and 2.5% methacholine
Associated diminished deep tendon reflexes

▨ BOX 7-7

1 Metabolic disturbances do not alter pupillary size or reactivity.

2 Unilateral cerebral hemispheric lesions cause an unilateral dilated and poorly reactive pupil if an uncal (transtentorial) herniation has occurred.

3 Midbrain lesions cause bilateral dilated and fixed pupils.

4 Pontine lesions cause bilateral miotic but reactive pupils.

It the patient has a fixed dilated pupil without ptosis or extraocular muscle paresis, this may have resulted from local application of sympathomimetic (dilating) drug. Failure of the dilated pupil to constrict following local application of 1% pilocarpine indicates pharmacologic blockade because pupillary constriction occurs with neurologic disorders. If the patient has a miotic pupil, there can be an oculosympathetic chain lesion (Horner's syndrome), or this can represent a normal variant. In Horner's syndrome, the miotic pupil does not respond (dilate) as well as a normal pupil to ocular instillation of cocaine solution, whereas if miosis represents normal asymmetry, the response in both eyes should be equal. Sympathetic fibers originate in the hypothalamus and traverse the brain stem to the spinal cord (C7–T2), then travel to superior cervical ganglion. Postganglionic sympathetic fibers traverse the carotid artery sheath, cavernous sinus, and orbit. Lesions at these locations cause Horner's syndrome (Box 7-8).

Determining the location of the lesion causing Horner's syndrome is simplified by the presence of certain accompanying findings, for example, radiographic evidence of a mediastinal mass or neurologic

BOX 7-8   Etiologies of Horner's Syndrome

First Neuron
Hypothalamic lesion
Pituitary-chiasmal lesion
Basal meningitis–arachnoiditis
Brain stem lesion
Cervical cord lesion
Second Neuron
Cervical rib
Apical lung lesion (Pancoast tumor)
Aortic aneurysm
Cervical adenopathy
Brachial plexus lesion
Third Neuron
Carotid artery lesion
Cavernous sinus lesion
Paratrigeminal syndrome
Orbital lesion
Cluster headache

signs of brain stem involvement. Pharmacologic agents can be used to differentiate central (hypothalamus, brain stem, and spinal cord) and preganglionic (mediastinum) causes from postganglionic (carotid artery sheath, cavernous sinus, and orbit) lesions causing Horner's syndrome. If the postganglionic system is involved, there is denervation hypersensitivity; the pupil dilates in response to local application of 1:1000 epinephrine solution. If the postganglionic system is intact (neurons from superior cervical ganglion in the neck to pupillodilator fibers in orbit), hydroxyamphetamine (Paredrine), which releases norepinephrine from postganglionic vesicles, causes pupillary dilation. Failure to obtain this dilation with Paredrine indicates postganglionic lesions as the cause of Horner's syndrome.

Conjugate gaze can be tested for command (ask the patient to look to right, left, upward, downward) and pursuit or slow tracking eye movements (ask the patient to follow the pointer). The pathway for supranuclear control of gaze for the saccades (rapid eye movements) begins in frontal lobe (area 8) and descends through the internal capsule and diencephalon to reach midbrain, where it crosses in paramedian pontine reticular formation (lateral gaze center). Cortical lesions can be irritative (neoplasm or abscess) or destructive (infarction or hemorrhage). These lesions cause differential effects on lateral conjugate gaze; certain lesions, for example, glioma and meningioma, can act as both destructive and irritative lesions. A destructive lesion above decussation causes paresis of horizontal conjugate eye movements to the contralateral side; lesions below decussation cause ipsilateral paresis. During simple partial seizures caused by irritative lesions originating in the left frontal region, frontal eye fields are stimulated with the eyes deviating to right side. Following a left-hemispheric destructive lesion, horizontal eye movement to right is impaired and eyes deviate to left (in the direction opposite the hemiparesis) such that eyes look toward the lesion. When lesions located below the oculomotor decussation, there is paralysis of conjugate gaze to the side of the lesion such that eyes deviate away from the brain stem lesion.

Another type of disorder involving horizontal (lateral) conjugate gaze is internuclear ophthalmoplegia caused by a lesion of medial longitudinal fasciculus that is located in the brain stem. This disorder causes impaired medial (adduction) movement of eye ipsilateral to the lesion with horizontal nystagmus in the abducting opposite eye. In resting state the eyes are conjugate and convergence movements are normal; this indicates that the medial rectus muscle functions normally. Bilateral internuclear ophthalmoplegia occurs most frequently in patients with multiple sclerosis. Other causes include brain stem tumors and ischemic vascular disease; these usually cause unilateral internuclear ophthalmoplegia.

Using a red lens placed over one eye (by convention, the right eye) helps clarify defective extraocular muscle(s) and/or cranial nerves in patients with diplopia. Box 7-9 lists some of the causes of extraocular nerve lesions. Two rules are inviolate: one, diplopia is maximal with the greatest separation of images in field of gaze of the involved muscle; and two, an image belonging to the paretic muscle projects peripherally. For example, in an isolated right lateral rectus lesion with abductor muscle paresis, diplopia is horizontal and maximal on the far gaze. With a red lens placed over the right eye, two images are seen on gaze to the right side with the red image (caused by the right lateral rectus) projecting peripherally to right (uncrossed diplopia). In right third-nerve lesions with adductor muscle paresis there is maximal separation of the two horizontal images on gaze directed to the left with the red image (with a red glass held over right eye) projecting peripherally (crossed diplopia). Muscles functioning as torters (rotation of globe) are tested by noting the degree of separation of objects when the head is tilted. For

BOX 7-9   Etiologies of Extraocular Nerve Lesion

Isolated Oculomotor Lesion

Painful   Carotid aneurysm
      Parasellar lesion
      Ophthalmoplegic migraine

Painless   Ischemic (diabetic) disease
      Head injury
      Basal meningitis
      Parasellar lesion
      Nasopharyngeal lesion
      Multiple sclerosis
      Myasthenia gravis
      Thyroid ophthalmopathy
      Wernicke's syndrome

Isolated Trochlear Paresis

      Head injury
      Multiple sclerosis
      Myasthenia gravis
      Thyroid ophthalmopathy
      Wernicke's syndrome
      Ischemic diabetic syndrome
      Neoplasm
      Orbital lesion

Isolated abducens paresis

Nonlocalizing

      Intracranial hypertension
      Lumbar puncture
      Head trauma
      Basal meningitis–arachnoiditis
      Myasthenia gravis
      Wernicke's syndrome

Localizing

      Brain stem (pontine)
      Clivus
      Temporal bone
      Parasellar region
      Cavernous sinus
      Superior orbital fissure
      Orbital lesion

example, with right superior oblique palsy, images are closer together when the head is tilted to the left and further apart when the head is tilted to the right. If the patient reports diplopia, ocular deviation can be due to muscle paresis or muscle restriction (as in thyroid ophthalmopathy). In restrictive disorders (such as thyroid eye disease) the forced duction test is performed with forceps to move the eye, and the eye cannot be moved because of eye muscle restriction by the pathologic process. Determination of paretic muscles in patients with diplopia can be very complex if multiple extraocular muscles are paretic.

If there is abduction defect (lateral rectus is innervated by sixth nerve), the underlying pathologic process can be myopathic (thyroid myopathy, myasthenia gravis) or neuropathic (such as caused by cranial nerve dysfunction). If neuropathic, sixth-nerve palsy can be caused by the effects of increased intracranial pressure or meningitic process (neoplastic, infectious-inflammatory) at the skull base. The sixth nerve may be damaged anywhere along its intracranial (e.g., midpons, cerebellopontine angle, clival or skull base, parasellar or cavernous sinus) or extracranial (superior orbital fissure, orbit) course. If there is hypertropia in adduction, the superior oblique muscle is usually involved. This nerve is susceptible to traumatic injuries; other causes (vascular, neoplastic) are less common. A droopy eyelid with only preserved lateral (abduction) movement is characteristic of oculomotor nerve paresis. This nerve may be damaged along its intracranial (midbrain, parasellar or cavernous sinus, tentorial notch) or extracranial (orbital) course. If the pupil is involved, a compressive lesion should be considered, whereas if the pupil is spared, there is usually ischemic process.

▨ CLINICAL SYNDROMES

The following clinical syndromes are best understood when the symptoms, acuity, visual field, funduscopy, pupils, motility, and etiology are all analyzed and taken into consideration.

Optic Neuritis

Symptoms. Loss of vision may worsen over several days; orbital or ocular pain especially moving eyes. Visual loss is usually unilateral but can be bilateral; however, this rarely develops simultaneously.

Acuity. Usually substantial impairment.

Visual field. Central scotoma(s).

Funduscopy. Blurring of disc margins, presence of hemorrhages and exudates; if involvement is retrobulbar, disc can initially appear normal and later show optic atrophy.

Pupils. Equal in size; the involved pupil responds more rapidly and briskly to consensual than direct light stimulation.

Motility. Normal.

Etiology. Demyelinating disease; less commonly, syphilis, systemic lupus, infections, including sinus disease. "Chronic" or slowly progressive optic neuritis can be incorrectly diagnosed when visual loss is actually due to juxtasellar mass lesion and there is usually unilateral visual impairment.

Associated findings. Can be none or other signs of multiple sclerosis (cerebellar, brain stem, corticospinal) or juxtasellar involvement.

Diagnostic studies. Visual evoked potentials, cerebrospinal fluid analysis with gamma-globulin content, skull roentgenogram with sella tomography and optic foramen views, orbital computed tomography or magnetic resonance imaging, serology (VDRL and fluorescent treponemal antibody), and studies for systemic lupus (LE prep and antinuclear antibodies).

Optic Neuropathy

Symptoms. Loss of visual acuity is characteristic. This can be sudden in ischemic lesions and slow in compressive (mass) lesions or hereditary, toxic, or metabolic deficiency conditions. (Visual loss is usually unilateral with compressive and vascular lesions and bilateral with hereditary, toxic, and metabolic deficiency conditions.)

Acuity. Can vary from minimal reduction to severe impairment. Color vision is usually severely impaired.

Visual fields. Central or ceocentral scotomas in hereditary, toxic, or metabolic deficiency. In compressive optic neuropathy, it is imperative to check carefully the visual fields in the eye with normal acuity for a possible temporal defect that suggests chiasmal extension. In ischemic optic neuropathy there can be an altitudinal visual defect.

Funduscopy. In ischemic and toxic lesions there is acute disc swelling. In hereditary optic neuropathy there is optic atrophy. In compressive lesions the disc can appear normal or atrophic.

Pupils. Equal in size. In bilateral conditions, pupillary response can be symmetric. In unilateral (ischemic, compressive) lesions there can be an afferent pupillary defect.

Motility. Normal.

Etiology. Ischemic (collagen vascular disorders, temporal arteritis, syphilis, diabetes mellitus); toxic (ethambutol, isoniazid, tobacco-alchohol, disulfiram);

metabolic (vitamin B_{12} deficiency); compressive (optic glioma, meningioma); hereditary (Leber's optic atrophy).

Associated findings. Can be none.

Diagnostic studies. Same as for optic neuritis. To include investigation for metabolic, infectious, collagen vascular disease.

Papilledema

Symptoms. Headache, nausea, vomiting, horizontal diplopia caused by lateral rectus paresis, and transient visual obscurations caused by intermittent optic nerve dysfunction.

Acuity. Usually normal until late in course; however, more sensitive vision parameters, including tests of contrast sensitivity, can show abnormalities.

Visual field. Enlargement of blind spots, constriction of visual fields, and inferior nasal quadrant defect.

Funduscopy. Loss of spontaneous venous pulsations; loss of physiologic cup, hemorrhages, and exudates; blurring of disc margins; venous engorgement with disc hyperemia; and blurring of retinal nerve fiber layer.

Pupils. Normal.

Motility. Can demonstrate lateral rectus paresis.

Etiology. Intracranial hypertension caused by mass lesion or idiopathic intracranial hypertension.

Associated findings. Related to underlying cause of the intracranial hypertension.

Diagnostic studies. Skull roentgenogram, computed tomography/magnetic resonance imaging (CT/MRI), angiogram, and cerebrospinal fluid analysis are necessary to exclude space-occupying mass lesion, hydrocephalis, or infectious-inflammatory disorders.

Prechiasmal Lesions (Optic Nerve–Optic Chiasm Junction)

Symptoms. Progressive dimming of vision in only one eye is usually initial disorder.

Acuity. Ipsilateral impairment of visual acuity.

Visual field. Contralateral monocular temporal hemianopia, and ipsilateral central scotoma.

Funduscopy. Optic atrophy is late sign.

Pupils. Delayed and incomplete constriction in ipsilateral eye in response to direct light stimulation with brisk consensual response (afferent pupillary defect).

Motility. Normal.

Etiology. Chromophobe adenoma, craniopharyngioma, parasellar meningioma, aneurysm.

Associated findings. Can be none or signs of pituitary dysfunction.

Diagnostic studies. Skull roentgenogram with sella turcica tomography and optic foramen views, CT/MRI scan, and carotid angiogram to detect tumor and exclude aneurysm.

Chiasmal Lesions

Symptoms. Gradual onset of visual blurring that progressively worsens; impaired peripheral vision and abnormal depth perception.

Acuity. Unilateral or bilateral visual loss, or can be normal.

Visual field. Bitemporal defect: if optic chiasm is compressed from undersurface, superior quandrantanopsia results; if the chiasm is compressed from above, inferior quadrantanopsia results.

Funduscopy. Optic atrophy or can be normal.

Pupils. Usually normal, but can see unilateral afferent defect.

Motility. Diplopia caused by extraocular muscle involvement as the lesion extends laterally into cavernous sinus.

Etiology. Chromophobe adenoma, craniopharyngioma, tuberculum sella meningioma, aneurysm.

Associated findings. Hypopituitarism with amenorrhea, infertility, hypothyroidism, hypoadrenalism; hyperpituitarism as expressed by amenorrhea-galactorrhea, acromegaly, or Cushing's syndrome.

Diagnostic studies. Skull roentgenogram, sella to-mography, CT/MRI scan, and angiography. Hormonal studies to detect hypothalamic-pituitary dysfunction.

Postchiasmal Lesions

Symptoms. Occasional difficulty seeing in involved visual field; more commonly no awareness of visual field abnormality occurs.

Acuity. Normal, but may ignore involved hemifield of eye chart.

Visual field. Homonymous defects: Temporal lobe: Superior homonymous quandrantanopsia Parietal lobe: Inferior homonymous quandrantanopsia Occipital lobe: Homonymous hemianopsia with or without macular sparing.

Funduscopy. Normal for postgeniculate lesions. Can see optic atrophy with pregeniculate lesions (optic tract and lateral geniculate body).

Pupils. Normal with postgeniculate lesions, or can have hemianopic pupillary afferent defect with optic tract lesions (e.g., when point source of light is directed into hemiretina corresponding to hemianopic field, diminished light response is present).

Motility. Normal.

Etiology. Vascular, neoplasm, trauma, and inflammatory.

Associated Findings

Temporal lobe: Partial complex seizures, aphasia, hemiparesis, hemianesthesia.

Parietal lobe: Aphasia, extinction of sensory stimuli, agraphia, acalculia, right-left confusion, and finger agnosia.

Occipital lobe: Usually none.

Diagnostic Studies.

EEG, CT/MRI scan, carotid angiogram.

Hysterical Blindness

Symptoms. Decreased vision or blindness; however, patient has no difficulty walking and does not bump into objects.

Acuity. Impaired, but severity of visual loss is constant and does not change at varying distances.

Visual field. Tubular with no change in size of the field with increasing distance from target (tunnel vision).

Funduscopy. Normal.

Pupils. Normal.

Associated findings. If a patient with unilateral visual loss is asked to read red letters with a red lens over the normal eye and a clear lens over the "blind eye," this can only be accomplished with the blind eye. This is because it is not possible to see red letters with a red lens over the eye; therefore, vision must originate from the eye alleged to be blind.

▨ SUMMARY

Diminished vision is a sign that the afferent (sensory) visual system is impaired, whereas diplopia (double vision) caused by abnormal ocular motility is a manifestation that the ocular motor (efferent) system is impaired. In patients who report visual loss it is important to assess the primary visual apparatus (ophthalmological system). If this is not the cause of the visual impairment, it is necessary to assess the optic nerve, optic chiasm, and visual pathways traversing the parietal and temporal lobes and their termination in the occipital lobe, which is the final common pathway for the visual system as the suspected cause of the visual impairment. Adequate visualization of the optic nerve head (papilla) is mandatory as the funduscopic findings can reflect the presence of normal or increased intracranial pressure as well as showing inflammation or demyelination of the optic nerve. The visual field examination is crucial to determine if the abnormality involves the retina, optic nerve, or pre- or postchiasmal region. Patients with ocular motility disturbances usually report double vision or the feeling of objects moving in the environment (oscillopsia); however, it is possible for patients with ocular motility disturbances to have no symptoms. Evaulation of the patient's eye movements as well as the eyelids, orbital region, and facial movements is necessary to determine whether the pathological process involves the extraocular muscles or cranial nerves supplying these muscles or is due to CNS dysfunction.

Suggested Readings

Neuro-Ophthalmologic Examination

Barrios RR, Bottinelli MD, Medoc J: The study of ocular motility in the comatose patient, *J Neurol Sci* 3:183, 1966.

Fisher CM: Some neuro-ophthalmological observations, *J Neurol Neurosurg Psychiatry* 30:383, 1967.

Glaser JS: *Neuro-ophthalmology,* ed 2, Philadelphia, 1990, JB Lippincott.

Afferent Visual System

Bradley WG, Whitty WM: Acute optic neuritis, *J Neurol Neurosurg Psychiatry* 30:531, 1967.

Chutorian AM and Schwartz JF: Optic gliomas in children, *Neurology* 14:83, 1964.

Jamieson M: Loss of vision, *Br Med J* 288:1523, 1978.

Knight CL, Hoyt WF, and Wilson CB: Syndrome of incipient prechiasmal optic nerve compression, *Arch Ophthalmol* 87:1, 1972.

Thompson HS: Afferent pupillary defects: pupillary findings associated with defects of the afferent arm of the pupillary light reflex, *Am J Ophthalmol* 62:860, 1966.

Wray SH: The management of acute visual failure, *J Neurol Neurosurg Psychiatry* 56:234, 1993.

Bruno A, Corbett JJ, Biller J: Transient monocular visual loss patterns and associated vascular abnormalities, *Stroke* 21:34, 1990.

Burger SK, Saul RF: Transient monocular blindness caused by vasospasm, *N Engl J Med,* 325:870, 1991.

The Pupil

Loewenfeld IE, Thompson HS: The tonic pupil: a reevaluation, *Am J Ophthalmol* 63:46, 1967.

Selhorst JB: Pupil and its disorders, *Neurol Clin North Am* 1:859, 1983.

CHAPTER

Episodic Loss of Consciousness

8

▨ DEFNINTION AND INCIDENCE

Syncope is the cause of 3% of emergency room visits and 6% of general medical hospital admissions. The term "faintness" includes the sensations of lightheadedness, dizziness, and weakness. This can be referred to as "presyncope." Syncope literally means "a cutting short." It is defined as a sudden, brief loss of consciousness and postural tone. There is immediate recovery after the period of unconsciousness. There is no postepisode confusion, although patients can briefly appear dazed. The majority of attacks are benign; however, trauma can result from falls, especially in elderly patients. Syncope can be experienced by normal subjects when transient reversible decreased cerebral blood flow or metabolism occurs.

The mechanism of syncope and patient outcome are closely linked. In 50%, no cause is delineated despite complete medical, cardiac, and neurologic evaulation; however, if the cause is cardiac (arrhythmias, valvular, cardiomyopathy), sudden death can occur in 20% to 30% of patients without treatment.

Syncope should be taken serously in elderly patients because the survival rate is reduced even if attack is of noncardiac origin. Syncope occurs in 7% of elderly patients and recurs in 30% of those.

■ HISTORY

The patient and observers of the episode should be carefully questioned regarding the following:

- Precipitating factors: emotional stress, fasting state, exercise, cough, swallowing, urination, defecation, position (prolonged standing, occurrence of episode immediately on assuming standing position). Syncope associated with physical exertion suggests cardiac disease.
- Warning symptoms: palpitations, chest pain, headache, visual blurring, dizziness, lightheadedness, paresthesias. Abrupt onset of syncope without warning symptoms suggests cardiac arrhythmia. Determine the initial symptom.
- Level of consciousness during the episode: twilight state, unconsciousness, aware of surroundings but unable to respond?
- Motor dysfunction: loss of muscle tone, tonic spasm, paralysis, myoclonic jerks.
- Evidence of injury as consequence of the episode.
- Sphincter incontinence.
- Postepisode (postictal) neurologic abnormalities: confusion, amnesia, focal neurologic deficit, myalgias, headache.
- Duration of episode.
- Autonomic disturbances: skin pallor, diaphoresis, flushed or cyanotic appearance, heart rate or rhythm disturbances.
- Detailed medication history: vasodilators such as nitroglycerin, antihypertensives, phenothiazines,

cardiac antiarrhythmic agents, dopaminergic medication, calcium channel blocking agents, tricyclic or tetracyclic antidepressants.

In syncopal attacks there is usually a brief warning including a sensation of lightheadedness, objects moving relative to the patient, visual dimming or blurring, spots in front of the eyes, nausea, ringing in ears, sweating, coldness, skin pallor, or weakness. If the patient is standing or sitting, symptoms can be aborted by lying down. During syncopal attack, certain patients are not arousable for several minutes, whereas others awaken immediately because recumbent position restores central nervous system circulation. Certain patients are completely unresponsive; others appear dazed and unable to respond appropriately to verbal stimuli. Recovery of consciousness is usually rapid, but brief amnesia can remain. Smelling salts or ammonia can be used to hasten recovery; however, they are unnecessary as full recovery occurs rapidly and spontaneously. The patient is usually able to describe presyncopal symptoms but is an unreliable observer for actual episode details. Postictal confusion does not occur in syncope, but the patient can remain weak or dazed for several minutes. As the patient recovers these changes occur: the pulse rate becomes strong and regular, blood pressure normalizes, skin pallor recedes, and the respiratory pattern normalizes.

▧ EXAMINATION

Attention is directed toward five specific areas:

- Blood pressure and pulse are monitored in both supine and standing positions; there should not be drop in blood pressure exceeding 10 mmHg in systolic or diastolic component; a greater drop is postural orthostatic hypotension. Measure blood pressure in both arms; unequal pressure suggests subclavian steal syndrome. Listen for bruits in carotid, supraclavicular (subclavian artery), supra-orbital, and temporal regions.

■ Gentle and careful carotid massage is performed with electrocardiographic (ECG) monitoring to exclude carotid sinus hyperactivity or hypersensi-tivity. Apply pressure to each carotid artery sepa-rately for not more than 5 seconds while monitor-ing blood pressure and ECG. A cardiac pause lasting longer than 3 seconds or a systolic blood pressure drop of more than 30 mmHg with synco-pal symptoms is diagnostic of carotid sinus syn-cope. Do not apply carotid pressure if the patient has carotid bruit, is known to have carotid steno-sis, or has suffered prior stroke syndrome.

■ The carotid artery is palpated and auscultated for bruits. Cardiac auscultation is performed to ascetain evidence of conditions causing left-ventricular out-flow obstruction (aortic stenosis, hypertrophic subaortic stenosis, obstructive cardiomyopathy).

■ The patient is hyperventilated for 3 minutes or to point of giddiness to reproduce syncope.

■ A neurologic examination is performed to exclude disease causing muscle weakness and wasting (e.g., myopathy, motor neuron disease, neuropathy with autonomic component).

▧ PATHOPHYSIOLOGY

Transient disruption of cerebral blood flow for 8 to 10 seconds results in loss of consciousness. If systolic blood pressure falls below 70 mm Hg or to a mean pres-sure of 30 to 40 mm Hg, syncope can result. Several pathophysiologic disturbances that decrease cerebral blood flow and metabolism cause syncope (Box 8-1).

CLINICAL SYNDROMES

Cardiac Disorders

Cardiovascular conditions (cardiac arrhythmias, neurocardiogenic disorders) are the most common causes of syncope. In these cases reduced cerebral perfusion results from decreased cardiac output and peripheral vasodilatation. Cardiac arrhythmias causing syncope occur in patients with heart disease but rarely occur without prior cardiac abnormality. Ventricular tachycardia is the most common and serious arrhythmia; this can cause syncope and sudden unexplained cardiac death. Ventricular tachycardia can be precipitated by a metabolic abnormality, such as hypokalemia or hypomagnesemia, or certain drug effects, such as antiarrhythmic medication or tricyclic antidepressants. Syncope caused by heart block (Strokes-Adam attacks) can occur abruptly without warning or when patient is recumbent as contrasted with other types of syncope that occur when the patient is standing. In other cardiac syncopal episodes palpitations or

---

BOX 8-1

1 Cardiac abnormalities leading to decreased stroke volume and inadequate cardiac output (arrhythmias, valvular obstructive lesions, cardiomyopathies)

2 Peripheral circulatory impairment caused by decreased blood volume, increased vasodilatation, decreased venomotor tone

3 Cerebral blood flow impairment (hyperventilation, pulmonary embolism)

4 Central neural inhibition (neurocardiogenic syncope, carotid sinus hypersensitivity)

5 Insufficient brain energy metabolism (hypoglycemia, anemia, hypoxia)

chest discomfort precede syncope. Left-ventricular outflow obstruction and myocardial disease can result in impaired cardiac output; in such patients, syncope commonly develops during physical exertion.

Peripheral Circulatory Impairment

Syncopal attacks from peripheral circulatory impairment characteristically occur when the patient arises from a recumbent position or after the patient has been motionless for prolonged time. Orthostatic syncope occurs most commonly in those patients who have the conditions described in Box 8-2.

In orthostatic syncope tachycardia reflexively develops in response to decreased blood pressure. In primary orthostatic hypotension blood pressure rapidly decreases when the patient stands, and compensatory tachycardia does not occur because of impaired autonomic reflexes.

Cerebral Blood Flow Impairment

Hyperventilation results in decreased carbon dioxide tension, which stimulates cerebral vasoconstriction. Syncope results from two mechanisms: anxiety

---

 BOX 8-2

1 Severe muscle wasting of any cause
2 Varicose veins causing peripheral blood pooling and impaired venous return
3 Prolonged bed rest impairing venomotor tone
4 Medication (antihypertensives, phenothiazines, diuretics, nitrates)
5 Postsympathectomy operations
6 Adrenal cortical insufficiency resulting in hypovolemia
7 Primary orthostatic hypotension

causes release of epinephrine, and hypocapnia causes cerebral vasoconstriction and peripheral vasodilation. Prodromal symptoms of hyperventilatory syncope include paresthesias and numbness (hands, feet, perioral), headache, dry mouth, breathlessness, and chest pain. Hyperventilatory attacks are provoked by emotional stress. These episodes can occur when the patient is sitting or recumbent; symptomatology is not relieved by recumbency. The diagnosis is established by reproducing the symptoms by hyperventilation. Panic attacks can also cause syncope and are not provoked by hyperventilation.

Carotid Sinus Hypersensitivity

This can be of two types. The first is cardioinhibitory, causing bradycardia as a result of atrioventricular block. This is the most common form (70%). Symptoms are reproduced by slight carotid digital compression producing a sinus pause of longer the 3 seconds. This condition is treated by atropine. The second is the vasodepressor type, in which hypotension can occur with or without bradycardia. Symptoms are induced by gentle carotid massage. This is blocked by vasopressor agents such as epinephrine. Pure vasodepressor syncope is uncommon (5%). The mixed pattern can include cardioinhibitory and vasodepressor types (25%).

Neurocardiogenic Syncope

Other terms for this disorder include "vasovagal syncope," "vasodepressor syncope," or "neurally medicated cardiac syncope." Patients initially report presyncopal symptoms including dizziness, lightheadedness, visual blurring, and generalized weakness. It is believed that this occurs with the following sequence of events. Initially, there is peripheral blood venous pooling, which results in decreased venous return and decreased left-ventricular blood volume. This *should* trigger compensatory cardiovascular reflexes (baroreceptor stimulation in the aortic arch and carotid sinus), resulting in tachycardia and enhanced peripheral vascular resistance, which increase blood pressure and cardiac output. If this occurs, cerebral blood flow is maintained and syncope does not occur. This mechanism is impaired in patients with neurocardiogenic syncope. In this disorder decreased left-ventricular volume causes increased left-ventricular contractility to result in myocardial sympathetic C fiber stimulation. The C fiber stimulation activates the medullary vasomotor center with enhanced vagal tone and peripheral vasodilation; this results in hypotension and asystole. This is the consequence of inhibition of efferent sympathetic tone (resulting in hypotension) and increased efferent parasympathetic tone (resulting in asystole). Myocardial C fiber sympathetic stimulation can be antagonized with beta-adrenergic receptor blocking agents (propranolol, metoprolol) or with theophylline and disopyramide; however, the exact mechanism of the two drugs is not clearly established. Although it would seem logical that beta-adrenergic blocking agents would worsen the situation because they cause heart rate slowing and reduced cardiac output, these drugs are effective in neurocardiogenic syncope because they inhibit myocardial C fiber sympathetic stimulation. Neurocardiogenic syncope is most common in young patients and is uncommon in patients with impaired cardiac function, possibly because of the myocardial C fibers being affected by cardiac disease. If these fibers are impaired, they cannot trigger the effect leading to syncope. Neurocardiogenic syncopal attacks are recurrent and can be precipitated by multiple stimuli such that patients can faint in varied emotional or physical situations.

Reflex Syncope

This results from peripheral vascular blood pooling and decreased venous return. There is reduced peripheral vascular resistance, and the normal compensatory increase in cardiac output does not occur. This usually occurs when the patient is in standing or, less commonly, in sitting position. Reflex syncope is precipitated by a response to emotional discomfort, painful stimulation, anxiety, or fear. In situational syncope there is mediation through stimulation of the central medullary vagal center; this leads to bradycardia and hypotension. Examples of precipitating factors for reflex syncope include urination, defecation, coughing, swallowing, sneezing, weight-lifting, diving, trumpet playing, and valsalva maneuver.

Insufficient Energy Substrates

If the systemic concentration of glucose or oxygen is decreased, brain metabolism can be impaired. If compensatory mechanisms (cerebral vasodilation) are not adequate to maintain brain function, syncope results. Hypoglycemia can result from endocrine (pancreatic, adrenal, and pituitary) or hepatic (impaired glycogen storage) disease. It occurs in diabetics taking insulin or can be reactive, occurring 2 to 5 hours after meals. Initial symptoms include headache, diaphoresis, pallor, tremor or shakiness, sense of hunger, abdominal cramps, mental irritability, and weakness. If this condition is not corrected, confusion and disorientation develop; more severe hypoglycemia results in loss of consciousness, sometimes with abnormal neurologic findings (decerebration, clonus, and Babinski signs). Attacks are aborted by glucose administration. Following attacks the patient frequently complains of severe headache caused by cerebral vasodilation. Diagnosis of hypoglycemia is established *only* when blood sugar is lower than 40 mg/dl and there are accompanying sympathetic hyperactivity features (unless these are suppressed by adrenergic blocking medication). In patients with pheochromocytoma, increased sympathetic activity (diaphoresis, hypertension, palpitations, tremor anxiety) are common. In patients with carcinoid syndrome or mastocytosis, flushing and gastrointestinal symptoms (nausea, vomiting, diarrhea) may be prominent.

Hypoxia (anoxia) causes syncope because of inadequate brain oxygen. Anoxia can occur because of cardiac or respiratory disorders or during high-altitude exposure. It occurs in anemic patients or in those with hemoglobinopathies impairing oxygen transport. Syncope caused by anoxia occurs during physical exertion and is usually preceded by presyncopal symptoms. In anoxic syncope brief *random* myoclonic jerking movements can occur. Hypoxia can cause cerebral vasodilation; this can result in headache, unusual for syncope but common in convulsion. The brief duration of anoxic syncopal disorder and lack of postictal phase should allow differentiation from generalized tonic-clonic convulsion.

▨ DIFFERENTIAL DIAGNOSIS

Epilepsy

The characteristic clinical features helping to differentiate fits from faints are listed (Table 8-1). In grand mal seizures, patients experience prodrome consisting of vague and uneasy feelings that warn of an impend-

TABLE 8-1	**Differentiating Features of Seizures and Syncope**	

Finding	Seizure	Syncope
Occurance in sleep	+*	−
Premonitory symptoms	+	+
Aura	+	−
Ictus		
Position	Opisthotonic	Limp (hypotonic)
Movement	Rhythmical jerking	Irregular myoclonic
Tongue biting	+	−
Incontinence	+	Can rarely occur
Postictal state		
Duration	Can be prolonged	Brief
Confusion	+	−
Focal deficit	+	−
Amnesia	+	−
EEG during episode	Spikes and slow waves	Diffuse slowing
Clinical pattern	Variable	Stereotyped
Autonomic disturbance		
Skin color	Flushed, cyanotic	Pallor
Perspiration	Hot and wet	Cold sweat
Headache	+	−
Myalgia	+	−

*+, Can occur; −, not present.

ing episode. These are feelings that patient has learned come with seizures, and they must be differentiated from feelings such as lightheadedness, nausea, pallor sweating, and weakness that patients have before fainting. In generalized grand mal seizures, the patient has no warning (aura) and can be injured.

Falls with injury occur as the patient is in the rigid (tonic) phase; however, this injury is rare in syncope because the patient falls limply or has adequate warning to avoid falling. In syncopal episodes in elderly patients trauma frequently occurs. In syncope patients can bite their tongues; however, tongue maceration occurs only in seizures. Incontinence occurs more frequently in seizures than syncope. In both conditions incontinence results from loss of sphincter tone if the patient has a full bladder. Random, diffuse, myoclonic jerks are common in syncope caused by cerebral hypoxia. Following syncope the patient may be dazed for several minutes, but disorientation—as seen commonly following seizures—does not occur. Convulsive syncope is defined as syncope with convulsive features of which tonic extensor spasms and random myoclonic jerks are most common. Rhythmic clonic jerking does not occur in convulsive syncope. The EEG shows diffuse slowing but does not show spike discharges in convulsive syncope. It is not known why only certain patients develop convulsive features with global cerebral ischemic anoxia. This condition represents primary syncope disorder and *not* a seizure; therefore, anticonvulsant medication is not indicated. It has been reported that 33% of patients initially diagnosed as having epileptic seizures were later diagnosed as having syncope. If there is any doubt in the clinical differentiation, use of the tilt-table test (p. 217) with ECG, blood pressure, and EEG monitoring should settle the issue.

Cerebrovascular Disease

With subarachnoid hemorrhage (SAH) caused by ruptured aneurysm there can be sudden transient loss of consciousness. In SAH there is usually severe headache, and the patient does not usually fully regain consciousness and can have residual neurologic deficit. In migraine autonomic instability leading to syncope is quite common. When loss of consciousness occurs in migraine, it can be difficult to differentiate syncope from seizure because both conditions can be associated with migraine. Transient ischemic attacks, which are caused by carotid artery ischemia, do *not* cause syncope. Drop attacks caused by vertebrobasilar insufficiency with ischemia involving ventral pons cause patients to fall to the ground, but these attacks are not associated with loss of consciousness. Drop attacks usually occur in middle-aged or elderly patients. Because these vascular episodes occur without warning and are brief in duration, the patient may not actually be able to report accurately if consciousness has been lost; therefore, these can be confused with syncopal attacks.

◼ DIAGNOSTIC ASSESSMENT OF SYNCOPE PATIENT

Diagnostic studies (in addition to attempting to provoke the episode) that are indicated in evaluating patients with syncope include the following:

- Complete blood count
- Fasting blood glucose content and 5-hour glucose tolerance test
- Plasma cortisol and thyroid hormone levels
- Serum electrolytes
- Electrocardiogram
- 24-hour Holter cardiac monitoring
- Echocardiogram
- Alcohol and drug screen
- Cardiac enzymes (to exclude myocardial infarction)

- Catecholamine screen for pheochromocytoma (24-hour urine sample for metanephrines and vanillyl-mandelic acid)
- 24-hour urine sample for 5-hydroxy-indole-acetic acid for carcinoid
- Pregnancy test
- Tilt table test
- Invasive cardiac electrophysiologic monitoring

This list represents a complete battery from which needed tests should be selected depending on clinical status. For example, not all studies would be necessary for a teenage patient who faints on one occasion while standing motionless for a prolonged period in church. A cardiologist should be consulted to analyze possible role of arrhythmias and myocardial or valvular dysfunction and should determine the need for cardiac physiological (noninvasive or invasive) testing. Because the major risk in syncopal patients is the presence of serious cardiac arrhythmia, ECG and Holter monitoring are essential parts of baseline evaluation. Invasive electrophysiological cardiac testing is warranted in patients when cardiac causes are suspected. This is becoming more routine because of several instances of sudden and unexplained deaths of famous healthy athletes. In women of child-bearing age, always perform a pregnancy test. Syncope can occur in early stages of pregnancy for undetermined reasons or also in later stages because of the compressive effect of the fetus on venous return.

In syncopal patients in whom diagnosis cannot be established by clinical history or the listed diagnostic tests, the tilt table test should be performed. The patient is positioned on a tilt table that has a footboard for weight bearing. The table is tilted 60 to 80 degrees from a horizontal position for 15 minutes while ECG, EEG, and blood pressure are continuously monitored. If syncope occurs, the test is immediately discontinued. If syncope does not occur, patient is placed in horizontal position and isoproterenol is infused intravenously (1 to 2 mg/min) to increase heart rate by 20% over the baseline, and the tilt is repeated. Positive response consists of reproduction of symptoms, usually accompanied by hypotension and bradycardia. Positive tilt table tests confirm the diagnosis of neurocardiogenic syncope, and these patients respond to appropriate treatment with beta-adrenergic blocking agents. Further neurodiagnostic and cardiologic tests are not necessary in these patients with positive tilt table responses. Certain normal patients without syncope develop hypotension and bradycardia on the tilt table; however, positive tilt table response is usually accepted as diagnostic for neurocardiogenic syncope.

Because intracranial lesions are rarely responsible for syncope, neuroimaging studies (CT/MRI) are not usually necessary; *however*, they are frequently performed with very low yield. For example, skull roentgenography, CT, and MRI might be performed if the patient has adrenal insufficiency, documented by laboratory studies such that a pituitary lesion is suspected. This would be a most unusual cause for syncope, and in almost all other cases CT/MRI would be unnecessary. In a patient who has suffered episodic loss of consciousness, clinical history is usually adequate to differentiate syncope from seizure; however, an EEG should be routinely performed. This is because in certain young patients with classical syncopal attacks there is EEG evidence of generalized (nonfocal) bursts of abnormal waves such as spikes or slowing. This condition would be classified as generalized seizure disorder. These would almost never be associated with structural brain lesions, and the neurologic examination would be expected to be normal; therefore, CT/MRI would not be necessary. These patients may clinically respond to anticonvulsants. Because 10% of normal persons without brain disease have nonspecific EEG abnormality, and therefore 10% of syncopal patients have nonspecific EEG abnormality, clinical history and EEG pattern should be carefully analyzed before considering treatment with anticonvulsants for any syncopal patients.

▦ TREATMENT

Treatment of syncopal disorders requires an understanding of underlying pathologic mechanism. If the patient is observed during the episode, the physician should place patient in a recumbent position, monitor vital signs, and, if necessary, secure a patent airway. If facilities are available, an intravenous line should be established and a blood specimen obtained to determine fasting glucose, hemoglobin, and electrolyte values. If hypoglycemia is suspected and the patient does not have rapid and immediate improvement when placed in recumbent position, glucose-containing substances should be administered. Oral intake is dangerous until the patient is alert because aspiration can occur. Inhalation of ammonia salts is frequently used, but this is not necessary. The patient should remain recumbent until steady and fully alert. The episode can recur if the patient stands up rapidly before cardiovascular reflexes have stabilized or before the underlying disorder has been corrected.

In young patients, vasovagal responses and hyperventilation are the most common causes of syncope; these attacks are triggered by emotional factors, and, if possible, these should be avoided. In patients with carotid sinus hypersensitivity rapid neck movements are to be avoided. In postural hypotension the patient should be instructed to stand up slowly, and when sitting or standing for prolonged duration the patient should massage the calves. Use of support stockings in patients with impaired venomotor tone decreases the effect of peripheral venous pooling. Avoiding drugs that cause peripheral vasodilation is necessary. Treatment of neurocardiogenic syncope with beta-adrenergic blocking agents is warranted. If syncopal attacks are preceded by presyncopal symptoms, the patient should assume a sitting or recumbent position as soon as these symptoms occur. Treatment of cardiac-mediated syncope depends on the underlying cardiac disorder.

▪ SUMMARY POINTS

Paroxysmal and completely reversible episodes of loss of awareness and consciousness are common medical disturbances. The most common mechanism of these episodes is transient reduction in cerebral blood flow and metabolism. This episode is called syncope. The multiple causes of syncope are reviewed in this chapter. Most are benign; however, certain cardiac etiologies must be recognized and treated to prevent sudden unexpected death. The most common neurologic cause of reversible loss of consciousness is a seizure. Based upon a carefully obtained history of the episode, it is usually possible to differentiate syncope (faint) from seizure (fit). EEG use can be helpful in certain selected cases, especially if epilepsy is suspected, and the use of a tilt table examination is important in provoking a characteristic episode, especially if syncope is suspected. Differentiation of syncope from seizure is important because antiepileptic medication is only warranted in treating epilepsy and would not be beneficial for other conditions causing transient loss of consciousness.

Suggested Readings

Evaluation

Day SC, Cook EF, Funkenstein H: Evaluation and outcome of emergency room patients with transient loss of consciousness, *Am J Med* 73:15, 1982.

Dohrmann ML, Cheitlin MD: Cardiogenic syncope: seizure versus syncope, *Neurol Clin North Am* 4:549, 1986.

Grubb, BP, Gerard G, Roush K: Differentiation of convulsive syncope and epilepsy with head-up tilt testing, *Ann Intern Med* 115:871, 1991.

Kapoor WN: Diagnostic evaluation of syncope, *Am J Med* 90:91, 1991.

Kapoor WN, Brant N: Evaluation of syncope by upright tilt testing with isoproterenol, *Ann Intern Med* 116:358, 1992.

Kapoor WN, Karpf M: A prospective evaluation and follow-up of patients with syncope, *N Engl J Med* 309:197, 1983.

Manolis AS, Linzer M, Salem D: Syncope: current diagnostic evaluation and management, *Ann Intern Med* 112:850, 1990.

Noble RJ: The patient with syncope, *JAMA* 237:1372, 1977.

Shillingford JP: Syncope, *Am J Cardiol* 26:609, 1970.

Etiologies

Akhtar M, Jazayeri M, Sra J: Cardiovascular causes of syncope, *Postgrad Med* 90:87, 1991.

Engel GL: *Fainting,* Springfield, Ill, 1962, Charles C Thomas.

Lin JTY, Ziegler DK, Lai CW, Bayer W: Convulsive syncope in blood donors, *Ann Neurol* 11:525, 1982.

Sra JS, Jazayeri MR, Avitall B: Comparison of cardiac pacing with drug therapy in the treatment of neurocardiogenic (vasovagal) syncope with bradycardia or asystole, *N Engl J Med* 328:1085, 1993.

Young WF, Maddox DE: Spells: in search of a cause, *Mayo Clin Proc* 70:757, 1995.

Stupor and Coma

9

The patient with a reduced level of consciousness presents a complicated clinical problem that requires prompt yet careful evaluation and management. Pathophysiologically, stupor, and coma are most commonly produced when there is significant damage or dysfunction in the ascending activating system in the brain stem. The ascending activating system has its origin in the reticular formation of the pons and midbrain, with possible contributions from other nuclei such as the locus ceruleus and median raphe. The ascending axons project to the thalamus, to the limbic system, and eventually to widespread areas of the cortex.

Clinically, there are two main mechanisms by which this system is affected and consciousness compromised: one, by diffuse disruption of neuronal metabolism such as seen in drug overdose or metabolic disease (e.g., uremia, hypoglycemia), or two, by direct damage to the activating system in the brain stem. Such damage is caused by primary neurologic diseases such as head trauma, occlusion of basilar artery, hemorrhage into the brain parenchyma, subarachnoid hemorrhage, brain stem pressure from mass lesions, and a variety of less common conditions (e.g., brain stem encephalitis, Wernicke's encephalopathy, acute multiple sclerosis).

The focus of this chapter is one the neurologic rather than medical aspects of the comatose patient. The reader requiring a more extensive discussion of the medical evaluation and management of coma is referred to the excellent monograph by Plum and Posner.

▨ EVALUATION

Because of the urgent nature of the problem, the initial evaluation phase is carried out in conjunction with the management of the acute emergency. The initial phase of evaluation consists of brief history. If an accompanying relative or friend is available, the examiner should ask what happened. If this person does not know, as is often the case, the physician should inquire if the patient is diabetic, hypertensive, a drug or alcohol abuser, or epileptic or has any known medical diseases. After the historical information is assimilated, attention is immediately turned to the patient. The physician should briefly examine the patient for evidence of trauma or meningeal irritation (hemorrhage or meningitis), establish an airway, and obtain visual signs. A large-caliber intravenous line is placed, and blood is drawn for an emergency blood cell count and chemistries (sugar, blood urea nitrogen, alcohol, liver profile, and electrolytes, including calcium and magnesium). Next, 100 mg of thiamine (for Wernicke's syndrome) is administered intravenously, followed by 50 ml of 50% glucose solution (for hypoglycemic reactions). This can be lifesaving and will not worsen the condition in diabetic ketoacidosis. If the patient does not promptly revive, the physician should insert a urinary catheter, check the urine for sugar and acetone, and save a sample for toxicology screening (drugs often prove to be the explanation for the coma, and exact identification of the substance is very helpful in management).

At this point, a more extensive history can be obtained, and a full physical and neurologic examination can be performed. From this examination the physician is usually able to

- establish if the coma is caused by a neurologic lesion or a metabolic/toxic disorder (a very important factor in both management and prognosis);
- determine the depth of the coma and the presence or absence of brain stem reflexes (these correlate well with the prognosis), and
- establish a specific cause.

Observation

The first step is to observe the patient as he or she lies quietly on the stretcher. The examiner should look for spontaneous movements and assess if they are purposeful or reflex. In addition the patient is assessed for seizure activity, myoclonic jerks (common in metabolic encephalopathies), asterixis (irregular flapping movements of the hands), tremor, diffuse twitching (seen in hypoglycemia and hyponatremia), and unilateral twitching and fasciculations. Also note any asymmetries of motor activity.

Respiration

Changes in respiratory patterns are common in comatose patients and often have specific significance for the level of coma or structure involved.

Hypoventilation

Shallow regular respiration suggests an overdose of sedative medication or alcohol.

Hyperventilation

High-amplitude rapid respiration can be seen in many conditions, including metabolic acidosis, hypoxia from pulmonary disease, and occasionally midbrain damage (central neurogenic hyperventilation).

Cheyne-Stokes

Cheyne-Stokes respiration is a pattern in which periods of hyperventilation are followed by periods of apnea. The transition between the two is gradual with a crescendo/decrescendo pattern. This is commonly seen in metabolic disease and bilateral hemisphere disease and rarely with upper brain stem damage. Although definitely abnormal, it does not carry the ominous prognostic implications of the other abnormal patterns.

Apneustic

Apneustic breathing is a rare pattern in which the patient holds his or her breath for a few seconds on inspiration (inspiratory cramp), then exhales. It is seen in patients with lesions of the tegmentum of the lower pons and indicates serious brain stem dysfunction.

Cluster

Another uncommon pattern that has the same anatomic and prognostic implication as apneustic breathing is cluster breathing. The pattern is characterized by a cluster of three or four breaths followed by short periods of apnea.

Ataxic

Ataxic breathing is a very irregular pattern that signals dysfunction of the medullary respiratory centers. When this pattern is seen, it is wise to place the patient on assisted respiration.

Preapneic

There are several very ominous respiratory signs, such as gasping, expiratory push, and fish-mouthing (opening the mouth during inspiration), that are commonly seen before total apnea.

Level of Consciousness

Assessment of the level of arousability is important for two reasons: to determine the seriousness of the patient's condition and to establish a reliable parameter by which to follow the patient's progress. A number of standard terms are used to describe levels of consciousness (Box 9-1).

These terms are helpful in describing the patient's level of consciousness, but only in a very general way.

 BOX 9-1

- *Alert:* awake and normally responsive to environmental input.
- *Lethargic or somnolent:* sleepy and somewhat inefficient mentally but usually oriented; tends to drift off to sleep if not stimulated.
- *Obtunded:* aroused with loud voice or gentle shaking but when roused tends to be confusional.
- *Stupor or semicoma:* requires vigorous stimulation to arouse.
- *Coma:* either no response to painful stimulation (deep coma) or reflex movement only with painful stimulation (light coma).

Because of the imprecision in these definitions several objective systematic evaluation schemes have been devised. The basic principle of these evaluations is that both the stimulus necessary to rouse the patient and the level of response are graded, thus giving a more objective description of the patient's responsiveness. The clinician should begin by calling the patient's name; if this is ineffective, the stimulus is increased in intensity. The examiner should next shout and then gently shake the patient and call his or her name. Finally, a painful stimulus (firm pressure on sternum or supraorbital ridge, pinching the skin, tightly grasping the Achilles tendon) can be applied. The stimulus required for arousal is recorded, along with a full description of the motor response, the level of vocalization, and the ocular response. These are organized in ascending order of severity in Table 9-1.

TABLE 9-1 Patient Response to Arousal Stimulus

Level of Vocalization	Ocular Response	Motor Response
Normal conversation	Open with eye contact with examiner	Obeys commands
Confused discourse	Open but no contact	Purposeful movements
Incoherent mumbling	Open with dys-conjugate gaze	Restless movements
Groaning	No eye opening	Decorticate posturing
Grunting		Decerebrate posturing
No response		Flaccid quadriplegia

By using this scheme the level of arousal can be tested as often as necessary and has the advantage that different examiners can evaluate the patient and accurately assess progress or deterioration. One complicating factor that must always be considered in following patients with decreased level of consciousness is the underlying effects of the sleep-wake cycle. This cycle is often disturbed in brain-damaged patients; therefore, fluctuations in arousability may not always represent deterioration in the patient's condition but may merely be a form of sleep.

Motor Response

When observing motor response the examiner should carefully note asymmetries of movement and tone. Absence of movement on one side usually indicates a structural lesion on the opposite side of the brain or brain stem and will quickly turn the examiner's attention toward a primarily neurologic evaluation. The quality of movements is also important because different types of movements are seen at different levels of coma. Certain movement patterns can also localize damage within the brain stem. Qualitative levels of motor response include those listed in Box 9-2.

Brain Stem Reflexes

The adequacy of brain stem functioning is a critical factor in the overall assessment of the comatose patient. The loss of brain stem reflexes is usually a sign of a poor prognosis unless the loss is transient. It signifies either a major structural damage in the brain stem or a metabolic or toxic disturbance of marked degree.

BOX 9-2

1 *Obeys commands.* This is the highest level of motor response and indicates that higher cortical language centers as well as the motor system are functioning.

2 *Purposeful movements.* This term is usually employed when the stuporous patient localizes and attempts to fend off a painful stimulus. Such movements indicate a fairly high degree of sensorimotor integration.

3 *Restless movements.* These are random movements in response to a stimulus. They are not accurate in their localization of the stimulus or effective in attempts to prevent it. Such movements do involve abduction of the limbs and would thus be considered as purposeful in a rudimentary sense.

4 *Decorticate posturing.* This is a type of reflex posturing in which the arms are adducted and flexed and the legs extended. Decorticate posturing indicates a hemispheric lesion; when bilateral, it often represents the first stage in central herniation.

5 *Decerebrate posturing.* In this case the patient extends, adducts, and internally rotates the arms and extends legs. Teeth are clenched, although on occasion there is reflex protrusion of the tongue. This posturing can be seen spontaneously or can be in response to stimulation. When present, this is a more ominous sign than decorticate posturing and usually indicates bilateral pyramidal tract dysfunction at the midbrain or upper pontine level. Decerebrate posturing can be seen in a metabolic coma, so it does not necessarily indicate damage to the brain stem.

6 *Mixed posturing.* On occasion patients with pontine lesions will demonstrate a mixed picture with extended arms and flexed legs.

7 *Flaccid quadriplegia.* When the brain stem is completely nonfunctional, tone is completely lost.

Pupils

Pupillary size, symmetry, and reactivity to light are all important. The pupillary reflex is integrated in the midbrain through the second cranial nerve, Edinger-Westphal nucleus, and third cranial nerve. There is influence from the sympathetic system, which begins in the hypothalamus and descends through the brain stem to synapse in the superior cervical ganglia and then ascends to the orbit via the nerve plexus along the carotid artery. Pupillary size is determined by the relative influences of the parasympathetic and sympathetic systems (Box 9-3).

Horner's Syndrome (Miosis, Ptosis, and Unilateral Anhidrosis)

With a small reactive pupil on one side and loss of sweating on the same side of the face and body, it is likely that the patient has either unilateral (ipsilateral) hypothalamic damage from early herniation or an ipsilateral brain stem destructive lesion.

 BOX 9-3

1 *Very widely dilated (8 mm) nonreactive, particularly if unilateral:* Strongly suggests that cycloplegics have been used.

2 *Midrange, equal, and reactive:* This pattern in a comatose patient usually indicates a metabolic or toxic cause.

3 *Small and reactive:* Can be seen in the early stage of central herniation.

4 *Midrange (5-6 mm), possibly irregular and unequal, and unreactive:* Midbrain damage is very likely; this can also be seen with glutethimide (Doriden) toxicity.

5 *One pupil dilated and fixed:* There is damage to one oculomotor nerve, which in the comatose patient is most commonly caused by herniation of the temporal lobe and pressure either to the nerve in the subarachnoid space or to the nucleus and nerve within the midbrain.

6 *Bilateral pinpoint and reactive:* Pontine hemorrhage (sympathetic damage) or narcotic overdose (the constricted pupils can be dilated with narcotic antagonists, e.g., naloxone).

7 *Bilateral dilated (6-7 mm) and fixed:* This can be seen with brain stem death or atropine toxicity.

Eye Position and Movement

The examiner opens the patient's eyes and observes the primary position of the eyes and any spontaneous movement.

- *Roving dysconjugate gaze:* In most comatose patients, the eyes spontaneously move in a random fashion. The patients do not fix on objects in the environment, and eye position is often dysconjugate. With this type of movement the brain stem is functioning to some extent.

- *Forced lateral gaze:* The frontal eye fields (area 8) exert a tonic effect on horizontal eye movement. With focal seizures the gaze will be forced away from the active hemisphere. With a destructive lesion, such as a cerebral infarct, the tonic activity from the intact hemisphere usually forces the gaze toward the damaged hemisphere. Forced horizontal gaze can occur in brain stem lesions.

- *Forced downgaze:* This is seen usually with thalamic hemorrhage, mass lesions in the pineal region, or in some metabolic comas, particularly hepatic.

- *Nystagmus:* These rapid jerking eye movements can be seen with seizure, phenytoin toxicity, and pontine damage in which the vestibular nuclei are damaged.

- *Ocular bobbing:* This pattern—rapid downgaze followed by slow upgaze in a patient who is incapable of horizontal eye movement—is seen in low brain stem lesions.

- *Bilateral paralysis of abduction:* Bilateral abducens palsy is commonly caused by increased intracranial pressure from either cerebral hemisphere or posterior fossa masses.

- *Total oculomotor paralysis in one eye:* This is caused by damage to the second cranial nerve from herniation or a burst internal carotid aneurysm.

Oculocephalic Reflex (Doll's Head Phenomenon)

The oculocephalic reflex is tested by placing the patient's head at 30 degrees above horizontal and quickly flexing the head or rotating it to either side. (This should not be done in patients who are suspected of having sustained neck trauma.) In a comatose patient with normal brain stem function, head rotation stimulates the semicircular canals and also the proprioceptive fibers in the cervical spine. These stimuli enter the brain stem and travel up the medial longitudinal fasciculus to activate the third and sixth nuclei, thus initiating lateral eye movement. Before the head is rotated, the eyes will be staring directly up at the ceiling; with rotation of the head to the right the eyes will continue to look at the ceiling even though the head is now to the right. The reflex system in the brain stem has stimulated both the left sixth nerve to rotate the left eye left and the right third nerve to make the right eye also look left. If the head is rapidly flexed, the eyes will open and look up (positive doll's head phenomenon). This last maneuver is the original doll's head phenomenon. When brain stem damage has occurred and this reflex arc is impaired, the eyes continue to stare ahead in the same plane of the head, and no ocular rotation occurs (negative doll's head phenomenon).

Oculovestibular Reflex (Caloric Stimulation)

The oculovestibular reflex is similar to the oculocephalic reflex, except that the stimulus to the vestibular system is via cold or warm water on the eardrum and not head rotation. This test should be performed if the doll's head response is negative because the negative response can result if the stimulus (head turning) was not adequate. The examiner must first check to see that the external ear canal is clean and that the tympanic membrane is intact; then ice water is introduced into the ear canal with a small catheter. Ten milliliters is usually sufficient, but as much as 50 ml should be used before deciding that the reflex is absent. In a patient with a functioning brain stem the eyes will slowly turn toward the stimulated side. In patients taking barbiturates, tricyclic antidepressants, aminoglycodise antibiotics, and other vestibulotoxic drugs, this reflex can be absent secondary to vestibular dysfunction alone and not brain stem dysfunction.

Corneal Reflex

The corneal reflex is tested by holding the patient's eye open and then touching the corneas. If facial paralysis prevents eye closure, the examiner can observe for any change in eye position. There is a normal forced upgaze when the patient attempts to close the eyes (Bell's phenomenon).

Gag Reflex

The gag reflex is a medullary reflex that should only be tested if the patient has been intubated because it can cause reflex vomiting and aspiration.

Funduscopy

During funduscopy the clinician should search principally for papilledema or subhyaloid hemorrhages; the latter is a classic sign of subarachnoid hemorrhage.

Muscle Stretch and Pathologic Reflexes

Asymmetries and pathologic reflexes such as Babinski signs or clonus should be sought. The Babinski sign can be positive and clonus can be present (but is usually bilateral) in metabolic disease, so this is not a sine qua non of structural neurologic disease. The presence of clonus and a Babinski sign indicates the need for neurodiagnostic studies to exclude focal brain disease or injury in the setting of severe enough metabolic encephalopathy to impair consciousness. For example, hepatic encephalopathy can cause these signs, but diagnostic studies must be done to exclude an associated intracranial hemorrhage caused by impaired coagulation mechanism or brain abscess caused by impaired immune response.

Response to Pain

The patient's response to pain has basically been tested during assessment of the level of consciousness, but it is also important to look for asymmetries. For example, thalamic hemorrhage elicits a markedly decreased response to pain on the side of the body opposite the lesion.

▨ DIFFERENTIAL DIAGNOSIS

The proper management of a coma requires an exact diagnosis. Because there is a wide variety of causes it is useful to be familiar with the relative frequency of the conditions most commonly known to cause coma. In one series of 500 cases of nontraumatic coma the general classifications were reported (Box 9-4).

The findings on the neurologic examination alone will often permit the examiner to place the patient into one of these general diagnostic categories. Plum and Posner (1980) deserve considerable credit for elucidating these syndromes. Box 9-4 outlines the five general diagnostic categories of the coma patient.

BOX 9-4

Metabolic disorders	35%
Exogenous toxins (drugs primarily)	30%
Supratentorial lesions	20%
Intracerebral hemorrhage	(9%)
Subdural hematoma	(6%)
Infarct	(2%)
Tumor	(1.5%)
Abscess	(1%)
Other	(0.5%)
Subtentorial lesions	13.5%
Brain stem infarct	(8%)
Tumor	(2.5%)
Pontine hemorrhage	(2%)
Cerebellar hemorrhage	(1%)
Psychogenic unresponsiveness	1.5%

BOX 9-5

1 Metabolic or toxic coma.
   a No lateralizing neurologic findings
   b Pupils equal, mid range, and reactive to light
   c Eyes roving and dysconjugate; can be forced downgaze
   d Oculocephalic and oculovestibular reflexes intact
   e Tremors and multifocal myoclonic jerks

2 Coma caused by structural brain lesions. An expanding hemispheric lesion causes shifts (herniations) of brain tissue from one brain region of higher pressure to one of lower pressure. The cerebral hemispheric mass can exert a downward or lateral force through the tentorial notch thus damaging the brain stem
   a Frontal, parietal, or midline mass (central herniation).
      ▪ Stage 1 (diencephalic): hemiparesis with decorticate posturing
      ▪ Stage 2 (midbrain/upper pons): pupils mid range and fixed, respiration rapid, decerebrate posturing, oculocephalic reflexes absent
      ▪ Stage 3 (low pons): pupils fixed, extremities flaccid with possible leg flexion, and low, rapid respiration
      ▪ Stage 4 (medullary): pupils fixed, breathing irregular or apneic, flaccid quadriplegia.

Continued.

BOX 9-5—cont'd

b Temporal mass (uncal herniation): the incus or medial temporal lobe is displaced into the tentorial notch to compress and distort the midbrain.
  - Stage 1: subtle decrease in level of consciousness, pupillary dilatation (usually on the side of the lesion) caused by ipsilateral oculomotor nerve and midbrain effect
  - Stage 2: complete third nerve palsy, rapid decrease in level of consciousness, hemiparesis (caused by pressure on cerebral peduncle). The hemiparesis is usually opposite the lesion, but occasionally the midbrain is pressed against the opposite tentorial edge and an ipsilateral hemiparesis develops (Kernohan's notch phenomenon). The posterior cerebral artery extends around the brain stem; this artery can be compressed against the tentorium by the uncus to cause occipital lobe infarction and homonymous hemianopsia.

3 Subtentorial lesions. There are several main lesions in this group, but most are characterized by a rapid onset of coma with evidence of damage to the brain stem. Vascular lesions cause more rapid onset and nonvascular mass lesions can cause a slower onset of symptoms. The neurologic deficit can be caused by upward (ascending) transtentorial herniation by the subtentorial lesion, or by cerebellar tonsilar herniation with sudden death because of pressure on and damage to the respiratory centers in the lower medulla.

a Basilar artery occlusion: Acute loss of consciousness, bilateral pyramidal tract findings, evidence of primary brain stem dysfunction (variable cranial nerve and gaze abnormalities)

b Pontine hemorrhage: Acute loss of consciousness, irregular respiration, tetraplegia often with decerebrate posturing, frequently very small but reactive pupils, abnormalities in ocular rotation, abnormal oculocephalic, and caloric testing

c Mass lesion (including neoplasms, abscesses, and subdural hematomas): Gradual decrease in level of consciousness, vomiting, hyperventilation, loss of upgaze or lateral gaze; oculocephalic reflexes preserved

d Cerebellar hemorrhage: Headache, ataxia, small pupils, nausea and vomiting, vertigo, dysarthria, sixth and often seventh nerve palsies, stiff neck, nystagmus, and bilateral

BOX 9–5—cont'd

Babinski signs. These signs progress rapidly as consciousness is being lost, so early recognition (before consciousness is impaired) is critical if surgical evacuation is to be successful

4 Psychogenic unresponsiveness (hysterical coma). This exists, but should only be seriously considered in the diagnostic process after organic disease is quite certainly ruled out. Such patients basically do not appear ill and show no abnormal physical or neurologic findings except their unresponsiveness. They may not respond to pain, and oculocephalic responses can be difficult to interpret, but caloric testing will elicit prompt forced gaze with nystagmus to the opposite side. The gaze shows fixation, and dysconjugate roving eye movements are not seen. After a completely negative physical, neurologic, and laboratory investigation, it is usually safe to observe the patient. The examiner can ask a psychiatrist to talk to the patient. The use of an Amytal interview technique (amobarbital injected intravenously at 25 mg/min) is frequently effective in rousing the patient.

5 Other states resembling coma.

a Akinetic mutism: The patient is lethargic and can appear alert but not responsive; can have spontaneous eye movements and visual pursuit but shows no signs of mental awareness even when stimulated; is capable of producing speech but is mute; and has no voluntary motor movement but is not paralyzed. The patient's eyes can be open, can blink in response to threat, and can even visually track objects. The patient is inattentive and mute (never spontaneously speaking). Other akinetic mute patients appear wakeful with their eyes open, and some eye contact can be made with examiners and family (coma vigil). The electroencephalogram shows a marked generalized slow wave pattern. This condition can be caused by bilateral basal frontal lobe or midbrain lesions (damaging midbrain reticular formation).

b Chronic vegetative state: This term is used to describe patients who have survived severe head injury or diffuse hypoxic-ischemic brain injury. They have widespread brain lesions in cortical and subcortical regions, but the brain stem is usually spared. The patient lies in bed with eyes open, can occasionally utter sounds or moans, but does not speak or respond to commands. The patient

Continued.

BOX 9-5–cont'd

may blink in response to threatening stimulus or can have searching eye movements and may briefly fixate on the examiner or family member, but there is no real eye contact. Reflex movements (decerebration, decortication, myoclonic jerks) can occur. Depending on the specific damaged brain regions, the patient can show bilateral limb weakness, spasticity, Babinski signs, and an arousal response but no awareness of the environment. Respiratory and circulatory function is normal. The electroencephalogram can show alpha rhythm (not well sustained) sometimes with normal sleep pattern; this contrasts with a slowing or isoelectric pattern seen in other comatose patients.

c Locked-in syndrome: In this condition the patient is totally immobile with an inability to move the limbs and is not able to speak or swallow or show facial expression; the eyes, however, are spared. The patient responds to questions by opening and closing the eyes or moving the eyes horizontally or vertically. There is no impairment of awakeness or consciousness. The electroencephalogram is normal. This condition is also called deafferented state or pseudocoma. It can be caused by a lesion of the basis pontis (involving corticospinal and corticobulbar fibers) with sparing of ascending reticular activating fibers. This condition can occur in basilar artery occlusion, central pontine myelinolysis, or motor neuropathy involving peripheral and cranial nerves.

d Catatonia: The patient appears akinetic and mute. The neurologic examination shows normal respiration, normal pupillary response and extraocular motility, and intact motor function with no abnormal reflexes. The limbs may remain in the position they are placed (waxy flexibility) and appear rigid. The electroencephalogram is normal. This condition can be seen in manic depressive illness and schizophrenia, but many cases have an organic cause such as basal ganglion disease, encephalitis, drug reaction, and various other metabolic and structural lesions (Philbrick and Rummans, 1994).

MANAGEMENT

The management of the comatose patient has three basic stages. The first stage, discussed briefly in the evaluation section, consists of the nonspecific emergency procedures necessary to maintain vital functions. The second stage is the specific medical or neurologic treatment of the cause of the coma. This is an exhaustive subject that cannot be covered in this chapter. Specific medical treatment of toxic and metabolic disease is discussed in standard medical texts. The care of neurologic disease such as tumors, strokes, and infections is discussed in other chapters of this volume. The third stage involves specific preventive measures that are necessary in immobile patients:

- General skin care to prevent decubitus ulcers
- Antiembolic stockings and possibly heparin in small doses in appropriate patients to prevent thrombophlebitis and pulmonary embolism
- Ointment in the eyes and patching to prevent corneal ulceration or abrasion
- Sponge padding of elbows to prevent pressure neuropathy of the ulnar nerves

PROGNOSIS

Knowing the expected long-term outcome in the comatose patient is useful both in discussing the patient's condition with the family and in planning the patient's future care. An exact prognosis cannot be given for each patient, but there are some general observations and statistics available that the clinician can use as a guideline. In a study of 500 nontrauma patients who were comatose for at least six hours, Plum and Posner[2] reported that only 15% made a satisfactory recovery. Seventy-six percent had died within 1 month, and 85% had died within 1 year. In general, patients with comas from primary neurologic diseases will have a much worse prognosis than patients in metabolic comas. For example, a good recovery is expected in 25% of the patients in metabolic coma but in less than 5% of patients with coma secondary to subarachnoid hemorrhage. In metabolic disease, if the coma is long or brain stem function is abnormal, the prognosis worsens dramatically.

In patients with a toxic overdose the prognosis is good and the death rate can be as low as 5%, but the survival rate decreases with prolonged coma, concurrent medical illness, complications, or advanced age.

The case of coma after cardiac arrest deserves special mention. The best overall parameter for judging prognosis is the length of time from the arrest to the initial return of consciousness. If this time is short, prognosis is good. If the patient is not awake in 10 to 12 hours, there is only a 40% chance of functional recovery. The quality of movement is also a good indicator. If the patient is comatose 1 hour after cardiac arrest and has decorticate or decerebrate posturing, the prognosis is much better. If the patient remains comatose for 6 hours and does not initiate purposeful withdrawal, the possibility of a good recovery drops to below 5%. At 24 hours, if no purposeful movement has returned, most patients will die or live in vegetative state. Another poor prognostic sign is a loss of oculocephalic reflexes after circulation has been reestablished.

◾ BRAIN DEATH

Death can be declared either when heart function ceases or when the brain is nonfunctional and irreversibly damaged. Although it is usually the neurologist or neurosurgeon who is called on to make a legal pronouncement of brain death, it is important for all physicians to know the basic criteria required. Brain death can be declared when a patient has known structural brain disease (e.g., trauma, hemorrhage, and infarction) and over a period of 6 hours (some prefer to wait 24 hours) demonstrates no hemispheric or brain stem function. Pupils should be fixed to light, caloric testing with 50 ml of ice water should be negative, and the patient should be apneic for several (5 to 10) minutes immediately after 10 minutes of ventilation with 100% oxygen. If the coma is due to toxin, hypothermia, or a metabolic cause, the prognosis is less certain than with structural lesions, and brain death should be diagnosed with great caution. Deep tendon reflexes and spinal withdrawal reflexes can be present in brain-dead patients. An electroencephalogram is not necessary, but if it is obtained, it should not show any brain activity exceeding $2\mu V$. If the above criteria are met, the patient can be considered clinically dead. The legal status of the concept of brain death and irreversible coma varies from state to state and can even differ in hospitals in the same city.

▨ SUMMARY

Comas are usually produced by either toxic (medication or drugs) or metabolic problems or by structural lesions. The clinical examination differs depending upon the cause of the coma. A careful neurologic examination can usually establish the diagnosis and lead to appropriate management.

Suggested Readings

Evaluation

Bates D: The management of medical coma, *Neurosurg Psychiatry* 56:589, 1993.

Fisher CM: The neurologic examination of the comatose patient, *Acta Neurol Scand* 45 (suppl 36):1, 1969.

Plum F, Posner JB: *The diagnosis of stupor and coma,* ed 3, Philadelphia, 1980, FA Davis.

Strub RL, Black FW: *The mental status examination in neurology,* Philadelphia, 1993, FA Davis.

Teasdale G, Jennett B: Assessment of coma and impaired consciousness, *Lancet* 2:81, 1974.

Prognosis

Bates D, et al: A prospective study of nontraumatic coma: methods and results in 310 patients, *Ann Neurol* 2:211, 1977.

Bates D: Defining prognosis in medical coma, *J Neurol Neurosurg Psychiatry* 54:569, 1991.

Jennett WB, Plum F: Persistent vegetative state after brain damage, *Lancet* 1:734, 1974.

Levy DE, et al: Predicting outcome from hypoxic-ischemic coma, *JAMA* 253:1420, 1985.

Brain Death

American Neurological Association Committee on Ethical Affairs: Persistent vegetative state, *Ann Neurol* 33:386, 1993.

Halevy A, Brody B: Brain death: reconciling definitions, criteria and tests, *Ann Intern Med* 119:519, 1993.

Multi-society Task Force on Persistent Vegetative State: Medical aspects of persistent vegetative state, *N Engl J Med* 330:1499, 1572, 1994.

Report of the medical consultants on the diagnosis of brain death to the President's Commission: Guidelines for the determination of death, *Neurology* 32:395, 1982.

Specific Etiologies

Bass E: Cardiopulmonary arrest, *Ann Intern Med* 103:920, 1985.

Dougherty JH, et al: Hypoxic-ischemic brain injury and the vegetative state: clinical and neuropathologic correlation, *Neurology* 31:991, 1981.

Malouf R, Brust JCM: Hypoglycemia, *Ann Neurol* 17:421, 1985.

Philbrick KL, Rummans TA: Malignant catatonia, *J Neuropsych Clin Neurosci* 6:1, 1994.

Common
Neurologic Diseases

CHAPTER

Cerebrovascular Disease

10

DEFINITION

The term "stroke" is used to indicate the sudden onset
of focal neurologic deficit. This is most commonly due
to pathological changes in cerebral arterial or arteriolar
circulation and rarely due to venous occlusion. Maximal neurologic deficit is reached rapidly (minutes to
several hours), and subsequent delayed deterioration
does not usually occur. The deficit caused by stroke
stabilizes, and subsequently neurologic improvement
occurs; however, certain patients rapidly deteriorate and
die because of increased intracranial pressure and herniation. Death resulting from ischemic stroke is usually
due to carotid or basilar artery occlusion or, in hemorrhagic stroke, results from large intracerebral, subarachnoid, or pontine hemorrhages. Recurrence is a potential
risk after the initial stroke. In classifying a stroke, it is
important to determine pathologic process and delineate specific vessel(s), for example, thrombotic occlusion of the carotid system, embolic occlusion of the
middle cerebral artery, or hemorrhagic stroke caused by
a ruptured carotid aneurysm (Box 10-1).

BOX 10-1   Classification of Strokes

Ischemic (nonhemorrhagic) process

Transient ischemic attack (TIA)

Reversible ischemic neurologic deficit (RIND)

Stroke in evolution

Cerebral infarction (completed stroke)
  Thrombosis
  Cerebral embolism
  Other conditions (arteritis, hematologic disorders, and oral
    contraceptives)

Hypertensive encephalopathy

Lacunar infarcts, lacunar state

Binswanger's disease

Hemorrhagic processes

Hypertensive spontaneous intracerebral hemorrhage

Ruptured saccular aneurysm

Ruptured arteriovenous malformation

Amyloid (congophilic) angiopathy

Hemorrhagic disorders (leukemia, aplastic anemia, thrombotic
  thrombocytopenic purpura, anticoagulants)

Dural sinuses and cerebral venous thrombosis

INCIDENCE

Cerebral ischemia composes 80% and intracranial hemorrhage composes 20% of stroke cases. Of the 600,000 people who suffer stroke annually, 150,000 die as a result of the stroke. There is 35% risk for recurrent strokes, and these patients can develop neurologic and mental disability (vascular dementia) resulting from the cumulative effect of these multiple strokes. The frequency of stroke death is exceeded only by heart disease and cancer. Cerebrovascular disease is the major cause of disability in patients

---

**BOX 10-2   Potential Risk Factors for
Cerebrovascular Disease**

<u>Modifiable</u>	<u>Nonmodifiable</u>
Hypertension	Gender (male)
systolic	Race (black, oriental, hispanic)
diastolic	Age
Left-ventricular	Family history
hypertrophy	
Cardiac disease	
Glucose intolerance	
Lipid abnormalities	
Cigarette smoking	
Obesity	
Coagulation factors	
(elevated hematocrit and	
fibrinogen)	
Alcohol consumption	
Sedentary lifestyle	
Illicit drug use	

---

older than 40 years old. There are 2.5 million stroke survivors, of whom many have not regained functional or vocational independence.

There has been decline in stroke mortality, probably because of improved risk factor control, for example, good blood pressure management, diet, exercise, and decreased cigarette smoking (Box 10-2). With improved hypertension management there has been a marked decrease in the incidence of cerebral hemorrhage (ICH). There has been decreased incidence of clinical stroke episodes; however, with CT/MRI used routinely for neurodiagnosis, clinically silent (asymptomatic) cerebrovascular lesions can be detected during life that previously would have only been detected at autopsy. With CT, detection of ICH is always accomplished. With CT and CSF findings, diagnosis of subarachnoid hemorrhage (SAH) is established. For ischemic stroke diagnosis, infarction is not always visualized by CT or MRI; however, ischemic deficit that is not detected by CT/MRI can be visualized by SPECT/PET findings, and vascular obstruction can be detected by vascular imaging techniques (ultrasound, MR angiography, or catheter angiography).

▨ APPROACH TO DIAGNOSIS

Apoplectic presentation (sudden onset) can occur in certain nonvascular conditions including brain neoplasms, subdural hematomas, multiple sclerosis, and brain abscesses. The neurologic condition rapidly stabilizes, and subsequent clinical improvement usually occurs in cerebrovascular disorders. Gradual onset of neurologic deficit and progressive neurologic deterioration are more consistent with nonvascular lesions.

When confronted with a possible stroke patient, the physician should answer those question found in Box 10-3.

It is important to classify patients with cerebrovascular disease on the basis of clinical findings, anatomical neuroimaging findings (CT/MRI), physiologic cerebral blood flow studies (SPECT, PET) and blood vessel imaging findings (angiography). Given these patterns, determination of therapeutic options is possible.

Distinguishing between ischemic and hemorrhagic strokes is not always possible based on clinical features; however, CT/MRI is necessary to confirm clinical impressions. Although hemorrhagic lesions are less prevalent, they are more often fatal and can require surgical intervention. As a general rule hemorrhagic lesions begin during waking hours, usually during

BOX 10-3

1 Is this a stroke or strokelike presentation of nonvascular process?

2 Is this a transient ischemic attack (TIA)? What is the underlying vascular mechanism?

3 Is this a completed stroke? Is it ischemic or hemorrhagic?

4 What vascular territory is involved—carotid or vertebrobasilar, large vessel or small vessel disease?

5 Is lumbar puncture helpful in the diagnosis? Should it be done as an emergency?

6 Is a cerebral angiogram indicated? How soon should this be done? Will noninvasive vascular imaging procedures provide the diagnostic information?

7 How soon after the stroke will CT/MRI show an ischemic or hemorrhage lesion?

8 How fast and vigorously should hypertension be treated in an acute stroke patient with elevated blood pressure?

9 What type of medical of surgical strategies should be initiated and what is timing of these treatments?

some type of physical activity, begin with a severe headache ("worst headache I ever had") followed by the onset of focal deficit, and are associated with impaired consciousness. On the other hand, mild or no headache, preservation of consciousness, onset during sleep, and history of prior TIA before onset of focal deficit suggest ischemic stroke. These general guidelines are usually reliable; however, small intracranial hemorrhages can simulate cerebral infarctions. Definitive diagnosis is possible only with CT or MRI.

ATHEROSCLEROSIS

Atherothrombotic cerebral infarction (ACI) is due to progressive deposition of lipids within the arterial wall (plaque formation) to narrow the vessel lumen. The plaque can disrupt the intimal surface causing intraplaque hemorrhage or ulceration; the formation of these complicated plaques can suddenly occlude the arterial lumen to result in clinical stroke. The earliest atherosclerotic lesion is a fatty streak; this is visualized as yellowish area on the intimal arterial surface. This lesion consists of lipid-swollen macrophages (foam cells). It appears that low-density lipoprotein (LDL) cholesterol is taken up by macrophages and smooth muscle cells. Atherosclerosis is a multifocal process. Certain focal regions of intra- and extracranial branches of anterior (carotid) and posterior (vertebrobasilar) arteries have the predilection to develop arteriosclerotic changes. For example, the initial extracranial portion of internal carotid is most commonly narrowed by plaque. This is important because it is surgically accessible for carotid endarterectomy. Atherosclerotic plaque can narrow vessel lumen to reduce the blood flow or can cause irregularity in vessel walls on which platelet-fibrin material adheres and embolizes distally to intracranial vessels. The process by which thrombotic material embolizes from one artery to another is referred to as artery-to-artery embolism or tandem arterial embolic stroke. Another source of stroke is brain embolism due to thrombus formation within the cardiac system.

Although the cause of atherosclerosis is still debated, important risk factors predispose or accelerate this process (see Box 10-2); these include genetic composition, high levels of low or very low density lipoproteins (LDL, VLDL) and low levels of high density lipoproteins (HDL), excessive saturated fats in diet, inactivity, diabetes, and most important hypertension. High dietary cholesterol and saturated fatty acids cause high blood levels of total cholesterol and LDL. These patients are at risk for ACI and coronary artery disease (CAD). Risk factors for stroke and CAD are quite similar. Thus, the profile of the person at highest risk for cerebral infarction emerges as a middle-aged, overweight, sedentary, hypertensive, diabetic, heavy smoker who has family and personal history of cardiovascular disease. When used in moderation, alcohol reduces the incidence of death caused by CAD. However, alcohol abuse can contribute to stroke risk by induction of hypertension and cardiac arrhythmias, enhancement of platelet aggregation, and reduction of cerebral blood flow. Hypertension is the most deleterious factor contributing to stroke because it not only accelerates atherosclerosis but also is the underlying cause of small intracranial arteriolar changes (lipohyalinosis, fibrinoid degeneration) leading to intracerebral hemorrhage, lacunar infarcts, acute hypertensive crisis, and subcortical arteriosclerotic encephalopathy (p. 284).

■ ASYMPTOMATIC CAROTID ARTERY STENOSIS

Arterial bruits indicate that blood flow is no longer laminar but is turbulent. Bruits develop because of certain hemodynamic conditions (anemia, thyrotoxicosis, obesity) not associated with arterial stenosis; however, carotid bruits usually indicate arterial stenosis. Bruits occur in 3% to 4% of the population older than age 45 and in 8% older than age 75. Bruits can be the first sign of carotid stenosis; they occur when the arterial cross section lumen is reduced by 50%. Bruits become louder as stenosis increases but can disappear when the carotid artery is occluded. In patients with bruits it is possible to have high-grade stenosis without neurologic symptoms. The annual stroke risk for all patients with asymptomatic carotid bruits is 1%; however, for patients with carotid bruits who have greater than 75% carotid stenosis (as measured by Doppler duplex imaging), the annual stroke risk is 5%. In patients with carotid bruits who develop strokes, this does not always occur on the side of bruit, and the stroke can occur in vertebrobasilar (V-B) territory or in small vessels (arterioles). Asymptomatic carotid bruit patients with Doppler evidence of high-grade carotid stenosis have 30% incidence for CT/MRI evidence of silent (asymptomatic) cerebral infarction. Patients with asymptomatic carotid stenosis have increased cardiac risk (myocardial infarction, congestive heart failure, atrial fibrillation, ruptured aortic aneurysm). This indicates that the bruit is a marker of multifocal systemic arteriosclerotic disease, especially cardiac disease. In patients with asymptomatic carotid stenosis TIA is more likely to initially occur than completed stroke. Severity and rate of progression of carotid stenosis (as measured by duplex Doppler studies) are the best markers of risk for developing symptomatic cerebrovascular disease. Currently certain patients with asymptomatic carotid stenosis of at least 60% should undergo prophylactic carotid endarterectomy (CEA) because this intervention reduces the 5-year risk of ipsilateral stroke compared with those treated with the best medical management.

▨ TRANSIENT FOCAL DEFICIT

When patients develop single or multiple transient episodes of sudden onset of focal neurologic dysfunction, it is presumed that the mechanism is vascular (TIA) or electric disturbance (seizure, migraine). In focal seizures, there is rapid *spread* (usually occurring within several minutes) over involved body region (Jacksonian march), and clinical symptoms are characterized by *positive* (clonic motor jerks, sensory tingling, or paresthesias) symptoms. These represent cortical excitatory electrical activity. If focal seizure is suspected, an EEG can detect focal spike discharges. If onset and spread occurs over a longer interval (10 to 20 minutes), includes prominent positive visual disturbances (fortification spectrum, scintillating scotoma), and is followed by contralateral headache, consider migraine. In migraine the mechanism is believed to be spreading cortical electrical depressive (inhibitory) activity rather than vasospasm causing ischemia. The oligemia (reduced blood flow) seen in migraine is due to reduced cortical metabolism. Headache, spread of neurologic deficit, and positive types of visual disturbances are uncommon in TIAs. TIA episodes can result from embolism, hypoperfusion, hemodynamic crisis, vasospasm, or vascular thrombosis caused by hematologic or hemorheologic factors (Box 10-4).

BOX 10-4   TIA Differential Diagnosis

Migraine

Focal seizures

Syncope

Hyperventilation

Metabolic disorder

Drug intoxication

Vertigo

Transient global amnesia

Psychogenic conversion reaction

▨ TRANSIENT ISCHEMIC ATTACK

TIAs are episodes of focal neurologic dysfunction of sudden onset and transient duration occurring in specific arterial distribution. By definition an episode lasts less than 24 hours; however it is more common for TIA to last 24 minutes than 24 hours. These attacks can be single or recurrent. TIA patients should be evaluated for the underlying cerebrovascular disturbance because therapy needs to be initiated to prevent a stroke, which occurs in 30% to 35% of TIA patients.

Clinical Features

The physician must rely on patient history in arriving at TIA diagnosis because most episodes have resolved by the time patients are seen by the physician. Associated symptoms are important clues to TIA etiology. For example, cardiac symptoms including angina pectoris or palpitations preceding TIA suggest cardiac embolus; neck movements precipitating V-B TIA suggest a combination of vertebral artery occlusive disease possibly resulting from degenerative cervical spine disease; brain stem or cerebellar ischemia precipitated by arm exercise in patients with marked differences in blood pressure findings in the arms suggests subclavian steal syndrome.

TIA symptoms depend on whether carotid or V-B vessels are involved. With extracranial ICA occlusive disease, two patterns occur: one, cerebral (cortical) hemispheric symptoms including contralateral hemiparesis or monoparesis, contralateral hemisensory deficit of cortical type, aphasia if dominant hemisphere is involved; and two, ocular, monocular visual blurring or blindness (amaurosis fugax). If the patient has isolated motor hemiparesis or hemisensory deficit, this suggests subcortical TIA. The mechanism of "cortical TIA" should prompt a search for ICA stenosis or occlusion, whereas the mechanism of "subcortical TIA" usually suggests small-vessel arteriolar disease such as diabetes or hypertension. V-B TIA symptoms include vertigo usually associated with ataxia, diplopia, dysarthria, drop attacks, and dysphagia. Visual disturbances caused by posterior circulation TIA affect both eyes and consist of visual dimming or graying out of vision, scotomas, and visual field defects. Isolated vertigo is rarely a manifestation of TIA but is usually caused by vestibular dysfunction. V-B TIAs can be precipitated by changes in head, neck, or body position. If precipitated by head or neck position, consider cranial-cervical junction abnormalities. If precipitated by rapid change in position or exercise, consider postural hypotension or hemodynamic factors such as low cardiac output or cardiac arrhythmias.

Clinical Evaluation

Clinical evaluation should delineate the TIA mechanism. Routine blood chemistries and cardiac studies should be initially performed (Box 10-5). In TIA patients it is important to determine whether attacks involve carotid or V-B arteries. With carotid TIA initially screen with Doppler duplex study (Box 10-6). All TIA patients should have CT to exclude hemorrhage or nonvascular lesions. CT can show ischemic lesions, but MRI is more sensitive for early ischemic lesions especially those involving the brain stem (Figure 10-1). PET and SPECT can be useful as they can show focal perfusion (cerebral blood flow) deficits even if CT/MRI shows no ischemic lesions. If SPECT/PET show perfusion deficit, this indicates that cerebral blood flow to the ischemic region is not

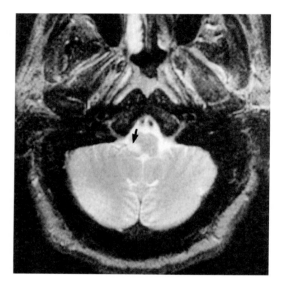

FIGURE 10-1. T-2 weighted axial MRI shows a high signal intensity lesion in the posterior-lateral brain stem (*arrow*) representing infarction.

adequate to protect brain tissue. This patient is at high risk for a major stroke. Angiography is indicated to demonstrate extra- and intracranial carotid and V-B circulation but does not detect small vessels (arterioles). If TIA involves V-B circulation, transcranial Doppler and angiography are indicated to delineate stenosis, occlusion, or blood vessel wall abnormality (dissection, fibromuscular dysplasia). In patients with TIA, lumbar puncture is not usually warranted unless headache is prominent, suggesting intracranial hemorrhage.

**BOX 10-5   Laboratory Evaluation
of TIA Patient**

1 Complete blood count including platelet count
2 Erythrocyte sedimentation rate
3 Activated partial thromboplastin time and prothrombin time
4 Lipid profile
5 Lupus anticoagulant and anticardiolipin antibodies
   (antiphospholipid syndrome)
6 Urine and serum toxicology
7 Syphilis serology
8 Plasma fibrinogen
9 Hemoglobin electrophoresis
10 Serum glucose
11 Urinalysis (for hematuria to suggest renal embolism and
    proteinuria to suggest hypertensive vascular disease)
12 Renal and hepatic function

 **BOX 10-6   Laboratory Studies in Selected
TIA Patients**

1 Protein S and C, and antithrombin III levels
2 Urine amino acid screen for homocystinuria
3 Immune complex screening studies including studies for
   systemic lupus erythematosus and rheumatoid arthritis
4 Serum and whole body viscosity
5 Platelet function studies
6 HIV, Lyme, and cysticercosis screening tests
7 Pregnancy test
8 Serum protein electrophoresis
9 Coagulation factor analysis
10 Chest radiogram for sarcoidosis

■ REVERSIBLE ISCHEMIC NEUROLOGICAL DEFICIT AND CEREBRAL INFARCTION WITH TRANSIENT SIGNS

Reversible ischemic neurological deficit (RIND) is focal neurologic deficit of vascular origin lasting more than 24 hours but less than 3 days or, by some definitions, 3 weeks. Evaulation and treatment should be identical to that for TIA patients. Complete neuroimaging and vascular imaging should be performed to delineate causal vascular lesions. Cerebral infarction with transient signs (CITS) is diagnosed when TIA symptoms rapidly resolve within 24 hours but CT/MRI shows a causal ischemic lesion. It is more likely that long-duration TIAs will show abnormal CT/MRI, whereas it is less likely that CT/MRI will show ischemic lesions with a short-duration TIA. It is not known if the risk of clinical stroke occurrence is greater if the CT/MRI shows an ischemic lesion. If the TIA deficit does not resolve within 1 hour, there is an 80% probability that neurologic deficit will not resolve within 24 hours. The term "minor stroke" has been used to describe stroke patients in whom minimal neurologic deficit remains after several weeks; this is similar to the definition of RIND. All ischemic stroke patients (TIA, RIND, CITS, minor stroke) have a 30% to 35% risk of subsequently developing a major stroke. It is more important to determine the underlying vascular mechanism than to classify these patients correctly on the basis of temporal pattern of neurological deficit.

MANAGEMENT OF REVERSIBLE ISCHEMIC VASCULAR EPISODE

Specific therapy is warranted in these conditions.

One, if TIA occurs in carotid distribution, vascular imaging is mandatory. Duplex ultrasound has 90% to 95% sensitivity for detecting angiographically proven 50% stenosis; however, it is my opinion that all carotid territory TIA patients should have conventional catheter angiography. This allows adequate assessment of extracranial and intracranial circulation. If the patient has severe symptomatic extracranial ICA stenosis plus an asymptomatic intracranial ICA aneurysm, this would certainly modify therapy. Considering the results of the North American Carotid Endarterectomy Study, surgery is beneficial for symptomatic patients with angiographically documented cervical carotid stenosis of at least 70%. With less than 30% stenosis, there is no evidence that CEA is beneficial, whereas in patients with 30% to 69% stenosis the value of CEA will not be established until the results of ongoing studies are available.

Two, for TIA patients with a cardiogenic cerebral embolic source, anticoagulation is indicated. In recently completed studies of patients with nonvalvular arterial fibrillation (NVAF) with or without neurologic symptoms, warfarin (Coumadin) significantly reduced stroke occurrence. In an ongoing study, aspirin is being compared with warfarin in patients with NVAF; however, given currently available data anticoagulation is an accepted treatment for stroke prevention in NVAF. If there are contraindications to warfarin, antiplatelet medication can be used.

Three, if TIA patients show antiographic evidence of high-grade stenosis of a large intracranial artery (carotid, middle cerebral, vertebral, basilar), the risk of stroke is quite high. In this circumstance neurologists frequently initiate intravenous heparin. This should be followed by oral Coumadin.

Four, if surgery and anticoagulation are not indicated in TIA patients, antiplatelet medication should be considered. There are several available drugs. Dipyridamole (Persantine) has not been proved to be more effective than aspirin alone. Pentoxifylline (Trental) is not actually an antiplatelet drug. It is believed to reduce blood viscosity, enhance erythrocyte flexibility, and increase tissue oxygen content. This medication has been shown to be effective in patients with peripheral vascular disease but has *not* yet been shown to be effective in cerebrovascular patients. Aspirin is effective in reducing cardiovascular and cerebrovascular events. It is associated with relative risk reduction of 30% for stroke, 22% for stroke death, and 15% for cerebro- and cardiovascular mortality. Multiple studies have demonstrated that doses of 325 to 1300 mg of aspirin are effective in stroke prevention; however, it is uncertain whether lower dose aspirin is equally effective in stroke prevention. Aspirin inhibits cyclooxygenase to prevent thromboxane A_2 formation (this substance has a proaggregatory and vasoconstrictive effect); and at high dosage, aspirin inhibits prostacyclin (this substance has a vasodilation effect and inhibits platelet aggregation). The theoretical advantage for low-dose aspirin is that prostacyclin inhibition is avoided at low doses; however, the enhanced effectiveness of low-dose aspirin has not been demonstrated in clinical trials. In fact, clinical studies have shown high-dose aspirin is more effective for stroke prevention in TIA patients. Despite this controversy most physicians use 325 mg of aspirin daily. It should be noted that although aspirin has been shown to be effective in stroke prevention in men, few clinical studies have shown demonstrable beneficial effects in women. Ticlid (ticlopidine) is another antiplatelet drug used for stroke prevention. Ticlopidine acts to reduce platelet-fibrinogen binding within plaque and reduces "white" (platelet-fibrin) clot size. Unlike aspirin, ticlopidine is not a cyclooxygenase inhibitor; therefore it does not reduce stomach prostaglandins. These substances protect gastric mucosa; therefore ticlopidine causes less gastric irritation than aspirin. The most effective dosage of ticlopidine is 250 mg twice daily. Clinical studies have used this dosage, and therefore controversy regarding the appropriate dose of ticlopidine has not been raised. Stroke reduction occurred for men and women TIA patients. In patients who suffered major strokes, ticlopidine has been shown to prevent *recurrent* strokes, and the evidence that aspirin is effective in preventing recurrent strokes is less certain. Potential side effects of ticlopidine include diarrhea, dyspepsia, hepatic dysfunction, and rarely irreversible neutropenia. Because of neutropenia risk, it is recommended that complete blood-count monitoring be performed biweekly for three months. Major side effects for ticlopidine and aspirin are 1% of all patients taking this medication.

▨ PROGRESSING OR DETERIORATING STROKE (STROKE IN EVOLUTION)

Progressing stroke (stroke in evolution) is a common circumstance when focal ischemia worsens and infarction extends. Most stroke syndromes reach maximal deficit within minutes to hours; however, in some cases there is delayed neurologic deterioration. Potential mechanisms for progression of neurologic deficit within the first week include hemorrhage within ischemic lesion, suggestive of embolic infarction;

increased size of ischemic lesion caused by continued cerebral perfusion deficit, distal clot propagation, or recurrent embolization; edema of vasogenic (caused by impaired blood-brain barrier) or cytotoxic (because of impaired cerebral perfusion inadequate to maintain cellular metabolism) type; seizure with prolonged postictal state; and systemic, hemodynamic, cardiac, or respiratory disturbances. Strokes most commonly associated with neurologic progression include large vessel (carotid, vertebrobasilar) disease with artery-to-artery embolism or distal clot propagation, cardiogenic cerebral embolism, lacunar infarct, and watershed territory infarction with reduced perfusion of arterial border zones especially if the patient develops systemic hypotension. When the stroke is due to intracerebral hemorrhage, progression is unlikely; however, this rare occurrence can be due to increased hematoma size resulting from continued blood extravasation from a ruptured arteriole, vasogenic edema, herniation, or hydrocephalus. Using serial CT/MRI studies it should be possible to delineate the mechanism of neurologic deterioration in progressing strokes of ischemic or hemorrhage stroke type. With carotid territory strokes further progression is unlikely if neurologic deficit has stabilized for 24 hours, whereas with V-B territory attacks further progression is unlikely if deficit has stabilized for 72 hours. Management depends on stroke progression mechanism. Neurologic progression that is delayed (after first week) is usually due to a recurrent stroke or systemic (cardiac, infectious, pulmonary, metabolic) complications.

CARDIOGENIC CEREBRAL EMBOLISM

Twenty to twenty-five percent of patients with TIA or stroke have a cardiac abnormality that can be the source of the stroke (Box 10-7). For example, patients with rheumatic mitral stenosis and atrial fibrillation have increased stroke risk (17 times more than control subjects); and patients with nonvalvular atrial fibrillation also have increased stroke risk. Certain cardiac disorders are definite high stroke risks, for example, prosthetic heart valves, whereas in others stroke risk resulting from cardiac conditions is less certain, for example, mitral valve prolapse.

In cardiogenic cerebral embolism (CCE), eight clinical features help establish this diagnosis: presence of a high-risk source of cardiac disease (see Box 10-7), evidence of systemic embolism, infarcts (visualized by

---

 BOX 10-7   Sources of Cardiogenic Cerebral Embolism

High Risk

Nonvalvular atrial fibrillation

Rheumatic valvular disease

Recent myocardial infarction

Atrial or ventricular thrombus

Atrial myxoma

Endocarditis

Mechanical prosthetic valve

Sick sinus syndrome

Dilated cardiomyopathy

Low Risk

Mitral valve prolapse

Mitral annulus calcification

Patent foramen ovale

Lone atrial fibrillation

Old myocardial infarction

Atrial septal aneurysm

CT/MRI) in more than one vascular territory, a clinical pattern of superficial cortical ischemic pattern (isolated Wernicke's aphasia, homonymous hemianopia, isolated facial or arm motor deficit) or top of basilar syndrome, minimal evidence of carotid atherosclerotic or small vessel arteriolar disease, CT evidence of hemorrhagic infarct, abrupt onset of neurologic deficit without progression, and no prior TIA. The initial CT can be normal or show nonhemorrhagic infarct in CCE patients; however, as the embolus is lysed (within 48 to 72 hours), the infarct can undergo hemorrhagic transformation as a result of reperfusion of an infarcted region that has lost its ability to autoregulate its blood flow. In CCE patients the risk of embolization recurrence can be as high as 1% per day in the initial two weeks after a stroke; however, the risk depends on the underlying cardiac disease. Embolization recurrence can be prevented by anticoagulation; however, this should be delayed for 72 hours after a clinical stroke, at which time the CT demonstrates that there has been no evidence of hemorrhagic transformation. In patients with cardiac conditions who are at high risk for developing cerebral embolus but who are currently neurologically asymptomatic, anticoagulation should be used prophylactically. For example, patients with valvular and nonvalvular atrial fibrillation should receive oral anticoagulants.

CEREBRAL ARTERIAL SYNDROMES

Internal Carotid Artery and Middle Cerebral Artery Syndromes

Neurologic findings in both internal carotid artery (ICA) and middle cerebral artery (MCA) ischemic stroke are hemiplegia associated with visual field defects, partial or complete sensory deficit, speech difficulties such as aphasia or dysphasia if the dominant hemisphere is

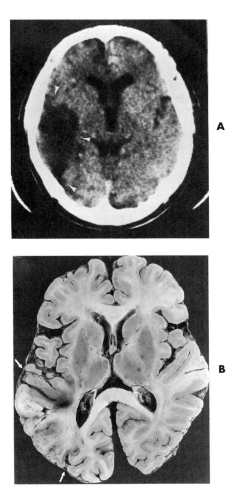

FIGURE 10-2. **A,** Horizontal section of the brain showing an infarct in the posterior portion of the left middle cerebral artery distribution (*upper and lower arrows*). **B,** CT scan of brain showing an infarct (*lucent area within arrows*) in part of the left middle cerebral artery.

involved, and anosognosia if the nondominant hemisphere is infarcted. All symptoms depend on the size of cerebral territory involved (Figure 10-2). With ICA occlusion the motor deficit usually involves the face and arm (MCA territory) as well as leg (ACA territory), whereas with MCA occlusive syndrome the leg is spared or less severely involved than the face and arm. There can be incomplete syndromes as a result of branch occlusions of distal branches of MCA, for example, Wernicke's aphasia caused by occlusion of the inferior branch of MCA or Broca's aphasia without hemiparesis or hemianesthesia caused by occlusion of the anterior parietal branch of MCA. With dominant hemispheric MCA ischemia aphasia develops; with nondominant hemispheric MCA clinical features can include anosognosia (denial of hemiplegia), unilateral spatial neglect, or inattention to the left side of the body such that the patient does not dress the left side or is not even aware of his or her left side. Ipsilateral blindness (caused by central retinal artery occlusion) with contralateral motor or sensory deficit is characteristic of extracranial ICA occlusion.

The initial portion of the extracranial portion of ICA is the most common site for atherosclerotic plaque formation. This can cause stenosis of the ICA and lead to TIA or completed stroke as a result of hemodynamic factors and reduced tissue perfusion. Platelet-fibrin clot or atherosclerotic plaque can dislodge from the stenotic artery to embolize distally to cause TIA or stroke (artery-to-artery embolus). Occlusion of MCA most commonly results from embolism originating from heart, aortic arch, or ICA (artery-to-artery embolus); however, less commonly thrombosis in-situ can involve the proximal (origin) portion of MCA.

🔲 ANTERIOR CEREBRAL ARTERY SYNDROME

Symptoms of anterior cerebral artery (ACA) ischemic stroke syndrome vary depending on the size of the lesion and whether there is unilateral or bilateral frontal ischemia. Weakness and sensory impairment in the lower extremity with mild or no involvement in the upper extremity or face suggests ACA territory ischemic lesion. Mental changes, apraxia, alterations in grasping and sucking reflexes, and problems with bowel and bladder incontinence can be due to ACA infarction especially if both frontal regions are supplied by one ACA through the anterior communicating artery.

Posterior Cerebral Artery Syndromes

Visual symptoms including poor vision, bumping into objects, and visual recognition of one side of objects or words in only one-half of the field of vision (indicating hemianopsia) are frequent complaints. The characteristic finding is the result of posterior cerebral artery (PCA) occlusion with occipital lobe ischemia; this is homonymous hemianopsia. Other findings may include hemianesthesia; hemiplegia is an unexpected finding. Impaired memory and confusion are reported in patients with hippocampal (temporal lobe) lesions. Reading disorders (alexia) and visual distortions of objects (metamorphopsia) can be found in patients with dominant hemispheric lesions.

Vertebrobasilar Syndromes

The basilar artery originates from paired vertebral arteries and is located on the ventral surface of the pons and midbrain. It terminates at the upper midbrain to bifurcate into paired posterior cerebral arteries that supply occipital lobes, medial temporal cortex, and medial thalamus. If there is atherosclerotic disease of the proximal subclavian artery before the vertebral artery origin, exercise of the arm can lead to vertigo and other manifestations of brain stem and cerebellar ischemia as blood is diverted from the brain stem and cerebellum in a retrograde pattern to the arms (subclavian steal syndrome). Although vertebral arteries are paired, one side is usually dominant and carries the majority of blood flow; therefore, if the dominant vertebral artery is occluded, there is high likelihood of brain stem and cerebellar ischemia. Thrombosis of the basilar artery usually involves the proximal portion supplying the pons, whereas with embolism there is occlusion at the top of the basilar artery, where it bifurcates into paired PCA arteries to cause ischemia involving midbrain, thalamus, occipital, and medial temporal cortex. The vertebral artery can be injured by neck manipulation or rotation, as well as rapid head movements. This can cause intimal tears and dissection of vertebral arteries and can lead to thrombus formation and vertebral artery occlusion.

The most characteristic V-B stroke syndrome is lateral medullary infarction caused by occlusion of vertebral or posterior inferior cerebellar arteries. Clinical features include sudden onset of vertigo and imbalance, ipsilateral cerebellar ataxia, ipsilateral facial hypalgesia and contralateral hypalgesia of trunk and extremities, ipsilateral Horner's syndrome, horizontal nystagmus, dysarthria, dysphonia, and dysphagia. Also, with vertebral artery occlusion cerebellar infarction can develop. Clinical features include gait or ipsilateral limb ataxia and limb dysmetria. With large cerebellar infarcts CT/MRI can show cerebellar infarction with marked mass effect; there can be compression of the fourth ventricle and brain stem with resultant hydrocephalus. Removal of the infarcted swollen cerebellar hemisphere may be necessary to decompress posterior fossa and prevent death. With top of basilar artery occlusion, pontine, midbrain, thalamic, and cortical (occipital, medial temporal) infarction can occur. These patients can have impaired consciousness, abnormal eye movements, miotic reactive pupils, and quadriplegia. This can simulate brain stem hemorrhage; however, a hemorrhage is excluded by a negative CT. In some cases there is thrombus propagation intracranially, and neurologic deficit can progress over 24 to 72 hours. This clot propagation can be prevented with intravenous anticoagulation. There are more than 30 syndromes with eponyms for infarction of different levels of brain stem. Box 10-8 lists the more common syndromes. MRI is a more reliable procedure than CT to detect brain stem ischemic lesions (Figure 10-1).

■ LESS CHARACTERISTIC (NONHEMIPLEGIC) STROKE SYNDROMES

Not all stroke patients are hemiplegic. It is important to be aware that focal neurologic deficit that results from stroke syndrome is not limited to classic hemiplegia or hemiparesis that most physicians equate with stroke. Sudden onset of many varied patterns of focal neurologic deficit are due to stroke. Examples of stroke syndromes without motor deficit are shown in Box 10-9.

BOX 10-8 Major Vertebrobasilar Ischemic Syndromes	
Artery Occluded	**Ischemic Region**
Vertebral artery Posterior inferior Cerebellar artery	Lateral medullary syndrome (Wallenberg's syndrome)
Anterior inferior Cerebellar artery	Lateral caudal pons
Paramedian branch of basilar artery	Inferior medial pons (Foville's syndrome)
Superior cerebellar artery	Lateral rostral pons and pons-midbrain junction
Paramedian branch of basilar artery	Superior medial pons
Basilar artery	Pons, midbrain, thalamus, occipital cortex
Paramedian penetrating midbrain basilar artery	Middle medial midbrain (Weber's syndrome)

EVALUATION AND MANAGEMENT OF ACUTE CEREBRAL INFARCTION

The first step is to regulate cerebral blood flow by correcting cardiorespiratory or systemic vascular abnormalities. Assess cardiac status to ensure optimal cardiac output. Vital signs and neurologic condition should be monitored carefully for the initial 72 hours to be certain that severe hypertension or hypotension do not occur and that no subsequent neurologic deterioration occurs. Rapid mobilization should be attempted to avoid decubitus, pneumonia, pulmonary embolism, and deep vein thrombosis as long as the

Clinical Manifestations

Ipsilateral cerebellar ataxia; Horner's syndrome; facial hemianesthesia; contralateral arm and leg hemianesthesia; vertigo; horizontal nystagmus; dysarthria; dysphagia; hiccups

Ipsilateral cerebellar ataxia; facial anesthesia; facial paresis; horizontal gaze palsy (towards side of lesion); deafness; contralateral body anesthesia

Horizontal gaze palsy towards side of lesion; ipsilateral abducens and facial paresis; contralateral weakness and hemianesthesia

Ipsilateral cerebellar ataxia; facial hemianesthesia, Horner's syndrome; contralateral hemianesthesia; superior oblique paresis (skew ocular deviation)

Internuclear ophthalmoplegia; palatal myoclonus; ipsilateral ataxia; contralateral hemiparesis

Abducens nerve paresis; internuclear ophthalmoplegia; impaired horizontal eye movements; ocular bobbing; miotic but reactive pupils; quadriplegia; coma if tegmentum involved; "locked in" if basis pontis involved

Ipsilateral oculomotor palsy and contralateral hemiplegia

patient's neurologic condition does not worsen with attempted postural change. Avoid oral intake until adequacy of the swallowing mechanism is determined. Left-ventricular hypertrophy on chest roentgenograms or ECG or arteriolar changes on funduscopy indicate that hypertensive cardiovascular disease preceded and probably caused the stroke rather than reactive hypertension being the consequence of the stroke. This reactive hypertension can occur as a result of transient catecholamine release or intracranial hypertension. Blood pressure control should be accomplished cautiously by reduction to levels not lower than 150/90 mm Hg. Extension of ischemic

BOX 10-9

1 Transient global amnesia (TGA) can be the result of an ischemic process in posterior cerebral artery territory. TGA is usually a benign syndrome characterized by the sudden onset of disorientation, inability to form new memories with preservation of consciousness and speech, and no other neurologic signs. This lasts from 15 minutes to 48 hours and is usually precipitated by exercise, sexual intercourse, or emotional stress. Recurrences are rare. In most patients with TGA, CT/MRI and vascular imaging procedures show no abnormality, but can sometimes show temporal ischemic lesions.

2 Temporal lobe dominant hemisphere vascular lesions can cause receptive (fluent) aphasia with minimal or no motor deficit. It is not uncommon to see patients with receptive fluent (Wernicke's) aphasia initially diagnosed as having psychiatric illness because speech is nonsensical, but because patients lack motor weakness, neurologic disease is not initially considered. If a nondominant temporal lobe vascular lesion occurs, the patient can develop an acute confusional state.

3 Acute onset of confusional states is caused by ACA territory involvement. This occurs if there is bilateral ACA ischemia as a result of the ACA being supplied by one ICA with flow through anterior communicating artery. Acute confusion with motor or sensory deficit can occur with right (nondominant) MCA involvement caused by temporal-parietal territory infarction.

4 With a lateral medullary infarct, the patient can experience vertigo and have unsteady gait, but no limb weakness.

5 Visual blurring because of homonymous hemianopsia is caused by PCA ischemia.

infarcts can be induced iatrogenically by lowering blood pressure too rapidly or to levels below that necessary for adequate brain perfusion. Cardiac arrhythmias, coronary artery disease symptoms, or cardiac valvular disease suggest potential CCE and potential need for anticoagulation. Occasionally, the stroke can be the initial manifestation of myocardial infarction (MI) caused by embolus following arrhythmia or mural thrombus. Monitor ECG and cardiac enzymes. Coagulation studies should be obtained in all stroke patients. Ocular signs associated with ICA stenosis or occlusion include intolerance of bright lights in the eye on the same side as stenotic ICA. Prominence and tortuosity of the ipsilateral temporal artery indicate increased external carotid artery collateral flow. In stroke patients chest roentgenograms can disclose unsuspected primary lung neoplasm and be the first indication of "strokelike" presentation of neoplasm.

CT/MRI should be obtained in all stroke patients because this not only localizes the lesion but also discloses unsuspected hemorrhages that can mimic ischemic lesion. As an emergency procedure CT is performed to exclude intracerebral hemorrhage; however, CT is less sensitive than MRI for detecting ischemic lesion. MRI can show ischemic lesions within 12 hours, whereas CT may not show ischemic lesions until 96 hours. CT can fail to show lacunar infarcts or brain stem infarcts, whereas these can be detected with MRI. Lumbar puncture in acute stroke is not necessary except if vasculitis is suspected (syphilis or other inflammatory process) or in selected cases before initiation of anticoagulants or thrombolytic medication. Cerebral angiograms or other noninvasive vascular imaging procedures (duplex Doppler, transcranial Doppler, MR angiography) determine underlying vascular lesions.

Therapeutic strategies for acute cerebral ischemia include prevention of cerebral thrombosis using anticoagulant and antiplatelet medication, reestablishment of cerebral blood flow (reperfusion) with thrombolytic agents (urokinase, streptokinase, tissue plasminogen activator), and cerebral neuronal protection. If there is evidence that thrombosis is propagating or embolizing intracranially (carotid, vertebral, basilar arteries) or there is a cardiac condition in which recurrent cerebral embolization is likely, anticoagulation is indicated. Initiate heparin in doses of 1000 units per hour to maintain partial thromboplastin time at 1.5 to 2 times normal controls. Several treatment strategies have been attempted to reestablish interrupted arterial circulation and reperfuse ischemic brain tissue. Thrombolytic agents are effective in coronary thrombosis; therefore it seems reasonable to attempt thrombolytic agents for acute ischemic stroke. Both intravenous and intraarterial thrombolytic agents have been evaluated, but efficacy has not been established in acute stroke, and intracranial bleeding is the potential complication. Hemodilution (isovolemic process performed by phlebotomy to reduce hematocrit and blood viscosity to enhance cerebral blood flow) or pentoxifylline (to enhance red blood cell deformability) has been used but has not improved outcomes. Cytoprotective agents (calcium channel blockers reduce intracellular calcium and reduce free radical formation, glutamate antagonists reduce neuronal excitatory processes, gangliosides enhance cellular repair) can prove useful to halt ischemia for several hours while reperfusion strategy is initiated. There is no evidence that glucocorticosteroids are effective in acute stroke because vasogenic edema is less important than cytotoxic edema and the latter is not prevented by glucocorticoids. Hyperventilation, glycerol, and mannitol are also not effective in reducing tissue damage caused by cerebral infarction but are used when intracranial hypertension and marked mass effects are suspected and risk of cerebral herniation is high.

■ NONATHEROSCLEROTIC ISCHEMIC STROKE

When the physician is confronted with a young, non-hypertensive, nondiabetic patient, nonatherosclerotic causes should be considered, including arteritides (collagen vascular disease, syphilis), spontaneous dissection of carotid arteries, fibromuscular hyperplasia, embolic lesions from atrial myxoma or congenital heart disease, hematologic disorders such as sickle cell disease or other hemoglobinopathies, and thrombotic thrombocytopenic purpura. In young females oral contraceptives or aortic arch syndrome (Takayasu's disease) can be considered. Also, in young patients with a history of migraine headaches, hemiplegic or ophthalmoplegic migraines can leave permanent deficits (migraine stroke). Recurrent unilateral headache associated with neurologic symptoms can incorrectly be diagnosed as migraines but can be a manifestation of aneurysm or vascular malformation. Antiphospholipid antibodies (lupus anticoagulant, anticardiolipins) are acquired circulating globulins (IgG, IgM) that have been found associated with cerebral or ocular ischemic symptoms. Those occur predominantly in young females. In young patients with stroke syndrome thorough evaluation for common and uncommon potential cardiac sources (patent foramen ovale, intraatrial aneurysm, atrial myxoma) must be undertaken (see Box 10-7). Also, blood and urine toxicology should be undertaken as illicit drugs are becoming increasingly common causes of strokes. Giant cell arteritis (temporal arteritis) usually involves branches of the external carotid artery and manifests as localized headache, scalp tenderness, and monocular blindness. The disease is extremely rare before age 60, and the erythrocyte sedimentation rate is constantly elevated.

■ HYPERTENSIVE ENCEPHALOPATHY

Hypertensive encephalopathy is reported in patients with recent-onset or longstanding hypertension and causes lethargy, weakness, headache, and vomiting, concomitant with a sudden rise in blood pressure and followed by coma and usually generalized or focal seizures. Transient focal neurologic findings are rare, and CSF pressure is usually elevated with otherwise normal CSF findings. Treatment should focus on rapid but careful blood pressure lowering. Cerebral infarction can result from too-rapid, aggressive lowering of blood pressure below cerebral perfusion pressure, which is higher in hypertensives than normotensives. The longer the blood pressure remains elevated, the greater the potential risk of intracranial hemorrhage.

■ LACUNAR INFARCTS–LACUNAR STATE

Lacunar Infarcts

Lacunar infarcts are small (less than 15 mm) infarcts seen in the putamen, pons, thalamus, internal capsule, and caudate nucleus. They are caused by occlusive arteriolar disease resulting from hypertension. Pathologically there is evidence of lipohyalinosis and fibrinoid degeneration, but lacunar infarcts can also be caused by microatheroma, microembolism, or rarely arteritis. Because of their location and size of vessels involved, an angiogram does not disclose arteriolar vascular lesions, but CT/MRI can demonstrate lacunar infarct. Lacunar syndromes include those in Box 10-10.

Lacunar State

Lacunar state is the end stage of severe and longstanding hypertensive arteriolar disease of the brain and

BOX 10-10

1 Pure motor hemiplegia without sensory deficit, aphasia, or cortical sensory deficit. This is due to lacune in pons or internal capsule

2 Pure sensory stroke is due to thalamic lesion

3 Brain stem syndromes:
   a Dysarthria-clumsy hand syndrome manifested by slurred speech and clumsiness of the arm
   b Ataxia and hemiparesis involving the arm and leg on same side of body

4 Sensorimotor stroke is due to posterior capsular lacunar infarct

5 Hemichorea-hemiballismus is due to basal ganglia lacunar infarct

consists of multiple and bilateral lacunes occurring in the basal ganglia or pons. Clinical features include bilateral hemiparesis, imbalance, incontinence, short-step shuffling gait, and pseudobulbar signs. Because of pseudobulbar signs, patients have difficulty in swallowing, talking, controlling salivation, and moving their tongues. Patients have emotional incontinence with frequent uncontrolled and unprovoked outbursts of laughing or crying (pseudobulbar affect). Neurologic deficit is due to the cumulative effect or multiple lacunar infarcts. Because lacunes are subcortical, dementia might be expected to be uncommon even in the presence of multiple lacunes; however, there is some evidence that the cumulative effect of multiple lacunar infarcts is dementia. Because the cause of lacunar infarcts is hypertension, this should be aggressively controlled to prevent development of hypertensive arteriolar disease.

◼ BINSWANGER'S DISEASE

Binswanger's disease is one form of vascular dementia that most commonly occurs in elderly hypertensive patients. Clinical features include disorders of cognition, memory, mood (depression), with apathy, impaired attention, and concentration also being prominent. Bilateral corticospinal and corticobulbar signs are usually present. Clinical findings that are due to subcortical white matter demyelination are caused by ischemia secondary to occlusion of white matter medullary penetrating arteries. The prominent demyelination is not due to multiple infarcts, and the exact pathophysiology of white matter demyelination is not established. The disease is frequently progressive and is often interrupted by apoplectic episodes. CT/MRI demonstrates white matter abnormalities (hypodense periventricular lesions on CT and high signal intensity lesions on MRI) in cerebral hemispheres. These white matter changes are referred to as leuko-araiosis (meaning white matter rarefaction). Leuko-araiosis is not specific for Binswanger's disease as the CT/MRI pattern can be seen in other dementias and also in normal elderly patients. The pathophysiology is unknown, so treatment is limited to aggressive control of hypertension.

◼ HEMORRHAGIC STROKES

Nontraumatic hemorrhage into brain parenchyma or subarachnoid space can occur from a variety of causes including hypertension, ruptured saccular arterial aneurysm, and ruptured arteriovenous malformations and a group of miscellaneous causes including blood dyscrasias, anticoagulants, drug abuse (e.g., cocaine, amphetamines, diet pills), bleeding into tumors, and angiopathies. Ictal episodes can vary from severe onset of headache with minimal altered consciousness as is characteristic of mild subarachnoid hemorrhage (SAH) caused by ruptured aneurysm to deep coma as found in large intracerebral or brain stem hematoma. In stroke patients with headaches, nausea, vomiting, altered consciousness, or seizures, hemorrhagic stroke is more likely than ischemic stroke; however, CT is required for a definitive diagnosis.

▨ HYPERTENSIVE INTRACEREBRAL HEMORRHAGE

This is the most frequent nontraumatic cause of intracerebral hemorrhage. Hemorrhages can be large or small. If large, mass effect and herniation can occur; the hemorrhage can extend into the ventricular system or subarachnoid spaces. The hemorrhage can originate in striatum (putamen) (Figure 10-3), thalamus, pons, or cerebellum. Certain hypertensive hemorrhages can arise from cerebral subcortical white matter (lobar hemorrhage), but alternate causes must be carefully excluded (e.g., aneurysm, angioma, tumor). The exact mechanism of hypertensive hemorrhage is not known, but sclerotic and necrotizing changes in deeply located arterioles such as lenticulostriate arterioles precede formation of miliary (arteriolar) aneurysms (Charcot-Bouchard aneurysms). Rupture of miliary aneurysms is believed to be the source of hypertensive hemorrhage. Multiple unruptured miliary arteriolar aneurysms can be found at autopsy in hypertensive patients and are almost never found in normotensives.

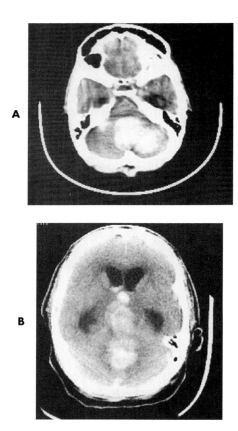

FIGURE 10-3.   CT scans of brain hemorrhage
A, Cerebellar hemorrhage
B, Brain stem hemorrhage extending upward into thalamus
and causing third ventricular hemorrhage

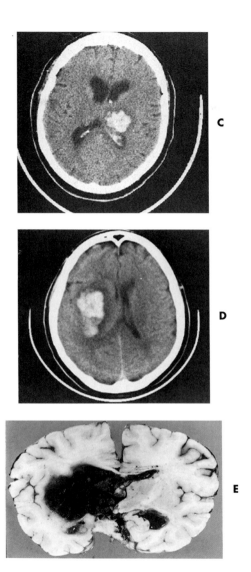

FIGURE 10-3, cont'd. C, Thalamic hemorrhage
D, Putaminal hemorrhage
E, Autopsy specimen of the brain showing massive left thalamic hemorrhage with intraventricular extension.

Clinical Presentation

Hemorrhages usually affect middle-aged hypertensives without previous neurologic deficit (no history of TIA). Initial symptoms are headache and focal neurologic deficit. If the hemorrhage is large or involves the brain stem, impaired consciousness occurs. These patients usually show longstanding hypertensive changes including retinal arteriolar changes and left-ventricular hypertrophy. This indicates that hypertension caused the hemorrhage rather than the hypertension being caused by the hemorrhage. Putaminal hemorrhage causes hemiplegia, hemianesthesia, hemianopsia, and horizontal ocular deviation toward the side of the hemorrhage (away from hemiplegic side) (Box 10-11). In thalamic hemorrhages similar findings can occur, but the eyes are usually deviated downward with paralysis of upward gaze. In pontine hemorrhages findings include coma, quadriplegia, pinpoint size but reactive pupils, absent oculocephalic and caloric responses, and respiratory disturbances. In cerebellar hemorrhages patients develop

---

BOX 10-11 Clinical Features of Hypertensive Intracerebral Hemorrhage

Putaminal	Thalamic
Hemiparesis or hemiplegia	Hemiparesis or hemiplegia
Hemianopsia	Hemisensory loss
Eyes look at the lesion	Downward deviation of eyes
	Paralysis of upward gaze
	Small but reactive pupils

dizziness, vomiting, and gait ataxia; the hemorrhage can enlarge to cause secondary brain stem dysfunction to simulate pontine hemorrhage.

Treatment

Treatment should be supportive with blood pressure control and maintenance of respiratory and cardiac functions. Prompt surgical evacuation of the cerebellar hematoma can prevent brain stem compression. Other than cerebellar hemorrhage there is no conclusive evidence that hematoma evacuation improves the prognosis in hypertensive hemorrhage. If the patient shows continued deterioration and is unresponsive to medical management of intracranial hypertension, hematoma evacuation is warranted, but the outcome is still usually poor. Monitoring of intracranial pressure with aggressive treatment (hyperventilation, mannitol, glycerol, corticosteroids) is warranted because elevated intracranial pressure indicates a poor prognosis. Corticosteroids reduce vasogenic edema, but their value is still controversial because

Cerebellar	Pontine
Nausea, vomiting	Quadriplegia
Ataxia	Pinpoint pupils
Facial weakness, coma	Absent horizontal eye movement
Decerebrate posturing	Bobbing of eyes
	Coma
	Respiratory abnormalities

there is no convincing evidence of improved outcome. If the headache is severe, use analgesics but avoid narcotic medications that depress respiration as resultant carbon dioxide retention worsens intracranial hypertension. Avoid aspirin-containing products for headache control as these exacerbate bleeding and hemorrhage expansion. If seizures occur, treat with intravenous phenytoin, but seizure prophylaxis is probably not warranted. The prognosis is poor in large pontine, putaminal, thalamic hemorrhages; however, in small hemorrhages the prognosis is good for recovery.

CEREBRAL AMYLOID (CONGOPHILIC) ANGIOPATHY

Primary cerebral amyloid angiopathy consists of infiltration of amyloid in cerebral blood vessels and is not associated with systemic amyloidosis. The diagnosis is suspected in cases of single or multiple intracerebral hemorrhages found in nonhypertensive patients usually over 60 years of age but can occur in younger patients in familial cases. Hemorrhages are predominately found at the junction of cortex and white matter in frontal, parietal, and occipital lobes ("lobar hemorrhages"). In one third of patients there is history of previous intracerebral hemorrhage. Treatment consists of supportive medical management or surgical evacuation.

SUBARACHNOID HEMORRHAGE CAUSED BY SACCULAR ARTERIAL ANEURYSM

The most frequent cause of primary nontraumatic subarachnoid hemorrhage (SAH) is rupture of arterial saccular aneurysm—the so-called berry, or congenital, type. Aneurysms are arterial dilatations found at bifurcations of large arteries at the base of the brain, usually in the anterior portion of the circle of Willis. They arise at sites where congenital medial arterial wall defects (the absence of muscular layer) are frequent. There is evidence that degeneration of the elastic layer occurs at the same places, so endothelium and fibrous tissue yield to intravascular pressure forming saccular dilatation. They are rarely seen in infancy or childhood and are more frequently symptomatic in young and middle-aged patients. In approximately 20% of patients aneurysms are multiple. Although hypertension is seen in 50% of patients in the acute symptomatic phase, this is not the cause of SAH. Asymptomatic aneurysms are found in approximately 5% of the general population, being detected at angiography (done for reasons other than bleeding episodes) or at autopsy. The clinical spectrum of aneurysms include the following:

- *No symptoms.* Aneurysm is found incidentally at autopsy or angiography. The most frequent site of unruptured aneurysm is MCA bifurcation.
- *Compression of adjacent structures.* The third nerve is the most frequently compressed neural structure. Third nerve palsy as a result of aneurysmal compression usually begins in acute fashion with orbital pain, ptosis, eye deviation outward and downward, and dilated paralytic pupil. Aneurysm usually arises from ICA at its junction with posterior communicating artery. Multiple cranial nerves (third, fourth, fifth, and sixth) can be compressed by aneurysms arising in the cavernous sinus portion of ICA. Aneurysms can enlarge sella turcica to simulate juxtasellar pituitary mass. Giant saccular aneurysms (larger than 3 cm) can

compress brain tissue, block CSF pathways, cause mass effect, or cause SAH. In giant aneurysms there is frequently evidence of partial or complete aneurysm thrombosis, but SAH can occur. Posterior fossa aneurysms can appear as expanding infratentorial mass lesions compressing the brain stem or cerebellum.

- *Rupture.* This is the most frequent complication of symptomatic aneurysms. The most frequent site of the ruptured aneurysm is the ICA junction with the posterior communicating artery, followed very closely by anterior cerebral–anterior communicating artery junction (Figure 10-4). Rupture of an aneurysm can produce pure SAH, SAH with intracerebral and/or intraventricular hematoma, SAH with subdural hematoma, SAH with infarction secondary to vasospasm, or microembolism from the aneurysmal sac.

Symptomatology of Ruptured Aneurysm

SAH causes severe headache ("worst headache I ever had") that can be associated with transitory loss of consciousness or weakness of the legs. This is described as "first and worst headache." It comes on as a "thunderclap" without warning and without the gradual build-up phase. This latter feature is characteristic of migraine headache and serves as an important differentiating feature. A stiff neck is not usually found early in SAH, but photophobia and miosis can be initial manifestations. Because no focal motor deficit is usually found, the patient is often misdiagnosed and released from the emergency department or physician's office with a prescription for analgesics and told that this is benign "vascular" or "tension" headache. This is a catastrophic mistake to fail to recognize the warning features of the "sentinel bleed" in

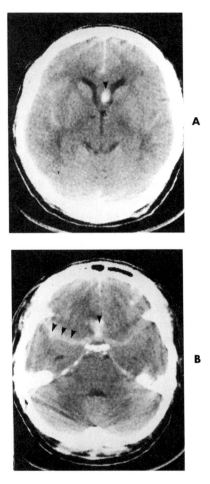

FIGURE 10-4. A, CT shows blood in the caval-septal region. B, Blood is seen in anterior interhemispheric fissure (*single arrow*) and extending into left middle cerebral artery cistern (*horizontal arrows*). This is characteristic pattern of ruptured anterior-cerebral-anterior communicating artery aneurysm that was subsequently demonstrated by angiogram.

SAH patients. The neurologically intact SAH patient is the patient in whom CT or lumbar puncture is mandatory to diagnose SAH; however, frequently the opportunity for early diagnosis of "sentinel" or "warning" leak caused by a ruptured aneurysm is missed because of failure to recognize the need for these diagnostic procedures, especially LP. Lumbar puncture is the most definitive study to diagnose recent SAH. If lumbar puncture is delayed for several days, red blood cells and xanthochromia can disappear from CSF, and diagnosis of SAH can be missed. This can be quite dangerous because mortality from an initial aneurysmal hemorrhage is 10%; however, mortality from a second hemorrhage is greater than 50%. CT is sensitive to detect subarachnoid blood if performed within 48 hours of bleed; however, CT sensitivity falls off significantly after this time. Early medical measures can prevent rebleeding. A second hemorrhage can occur, usually in the first week, and at that point an intracerebral hematoma can develop from the rebleeding aneurysm with severe deterioration in neurologic condition. Grading of patients according to their neurologic function helps surgical management and prognosis. Box 10-12 outlines the five grades.

Potential complications resulting from ruptured aneurysm include sudden and massive intracranial hypertension, mass effect and cerebral edema, hydrocephalus from mass effect or from blood in subarachnoid spaces or ventricular system, vasospasm and cerebral ischemia from subarachnoid blood, and rebleeding. Demonstration of aneurysm and associated vasospasm is established by angiography. CT/MRI can demonstrate an infarcted brain mass effect or hydrocephalus. Transcranial Doppler is an

BOX 10–12

Grade 1 Patients are asymptomatic or alert and oriented and have a mild headache and slight neck stiffness.

Grade 2 Patients have moderate to severe headache with major meningeal signs, mild alteration in sensorium, and no neurologic deficit other than cranial nerve palsy caused by direct aneurysmal compression.

Grade 3 Patients are drowsy, confused, or have mild focal deficit.

Grade 4 Patients show stupor, moderate to severe hemiparesis, possible early decerebrate rigidity, and vegetative disturbances.

Grade 5 Patients are in deep coma, with decerebrate rigidity and moribund appearance.

effective technique to follow noninvasively the increase or reduction of vasospasm without a repeat angiogram.

Treatment

Treatment of an aneurysm patient varies depending on the patient's clinical grade. Medical management consists of carefully controlling systemic arterial hypertension. Blood pressure should be monitored and stabilized according to clinical response. Sustained hypertension can be necessary to perfuse brain and prevent vasospasm. Total bed rest, sedation, and laxatives are used to avoid a sudden rise of blood pressure and development of intracranial pressure; both factors can cause rebleeding. It is important to treat headache, nausea, and vomiting; if these are not controlled, the patient can become agitated. Use of sedative drugs (phenobarbital, diazepam) can calm patients and prevent rebleeding. Cardiac arrhythmias are frequently detected in SAH patients and can be life threatening, so cardiac monitoring is warranted. Careful control of sodium and fluid balance is performed because hyponatremia can cause seizures. In managing fluids and electrolytes do not use severe fluid restriction because this can contract blood volume and increase hematocrit and blood viscosity. When these abnormalities occur, this can initiate vasospasm to cause cerebral ischemia. Administer 2 to 3 L of crystalloid fluids to maintain adequate intravascular volume. Use the central venous line or pulmonary wedge pressure monitoring to avoid fluid overload. Avoid intracranial hypertension, which can result in cerebral ischemia or herniation. If conventional treatment (hyperventilation, corticosteroids) is not effective, barbiturate coma, diversionary shunting, or surgical hematoma evacuation may be necessary to control intracranial pressure. Serial CT studies are necessary to determine if hydrocephalus is developing; if so, ventricular drainage or a diversionary shunt may be necessary. Recurrent bleeding and vasospasm are the most dreaded complications of ruptured aneurysms. Surgical aneurysm clipping is necessary to avoid rebleeding. Antifibrinolytic medication (aminocaproic acid [Amicar]) can be used before surgery to prevent lysis; however, deep vein thrombosis, pulmonary embolism, or ischemic stroke can be potential risks as a result of the effect of medication. To prevent vasospasm, volume expansion (supplemented by drug-induced hypertension) and calcium channel blocking agents (nimodipine) are effective.

▨ VASCULAR MALFORMATIONS

Vascular malformations are congenital lesions originating early in fetal life and varying in degree from dilatations of capillaries (telangiectasia, usually small and frequently found as incidental lesions at autopsy) to large cavernous arterial or venous dilatations that consist of arteriovenous malformations (AVM) or fistulas and can communicate without the intervening capillary bed. When these lesions are familial, they can be associated with neurocutaneous syndromes (phakomatoses).

Signs and Symptoms

Subarachnoid or intracerebral hemorrhage in a young patient with history of seizures is highly suggestive of vascular malformation. Seizure disorder can precede the onset of brain hemorrhage. Deep cerebral hemispheric, brain stem, or cerebellum malformations usually are not preceded by seizure disorder and can appear as intracranial hemorrhage. Once the hemorrhage has occurred, the probability of recurrent bleeding is high. Mortality from bleeding is less than that associated with ruptured aneurysm.

Diagnostic Studies

CT/MRI can demonstrate vascular malformation (Figure 10-5); prior episodes of hemorrhage are best demonstrated by MRI. Angiography is necessary to define supplying and draining vessels of the vascular malformation.

Treatment

Treatment varies according to the site and size of the lesion but is predominantly surgical if the lesion is in a resectable area. If AVM is large, embolization using particulate material introduced at the time of angiography through an arterial catheter can occlude supplying vessels to reduce AVM size. Medical management during the acute stage is similar to that of SAH

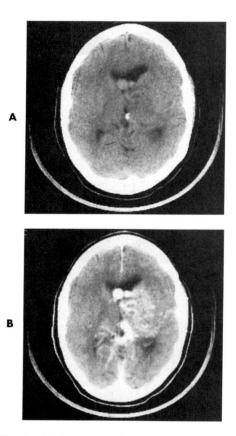

FIGURE 10-5. **A,** Noncontrast CT shows hyperdense noncalcified globular serpiginous areas representing abnormal vessels. **B,** There is dense contrast enhancement consistent with large arteriovenous malformation, confirmed angiographically.

caused by ruptured aneurysm. It is necessary to be able to surgically resect the vascular malformation because clipping supplying and draining vessels is not effective.

▦ INTRACRANIAL HEMORRHAGE— OTHER CAUSES

Other causes of intracerebral hemorrhage are uncommon, and there are usually clinical clues to the cause. Blood dyscrasias and anticoagulants can produce multiple intracranial hematomas. Multiple hemorrhagic lesions visualized by CT with a pulmonary lesion indicate metastasis; a history of drug abuse suggests vasculitis. Evidence of systemic manifestations (fever, arthritis, skin rash) suggests vasculitis or endocarditis. Anemia, visceromegaly, and retinal splinter hemorrhages suggest leukemia. Investigate carefully for history of substance abuse, for example, cocaine or amphetamines, as this can cause the hemorrhage.

▦ DURAL AND CORTICAL VEIN THROMBOSIS

Dural and cortical vein thrombosis can be septic. These are usually associated with pyogenic or fungal infections. This can occur as a complication of meningitis. Noninfectious or marantic thrombosis can occur as a complication of malnutrition, congenital heart disease, polycythemia, dehydration, head injuries, or coagulation disorders. The most commonly involved sinuses are superior sagittal, lateral, cavernous, and straight. Sinuses have a prominent role in CSF circulation; therefore venous sinus thrombosis leads to intracranial hypertension and hydrocephalus. In young females dural venous thrombosis is sometimes associated with oral contraceptive use. It also occurs during postpartum period or pregnancy and can be related to hypercoagulability. Clinical features can be increased intracranial pressure (headache and vomiting), seizures, and focal motor deficit. Angiography is the most specific diagnostic test for showing whether blood has filled veins and sinuses. CT/MRI can show thrombosed veins as well as hemorrhagic venous infarct. Treatment depends on the cause. Intracranial hypertension is frequently present and should be aggressively managed. For prevention of venous thrombotic process, anticoagulants have been used; however, they have potential to cause further bleeding if a hemorrhagic infarct is present. For septic venous thrombosis antibiotics are necessary to treat underlying infections.

SUMMARY

Cerebrovascular disease is most commonly one part of multifocal atherosclerotic (coronary artery disease, peripheral arterial vascular disease) or hypertensive vascular disease. Stroke is the most common cause of disability and the third leading cause of death in adults. Stroke can result from leakage of blood through the damaged arterial wall to result in intracerebral or subarachnoid hemorrhage or from occlusion of cerebral blood vessels to result in ischemia or infarction. Intracerebral hemorrhage is most commonly caused by hypertension and occurs within the putamen, thalamus, cerebellum, and pons. Subarachnoid hemorrhage most commonly is due to ruptured berry aneurysms or vascular malformations. Cerebral infarction can be due to occlusion of cerebral arteries as a result of cardiac disease with embolization of thrombus (clot) to the brain (cardiogenic cerebral embolism) or to occlusion of large (extracranial or intracrannial) or small (intracranial) arteries derived from the carotid or vertebral-basilar vascular system. It is important to recognize the warning symptoms of cerebrovascular disease, which are called "transient ischemic attacks," because one third of these patients subsequently develop strokes without appropriate medical or surgical treatment.

Suggested Readings

Cerebrovascular Risk Factors
Wolf PA, Kannel WB, Verter J: Current status of risk factors for stroke, *Neurol Clin North Am* 1:317, 1983.

Adams HP, Butter MJ: Nonhemorrhagic cerebral infarction in young adults, *Arch Neurol* 43:793, 1986.

Wolf PA, D'Agostino RB, Belanger AJ: Probability of stroke: a risk profile from the Framingham study, *Stroke* 22:312, 1991.

Sacco RL, Hauser WA, Mohr JP: One-year outcome after cerebral infarction in whites, blacks, and hispanics, *Stroke* 22:305, 1991.

Gorelick PB: Alcohol and stroke, *Stroke* 18:268, 1987.

Atherogenesis
Yatsu FM, Fisher M: Atherosclerosis: current concepts on pathogenesis and interventional therapies, *Ann Neurol* 26:3, 1989.

Adams RJ, Carroll RM: Plasma lipoproteins in cortical versus lacunar infarction, *Stroke* 20:448, 1989.

Amarenco P, Dukekaerts PT: The prevalence of ulcerated plaques in aortic arch in patients with stroke, 326:221, 1992.

Asymptomatic Carotid Stenosis
Ingall TJ, Homer D, Whisnant JB: Predictive value of carotid bruit for carotid atherosclerosis, *Arch Neurol* 46:418, 1989.

van Ruiswyk J, Noble H: Natural history of carotid bruits in elderly persons, *Ann Intern Med* 112:340, 1990.

Chambers BR, Norris JW: Outcome in patients with asymptomatic neck bruits, *N Engl J Med* 315:860, 1986.

Norris JW, Zhu CZ: Silent stroke and carotid stenosis, *Stroke* 23:483, 1992.

Hennerici M, Hulsbomer HB: Natural history of asymptomatic extracranial arterial disease, *Brain* 110:777, 1987.

Thompson JE, Patman RD: Long-term outcome of patients having endarterectomy compared with unoperated controls, *Ann Surg* 188:308, 1978.

Yatsu FM, Fields WS: Asymptomatic carotid bruit: stenosis or ulceration, a conservative approach, *Arch Neurol* 42:383, 1985.

Executive Committee for the Asymptomatic Carotid Atherosclerosis Study, *JAMA* 273:1421, 1995.

Transient Cerebrovascular Disorders

Caplan L: Transient ischemic attacks, *Neurology* 38:791, 1988.

Bogousslarsky J, Regli F: Ischemic stroke in adults younger than 30 years of age, *Arch Neurol* 44:479, 1987.

Hankey GJ, Warlow CP: Lacunar transient ischemic attacks, *Lancet* 337:335, 1991.

Treatment of Transient Cerebral Ischemic Disorders

Canadian Cooperative Study: A randomized trial of aspirin and sulfinpyrazone in threatened stroke, *N Engl J Med* 299:53, 1978.

Antiplatelet Trialist's Collaboration: Secondary prevention of vascular disease by prolonged antiplatelet treatment, *Br Med J* 290:320, 1988.

ESPS Group: European stroke prevention study, *Lancet* 2:1351, 1987.

Levy DE: How transient are transient ischemic attacks? *Neurology* 38:674, 1988.

Gent M, Easton JD, Hachinski VC: 1989. Canadian-American ticlopidine study (CATS) in thromboembolic stroke, *Lancet* 1:86, 1989.

Hass WK, Easton JD, Adams HP: A randomized trial comparing ticlopidine hydrochloride with aspirin for the prevention of stroke in high-risk patients, *N Engl J Med* 321:501, 1989.

Dutch TIA Trial Study Group: Comparison of two doses of aspirin (30 mgm vs. 283 mgm a day) in patients after TIA or minor ischemic stroke, *N Engl J Med* 325:1261, 1991.

North American Surgical Carotid Endarterectomy Trial Collaborators: Beneficial effect of carotid endarterectomy in symptomatic patients with high-grade carotid stenosis, *N Engl J Med* 325:445, 1991.

UK-TIA Study Group: The United Kingdom transient ischemic attack (UK-TIA) aspirin trial: final results, *J Neurol Neurosurg Psychiatry* 54:1044, 1991.

Treatment of Progressing or Completed Stroke

Grotta JC: Current medical and surgical therapy for cerebrovascular disease, *N Engl J Med* 317:1505, 1987.

Duke RJ, Bloch RF, Turpie AG: Intravenous heparin for the prevention of stroke in acute partial stable stroke, *Ann Intern Med* 105:825, 1986.

Marshall RS, Mohr JP: Current management of ischemic stroke, *J Neurol Neurosurg Psychiatry* 70:6, 1993.

Cardiogenic Cerebral Embolism

Boston Area Anticoagulation Trial for atrial fibrillation investigators: the effect of low dose warfarin on the risk of stroke in patients with nonvalvular atrial fibrillation, *N Engl J Med* 323:1505, 1990.

Cerebral Embolism Study Group: Cardioembolic stroke: immediate anticoagulation and brain hemorrhage, *Arch Intern Med* 147:636, 1987.

Conally SJ, Laupacis A, Gent M: Canadian atrial fibrillation anticoagulation study, *J Am Coll Cardiol* 18:349, 1991.

Kittner SJ, Sharkness CM, Price L: Infarcts with a cardiac source of embolism, *Neurology* 40:281, 1990.

Yatsu FM, Hart RG, Mohr JP: Anticoagulation of embolic strokes of cardiac origin, *Neurology* 38:314, 1988.

Lacunes

Mohr JP: Lacunes, *Stroke* 13:3, 1982.

Weisberg LA: Diagnostic classification of stroke, especially lacunes, *Stroke* 19:1071, 1988.

Bamford J, Sandercock P, Jones L: The natural history of lacunar infarction: the Oxfordshire Community stroke project, *Stroke* 18:545, 1987.

Weisberg LA: Racial differences for lacunar infarcts documented by CT: comparison of black and white patients, *J Stroke Cerebrovascular Dis* 3:157, 1993.

Nonatherosclerotic Causes of Stroke

Bevan H, Sherma K, Bradley W: Stroke in young adults, *Stroke* 21:382, 1990.

Levine ER, Welch KMA: Cerebrovascular ischemia associated with lupus anticoagulant, *Stroke* 18:257, 1987.

Bogousslarsky J, Regli F: Cerebral infarction with transient signs, *Stroke* 15:536, 1984.

Adams HR: Nonhemorrhagic cerebral infarction in young adults, *Arch Neuro* 43:793, 1986.

Bogousslarsky J, Pierce P: Ischemic stroke in patients under age 45, *Neurol Clin North Am* 19:113, 1992.

Kaku DA, Luwenstein DH: Emergence of recreational drug use as major risk factor for stroke in young adults, *Ann Intern Med* 113:821, 1990.

Levine SR, Welch KMA: Antiphospholipid antibodies, *Ann Neurol* 26:386, 1989.

Intracerebral Hemorrhage

Gilles C, Brucher JM, Khoubesserian P, et al: Cerebral amyloid angiopathy as a cause of multiple intracerebral hemorrhages, *Neurology* 34:730, 1984.

Weisberg LA, Stazio A, Shamsnia M: Nontraumatic parenchymal brain hemorrhages, *Medicine* 69:277, 1990.

Caplan L: Intracerebral hemorrhage revisited, *Neurology* 38:624, 1988.

Aneurysms

Kassell NF, Drake CG: Review of the management of saccular aneurysms, *Neurol Clin North Am* 1:73, 1983.

Biller J, Godersky JC, Adams HP: Management of aneurysmal subarachnoid hemorrhage, *Stroke* 19:1300, 1988.

Solomon RA, Fink ME: Current strategies for the management of aneurysmal subarachnoid hemorrhage, *Arch Neurol* 44:769, 1987.

Adams HP, Jergensen DD, Kassell NP: Pitfalls in diagnosis of subarachnoid hemorrhage, *JAMA* 244:794, 1980.

Vascular Malformations

Stein B, Wolpert A: Arteriovenous malformations of the brain, *Arch Neurol* 37:1, 1980.

Crawford, PM, West CR, Chadwick DW: Arteriovenous malformations of the brain: natural history in unoperated patients, *J Neurol Neurosurg Psychiatry* 49:1, 1986.

Jane JA, Kassell NF, Tonern JC: The natural history of aneurysms and arteriovenous malformations, *J Neurosurg* 62:321, 1985.

Venous Occlusive Disease

Ameri A, Bousser MG: Cerebral venous thrombosis, *Neurol Clin North Am* 10:87, 1992.

Bousser MG, Chiras J, Sauron B: Cerebral venous thrombosis, *Stroke* 16:199, 1985.

Averback P: Primary cerebral venous thrombosis in young adults: the diverse manifestations of an under-recognized disease, *Ann Neurol* 3:81, 1978.

CHAPTER

Seizures and Epilepsy

11

DEFINITION AND INCIDENCE

Hughlings Jackson defined epilepsy as a group of disorders characterized by excessive and paroxysmal neural discharges causing sudden alteration in neurologic function. The terms "epilepsy" and "seizure" refer to similar clinical conditions; however, epilepsy refers to *recurrent* seizures. It implies the presence of cerebral dysrhythmia (paroxysmal discharges of cerebral neurons indicating an underlying condition characterized by abnormal cortical excitability) for which there may be underlying genetic basis. Epilepsy implies recurrent seizures unprovoked by toxic, febrile, or metabolic conditions. The recurrent seizures can be symptomatic of an underlying microscopic or macroscopic brain lesion; but they can occur in the absence of identifiable pathologic or biochemical abnormality (idiopathic). Seizures are classified according to clinical manifestations of episodes and the EEG pattern.

Seizures affect almost 1.5 million persons in this country (6.5 people per 1000 are affected). One of every 10 or 20 patients will have one seizure during his or her lifetime, and 1 out of 200 develop epilepsy. The diagnosis of epilepsy should be established accurately on clinical and EEG features because of the adverse impact on the patient of an incorrect diagnosis, for example, the stigma of being diagnosed as "epileptic," the need to use potentially toxic antiepileptic medications, and restrictions imposed on the patient's lifestyle. Despite the importance of a high degree of accuracy, 10% to 25% of patients subsequently evaluated for medically intractable seizures actually have nonepileptic events.

■ CLINICAL HISTORY

The keystone to diagnosis and classification is accurate description of the clinical event. It is most important that observers (friends, family, and co-workers) be questioned because the patient may be amnestic and unable to provide a complete description or assess episode frequency. Clinical features of seizures are analyzed by the individual stages. Try to characterize these as carefully and completely as possible for each seizure.

Prodrome

This can last for several hours. There can be subtle changes in mood, behavior, or thinking, characterized by increased anxiety, depression, or an inability to concentrate or think clearly. Close observers can be cognizant of this change and able to predict subsequent seizure occurrence. There are no changes in EEG pattern during this stage. If prodromal pattern is stereotyped, occurs early, and lasts long enough, it is sometimes possible for patients to abort the attack with extra doses of medications, but medication does not take effect rapidly enough to be effective when taken in this manner only.

Aura

The aura is the *initial* portion of the seizure; the EEG pattern changes, signaling the localized seizure origin. The aura usually lasts several seconds to minutes. Aura occurs in *partial* seizures of simple partial type with elementary symptomatology (jacksonian motor march, spreading paresthesias) or complex partial seizures (foul odor, rising feeling in chest or stomach, bitter taste in the mouth, thought disorders). The aura frequently helps localize the origin of seizure discharge. In primary generalized seizures, patients experience *no* aura.

Ictus

Ictus refers to the seizure episode. Ictus begins abruptly; the patient can be normal then unconscious or unaware of surroundings and unable to respond appropriately seconds later. Individual attacks can last 15 to 30 seconds in absence of seizures, 2 to 5 minutes in major motor seizures, and 1 to 5 minutes in simple or complex partial seizures. The EEG is invariably abnormal if recorded during the ictus; however, rarely in certain partial complex seizures, the surface EEG is normal, but an abnormal pattern is seen if sphenoidal, nasopharyngeal, or depth electrodes are used (Figure 11-1). The EEG should be abnormal during major motor seizures, although EEG abnormalities can be obscured by muscle potential artifacts; therefore a normal ictal EEG is strong evidence that the "seizure" is *nonepileptic,* for example syncope or psychogenic seizure. The patient is amnestic for ictus in generalized (major motor, absence) and partial complex seizures but is not amnestic in simple partial seizures.

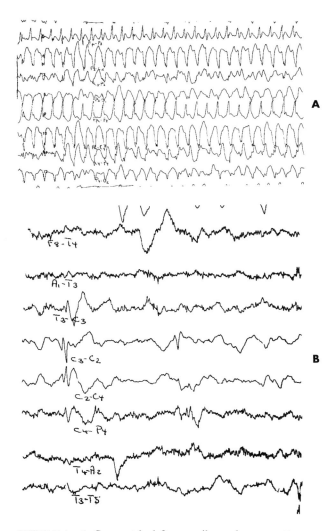

FIGURE 11-1. **A,** Symmetrical 3-cps spike and wave pattern in a child with absence seizures. **B,** Several bursts of spikes followed by slow wave in the interictal period of a patient with generalized seizures.

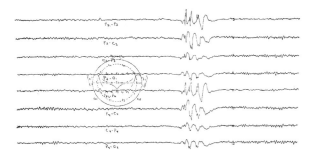

FIGURE 11-1, cont'd. C, Normal background rhythm followed by drowsiness (suppression of normal background) followed by a burst of spike and wave in a patient with generalized seizures.

Postictal Stage

This refers to events immediately after the seizure. Following absence seizures patients can be perfectly alert and resume speech or work at the point it was discontinued, whereas following major motor or partial complex seizures the patient can be dazed, confused, or disoriented. Family members may report that on certain mornings the patient awakens and appears "not to be quite right"; this suggests that a nocturnal seizure has occurred, and the patient has early morning postictal state. During the postictal period the patient should be examined carefully for Todd's postictal paralysis (hemiparesis, aphasia, anesthesia, reflex asymmetry, Babinski sign, visual field defect) neurologic deficit. This can be the diagnostic signature to lesion localization. In postictus the EEG can show diffuse or focal slow wave activity with suppression of normal background activity and then slowly normalize. Elevation of serum prolactin content can develop immediately following generalized tonic-clonic and partial complex seizure (within 30–60 minutes), rapidly normalizing in interictus. This prolactin elevation differentiates epileptic seizures from psychogenic nonepileptic seizures.

Interictal Period

Between attacks the patient appears entirely normal, especially if seizures are infrequent. Other patients have persistent focal deficit because of the presence of an underlying structural lesion.

▨ SEIZURE HISTORY

In patients with seizures the following information must be ascertained:

- Family history of seizures, episodes of sudden unexplained death, neurologic, or neurocutaneous diseases.
- Birth history, especially relating to perinatal hypoxia.
- Prior episodes of head trauma or CNS infection.
- Use of medication or drugs including alcohol, antihistamines, antipsychotics, antidepressants, and illicit drugs, especially phencyclidine and cocaine. These drugs and others can precipitate seizures.
- Precipitating factors for seizures including fever, sleep deprivation, menstruation, hyperventilation, emotional stress, and exposure to flashing lights (photic stress) as occurs with video games.

Description of the seizure should include a detailed account of the patient during each stage. The types of questions that should be asked are listed in Box 11-1.

A neurologic examination can be performed in the interictal or postictal phase. In the interictal stage

BOX 11-1

1 Was there any change in patient's personality, mood, or behavior before the seizure?

2 What were the circumstances in which the seizure occurred?

3 Was there an abrupt beginning to the episode, and how did the attack terminate including the postictal phase?

4 Were there premonitory symptoms? (Lightheadedness, visual blurring, weakness, dizziness indicate syncope.)

5 How did patient appear during the seizure?
   a Was there loss of awareness or responsiveness, or did patient completely lose consciousness?
   b Did patient lose postural control? Any evidence of patient injury?
   c What type of motor (rhythmical symmetrical tonic-clonic, diffuse myoclonic jerking, stereotyped repetitive semipurposeful) activity occurred?
   d Did tongue biting or maceration occur?
   e Did urinary or fecal incontinence occur?

6 What characterized the patient in the postictal stage?
   a Lethargy, disorientation, or focal neurologic deficit? How long in duration?
   b Autonomic disturbances? Hyperventilation and tachycardia can be seen following seizures; hypotension, bradycardia, and other cardiac arrhythmias are more common with syncope.
   c Other symptoms, including headache and myalgias?

7 When do attacks occur?
   a Pattern: single or bursts?
   b Duration of each attack?
   c Time of occurrence: diurnal or nocturnal?
   d Relationship to other precipitating factors?

8 Are attacks stereotyped or are there multiple clinical seizure patterns?

9 Are seizures controlled with medication?

10 Does patient comply with medication?

11 Is there medication toxicity?

attention is directed toward defining mental change (memory loss, behavioral change, dementia), focal neurologic deficit, and intracranial hypertension. Listen over the patient's head with a stethoscope for bruit caused by vascular malformation, and inspect the skin for evidence of neurocutaneous disorders (café au lait spots, neurofibroma, facial hemangioma, depigmented spots). Examination in postictal period should be made for Todd's motor paralysis, visual field or hemisensory defect, reflex asymmetry, Babinski sign, and meningeal signs suggesting meningitis or subarachnoid hemorrhage.

CLINICAL SEIZURE DISORDERS (Box 11-2)

Generalized Seizures

Tonic-Clonic Seizures (Primary Generalized, Major Motor, and Grand Mal)

Primary generalized seizures begin without an aura. Initially there is a sudden loss of consciousness. If standing, the patient falls to the ground like a wooden board in a hypertonic (rigid) position; the patient can be injured by falling. An initial tonic position is assumed: trunk and neck are hyperextended, shoulders and arms are extended and abducted, wrists are supinated, legs are extended, and feet are plantar flexed. An epileptic cry occurs as air is expelled forcibly through abducted vocal cords. The patient can become cyanotic, but apnea and respiratory arrest are infrequent unless the seizure is prolonged or status epilepticus occurs. The tongue can be macerated; urinary or fecal incontinence can occur.

The tonic phase is interrupted by the clonic phase, during which there are symmetrical and rhythmical

BOX 11-2   Classification of Seizures

Generalized Seizures

Tonic-clonic seizures

Absence seizures
   Simple
   Complex or atypical (with myoclonic jerks, change in
      postural tone, automatisms)
   Myoclonic seizures
   Infantile spasms
   Tonic seizures
   Atonic seizures

Partial Seizures

Simple partial (consciousness preserved)
   Motor symptoms
   Somatosensory symptoms
   Special sensory (visual, auditory) symptoms
   Autonomic features
   Psychic symptoms
Complex partial (consciousness impaired)
   Cognitive
   Affective

Secondarily Generalized Seizures

Simple partial evolving to generalized seizure
Complex partial evolving to generalized seizure
Simple partial evolving to complex partial, then to generalized
   seizures

jerking movements of head, body, and extremities.
Initially, these occur at 2 cps; they become irregular
and intermittent and then stop. The clonic jerking
never stops *abruptly* in epileptic seizure as this abrupt
cessation of clonic jerking is characteristic of pseudoseizures. Seizures usually last 2 to 5 minutes, but it is
not uncommon for observers to overestimate seizure
duration because of the anxiety engendered by the
attack. If the seizure occurs at night (nocturnal) and

the patient is alone, the only evidence that the seizure occurred may be that the patient awakens on the floor having violently been thrown off the bed by the motor activity, has a bloodied or macerated tongue, or has urinated in the bed.

Postictally, the patient is confused and drowsy; this can last several minutes to 24 hours. Because of intense muscle contractions during the seizure, myalgias can persist for several hours. Autonomic phenomena include pupillary dilatation, salivation, diaphoresis, tachycardia, and hypertension. Respirations are rapid and shallow as a result of lactic acidosis caused by intense muscle activity. Patients complain of headaches caused by vasodilation and muscle contractions resulting from seizure activity.

During the tonic phase the EEG demonstrates generalized symmetrical spike discharges; this changes to spikes interspersed with slow waves in the clonic stage. Because of intense muscle activity, the EEG can be obscured by muscle potential artifact. Postictally there is generalized slowing, and low-voltage pattern and background activity is suppressed. A normal EEG during the episode would be inconsistent with epileptic seizures; however, 25% of seizure patients have a normal interictal EEG. Patients with frequent seizures are more likely to have an abnormal EEG than patients with infrequent seizures. The more times that interictal EEG is performed, the more likely that EEG abnormality is detected because of increased EEG "sampling time." The "routine" EEG obtained during an awake state should be supplemented by an EEG obtained during hyperventilation (duration 2 to 3 minutes), during natural or drug-induced sleep, and following photic stimulation. Newer techniques including video monitoring (observing simultaneous EEG and patient activity during a "seizure") and ambulatory EEG monitoring (similar to cardiographic Holter monitoring) are useful in *selected* patients suspected of having seizures but in whom there is diagnostic uncertainty. Certain activation procedures using pharmacologic agents (short-acting barbiturates, Metrazol) or nasopharyngeal electrodes (to demonstrate temporal region spike discharges) can be indicated if diagnosis of epilepsy is uncertain. In patients with clinically witnessed generalized tonic-clonic seizures but in whom focal onset may not be observed, the EEG is crucial for detecting the electrical focality of the seizure. The presence of focal spike and slow wave discharge suggests an underlying pathological lesion, but focal spike discharge alone can occur without underlying lesions detected by CT/MRI.

Because diagnosis of seizure disorder is established clinically, the role of EEG in suggesting the diagnosis of "epileptiform activity" without any clinical evidence to support this impression should be discouraged. Because 5% to 15% of the normal population (without seizures) have nonspecific abnormal EEG patterns and even some nonepileptic patients have EEG spike patterns, overreliance on an EEG for establishing the epilepsy diagnosis should be discouraged. For example, a history of fainting spells occurring in a patient with a nonspecific EEG abnormality should not be used to make the diagnosis of epilepsy.

If the patient is evaluated *immediately* following the initial seizure, studies including complete blood count, urinalysis, blood sugar, calcium and phosphorus, serum electrolytes (including bicarbonate and magnesium), liver and renal function profile, toxicology screen, and urine porphyrins should be performed. If these are negative, lumbar puncture should be done to exclude subarachnoid hemorrhage or meningitis. Skull roentgenography is important to detect intracranial calcification as seen in certain congenital diseases (tuberous sclerosis, Sturge-Weber syndrome), infections (toxoplasmosis), neoplasms (meningioma, astrocytoma, oligodendroglioma), or vascular malformations. With high-resolution CT, intracranial calcification is readily detected. CT/MRI is indicated for patients with partial seizures and for patients with generalized seizures who have EEG evidence of focal discharge or focal postictal neurologic deficit. MRI is indicated for patients with partial seizures with negative CT as certain cortical abnormalities (cortical heterotopia, hippocampal sclerosis) are better visualized with MRI. CT/MRI are not necessary in patients with *primary generalized* epilepsy because of very low likelihood of an underlying structural abnormality being present.

Certain patients diagnosed *initially* as having primary generalized tonic-clonic seizures initially have no clinical or EEG findings to indicate focal onset; however, focal features can develop at a later time. This indicates the need for periodic reassessment of seizure patients. Specific indications for reassessment for epilepsy patients include the following: change in type of seizure pattern, increase in seizure frequency despite compliance with drug therapy and high anticonvulsant blood levels, and development of neurologic deterioration of generalized (dementia, memory loss) or focal type not explained by medication effect.

The onset of primary generalized tonic-clonic seizures is before age 25. There is increased familial incidence especially if seizures occurred in childhood; this familial tendency decreases in older patients. It has been speculated that the genetic pattern for primary generalized tonic-clonic seizures is autosomal dominant with incomplete penetrance.

Once a diagnosis of primary generalized tonic-clonic seizure has been established and diagnostic studies have not detected pathological or metabolic abnormality, decide whether to treat the initial seizure and make choice of the appropriate medication. Most physicians assume that the initial seizure is the harbinger of epilepsy attacks and requires prophylactic anticonvulsant therapy; however, 5% of the general population has single nonfebrile and nonprovoked seizure. If patient has seizure recurrence, this usually occurs within 1 to 3 years of initial seizure. Because certain patients do not have recurrence, the risk of treatment must be weighed against "watchful waiting" approach (danger of patient injury from the next seizure or possibility that status epilepticus will be next seizure). The decision to withhold treatment to determine if seizure is an isolated episode or is recurrent carries risk because there is suggestive evidence that early control is associated with low recurrence rate. Prophylactic therapy for a single seizure is warranted for the following situations: the initial seizure was long in duration with prolonged postictal Todd's paralysis, the interictal EEG shows specific epileptiform activity, a second seizure would interfere with the patient's life (financial, vocational, social, psychological), and prior history of neurologic injury that is the probable cause of the seizure, for example, head trauma, encephalitis. Drug treatment is not usually initiated if there is an obvious precipitating factor (e.g., emotional stress, alcohol or drugs, sleep deprivation) unless the seizure is the partial (simple or complex) type.

Certain general principles of prophylactic anticonvulsant management should be followed:

- Each drug has relative specificity for clinical and EEG seizure patterns (Tables 11-1 and 11-2). In general terms drugs that are effective against generalized tonic-clonic seizures exacerbate absence seizures (with exception of valproic acid).
- If the patient has several seizure types, including generalized tonic-clonic seizures, initial treatment is directed toward this seizure, which represents greatest risk to the patient. After major motor seizures are well controlled, drugs can be initiated to treat other seizure types if these persist.
- Treatment should be initiated with a single drug (monotherapy) at a low dose and gradually increased. Increase the dosage of a single anticonvulsant medication until seizures are controlled or side effects of medication occur. Adjust the dose administration schedule to accommodate patient's lifestyle but in accordance with drug half-life. With monotherapy, it is possible to avoid multiple drug interaction problems. Multiple drugs can interfere with other drug metabolism (see Tables 11-1 and 11-2), and this increases the need for frequent anticonvulsant blood levels. If adverse effects occur when the patient is treated with two drugs, it is not possible to know precisely which drug caused the adverse effect. The goal of treatment is to render the patient seizure free without causing drug toxicity. Attainment of blood level that is in the correct "therapeutic range" is important; however, the therapeutic blood levels represent a range of values at which normal individual patients achieve seizure control and at which, if exceeded, most patients become toxic. The effect

TABLE 11-1 Oral Administered Anticonvulsant Medications

Drug	Dose (mg/kg)	Frequency of Administration	Therapeutic Range (µg/ml)
Phenobarbital	0.5	Single, but usually divided with ⅔ in evening and ⅓ in morning	20–40
Phenytoin (Dilantin)	5	Single dose possible usually q 12 h or q 8 h	10–20
Primidone (Mysoline)	10–25	Divided doses q 8 h	8–12
Carbamazepine (Tegretol)	10–20	Divided doses q 6–8 h	4–8
Ethosuximide (Zarontin)	10–20	Divided doses q 12 h	40–100
Valproic acid (Depakene) (Depakote)	15–60	Divided doses q 6–8 h	50–100
Clonazapam (Clonipin)	0.1–0.2	Divided doses q 8 h	40–80
Diazepam (Valium)		Divided doses q 8 h	

Toxicity	
Dose-Related	*Idiosyncratic Reactions*
Sedation, nystagmus	Skin reaction, paradoxical hyper-kinesia (common in children)
Gingival hyperplasia vertigo, ataxia, EEG slowing, encephalopathy, neuropathy	Skin reaction, pseudolymphoma, systemic lupus, hepatitis, neutropenia, aplastic anemia
Sedation, nystagmus	Skin reaction
Sedation, nystagmus, dizziness, ataxia, slurred speech	Liver dysfunction, bone marrow suppression, skin reaction
Nausea, vomiting, sedation, dizziness	Pancytopenia, skin reaction
Nausea, vomiting	Liver dysfunction, tremor, amenorrhea, skin reaction
Sedation, dizziness	Skin reaction, drooling, hyperactivity
Sedation, ataxia	Skin reaction

Continued.

▨ TABLE 11-1 Anticonvulsant Medications—cont'd

Drug—cont'd.	Other Effects	Monitor	Drug Increases Plasma Concentration
Phenobarbital	Megaloblastic anemia	Blood level, CBC	Valproic acid
Phenytoin (Dilantin)	Megaloblastic anemia, hyper-glycemia, hirsutism, hypocalcemia, osteomalacia	Blood level, CBC, liver profile, calcium/phosphorus	Disulfiram Isoniazid Warfarin Phenobarbital Primidone Ethosuximide
Primidone (Mysoline)	Megaloblastic anemia	Blood level, CBC	Carbamazepine
Carbamazepine (Tegretol)		CBC, liver profile, blood level	Isoniazid Erythromycin Propoxyphene
Ethosuximide (Zarontin)		CBC, blood level	
Valproic acid (Depakene) (Depakote)		CBC, blood level, liver function tests	Aspirin Antacids Phenobarbital
Clonazapam (Clonipin)		CBC	
Diazepam (Valium)			

Interaction		
Decreases Drug Plasma Concentration	*Drugs Whose Plasma Concentration Is Reduced by the Anticonvulsant*	*Seizure Type*
Rifampin		Grand mal, complex partial, simple partial
Carbamazepine Ethanol Valproic acid Folic acid Loxapine Chloramphenicol	Digoxin Dexamethasone Vitamin D Oral contraceptives	Grand mal, complex partial, simple partial
Rifampin		Complete partial grand mal
Nicotinic acid		Complex partial
		Absence
Phenytoin		Lennox-Gastaut, complex partial, absence, grand mal
		Absence, Lennox-Gastaut
		Absence

TABLE 11-2 Anticonvulsant Medications

Drug	Dose (μg/ml)	Frequency of Route	Therapeutic Range	Dose-Related
Felbamate	2.5 to 7.5 1800–4800 mg daily supplied as 400 or 600 mg tablets	q 8 h	Not performed	Insomnia Fatigue Headache Fatigue Weight loss Gastro-intestinal
Gabapentin	8 to 14 600–1800 mg daily supplied as 300 to 400 mg tablets	q 8 h	Not performed	Somnolence Fatigue Ataxia Dizziness
Lomotrigine	1–4 50–300 mg daily	q h 8	Not established	Fatigue Diplopia Dizziness

for the individual patient can be quite different than the "average normal patient." If the individual patient continues to have frequent seizures with high blood levels but no clinical signs of toxicity, increase the anticonvulsant dosage until control is achieved or *signs* of toxicity occur. If control is not achieved with one drug and the patient shows signs of toxicity, switch to a second drug rather than initiate polypharmacy (using more than one medication). Two thirds of epileptic patients achieve seizure control with one medication; the addition of a second medication achieves increased seizure control in only 10% additional patients, and toxicity develops in 90% of those using two drugs. The potential for drug toxicity

Toxicity Idiosyncratic	Monitor	Use	Drug Interaction	
			Blood Level	Blood Level
——	None needed	Lennox-Gastaut Partial complex	Phenytoin Phenobarbital Valproic acid	Carbamazepine
pancreatic acinar carcinoma in animals	Renal function	Partial complex	No drug interactions as not metabolized by liver	
Rash	Liver function	Partial complex	Carbamazepine	Valproic acid

and adverse interactions between multiple antiepileptic drugs are two reasons to avoid polypharmacy. When changing the drug regimen, only modify one drug at one time so that if adverse effects occur it can easily be attributed to the most recent change. When changing drugs never *abruptly* discontinue an anticonvulsant medication because this can precipitate drug-withdrawal seizures.

- Patient noncompliance is the major reason for poor seizure control. This is defined as failure of patient to take medication in the manner prescribed by the physician. Ideally, frequency of drug administration should be based on pharmacokinetics (e.g., absorption time, drug half-life), but frequently patients alter the drug schedule to fit their lifestyles and to attempt to minimize drug toxicity (e.g., sedation of phenobarbital, epigastric distress of phenytoin). Patients are more likely to take morning and evening doses and to omit the midday dose while at work or school. Because anticonvulsants affect CNS function, they can adversely influence alertness, attention, thinking, concentration, and memory. Compliance with anticonvulsant treatment is best ensured by educating patients about seizures, goals of seizure control, the effects of medication, and their responsibility for monitoring the effects of treatment. It is futile to take medication only when the patient feels a seizure is about to occur as is attempted by some patients. All too often the physician hears about the seizure patient who completes prescription but never returns for follow-up evaluation until the seizure recurs. This is especially dangerous because blood levels of anticonvulsant medication fall rapidly and status epilepticus can develop as a result of this rapid fall. This occurs because the patient did not understand chronic and recurrent nature of epileptic disorder.

- Anticonvulsant blood level determinations are sometimes done "routinely" but are of real value in only certain circumstances. If seizure control is poor, blood levels are indicated. If they are low, possible explanations include noncompliance, poor absorption, drug interactions, abnormal plasma protein binding, rapid drug metabolism, or inactive outdated drug preparations. Noncompliance is the most common cause of low drug blood levels. Before increasing the dosage or changing medications, evaluate the patient under controlled circumstances (physician is certain that patient has taken drug). If the patient has adequate seizure control but low blood levels, it is not necessary to increase medication dose. Anticonvulsant blood levels are frequently necessary if patients are taking medications for other conditions (diabetes, hypertension, infections) or if patients receive multiple anticonvulsants (see Table 11-1).

Treatment of generalized tonic-clonic seizures. In adults, the initial drugs of choice include phenobarbital, phenytoin, valproic acid, or carbamazepine. Phenobarbital is a safe, cheap and effective anticonvulsant but it is sometimes poorly tolerated because of the sedative effect and cognitive impairment effect. Unfortunately, many patients cannot function competently when taking phenobarbital. Therapy is initiated with a dose of 0.5 mg/kg using a bedtime dose; this can be gradually increased to a maximal dose of 2.0 mg/kg daily. Because there is marked variation in individual phenobarbital tolerance, toxic level is difficult to predict. This drug can induce its own metabolism; therefore a stable dose of phenobarbital can give consistent blood levels for 4 weeks, then the blood level can drop rapidly as a result of increased hepatic metabolism. Because of the half-life of phenobarbital, it is acceptable to give the entire dose at bedtime; the alternative approach is to administer phenobarbital twice daily, with two thirds of total dose at bedtime if patient awakens too tired in the morning on once-a-day dose schedule.

Phenytoin (Dilantin) is the most widely used anticonvulsant. It does not cause sedation at usual therapeutic doses. Because absorption is slow and its half-life ranges from 12 to 24 hours, divided doses (twice daily) are usually used, although in some patients the drugs can be administered only daily and adequate seizure control is still obtained. The usual starting dosage is 300 mg daily (4.5 mg/kg). When therapy is initiated at this level, therapeutic blood levels are attained in 7 to 10 days. Rapid attainment of therapeutic blood levels ("dilantinization") within 2 days is achieved by loading dose (i.e., initial dose of 1 g, followed by 800 mg and 600 mg on second and third days). The therapeutic range of phenytoin is 10 to 20 µg/ml; horizontal nystagmus is usually present at this level, and its demonstration on neurologic examination is a rough estimate of "normal" therapeutic blood level. At blood levels higher than 20 µg/ml vertical nystagmus and ataxia develop; at levels greater than 50 µg/ml encephalopathy can develop. Phenytoin has a narrow therapeutic range; seizures can be a toxic manifestation of high blood levels or a consequence of low blood level. Phenytoin causes gingival hyperplasia. Gum disease is prevented by careful oral hygiene including frequent dental check-ups. Because phenytoin can cause hirsutism and gingival hyperplasia, it is not well accepted in young patients, especially females. Valproic acid and carbamazepine have more side effects than phenobarbital and phenytoin but are also excellent anticonvulsants (Table 11-1).

Treatment of an active single generalized tonic-clonic seizure. During an active seizure, protect the patient from injury, then administer medication to stop the seizure if the seizure has not stopped spontaneously. Almost all seizures stop spontaneously after several minutes, and an individual single seizure does not cause permanent CNS damage; however, this is different from potential brain damage that can occur as a result of status epilepticus. To protect the patient, place the patient's head on a soft pillow to prevent head injury. A soft, padded tongue blade is inserted in the mouth to prevent tongue biting, but care must be taken not to force the tongue blade into the mouth against clenched teeth. A metallic spoon should never be used because of the risk of breaking teeth that can be aspirated. Respiration can become labored and irregular, and there can be short apneic periods, but usually no respiratory support is necessary. No attempt should be made to restrain patients because this effort can cause orthopedic injuries. If an intravenous line is in place, the seizure can usually be aborted clinically and electrically by administrating 5 mg of diazepam (Valium) or 1 to 2 mg of lorazepam (Ativan). The seizure usually stops spontaneously within 2 to 5 minutes even without medication, therefore it is unnecessary to try to establish an intravenous line in an acutely seizing patient. If the patient is a known epileptic under treatment, administrating an additional dose of medication is frequently sufficient treatment, although probably not necessary, and the patient should be observed until fully conscious. Do not attempt to administer oral medication if the patient is not fully awake. Although the patient is quiet in the postictal state, an intravenous route should be established because it is possible that another seizure will occur and intravenous anticonvulsant medication would be necessary.

Absence Seizures (Petit Mal)

Absence seizures occur without prodrome or aura. There is sudden loss of awareness during which the patient appears dazed and unresponsive. In simple absence seizures there is no observed change in body tone and no myoclonic or stereotyped semipurposeful (automatic) movements. If these patients are carefully monitored by videotape recordings, clonic eye blinking, mild myoclonic jerks of extremities, slight hypertonia of neck or trunk, slight hypotonia with head drooping, or semipurposeful automatisms can be detected. When these occur, this is defined as complex absence seizures. During an absence attack calling or shaking the patient does not interfere with the trancelike state. If the patient is talking, speech abruptly stops in midsentence. If the patient is standing, posture is maintained, but loss of awareness can lead to injury if the patient is riding a bicycle or driving a car. Attacks last 10 to 45 seconds or sometimes even longer. Awareness abruptly returns, and the patient continues activities performed before the "spell." Postictally, patient is only aware of a "blank period." Initially these patients are sometimes thought to be daydreamers or to have behavior problems in school or at work before the correct diagnosis of absence seizures is established.

Attacks can occur so infrequently that they are not detected or as often as several hundred times daily and interfere with the patient's daily living and school activities. Absence seizures are provoked by hyperventilation and worsened by anxiety and exercise. These seizures begin in childhood, decrease in frequency in adolescence, and occasionally persist into adulthood. Fifty percent of patients with absence attacks subsequently develop generalized tonic-clonic seizures, and this usually occurs in the early teenage period with maximal vulnerability for girls during menarche. During an absence attack the EEG shows an abrupt change from normal background to a 2- to 3-cps spike and wave pattern. The patient does not have a clinical episode every time this EEG pattern occurs unless electrical dysrhythmia persists for longer than 5 to 10 seconds. In patients with absence attacks an underlying lesion is rarely present; therefore CT/MRI is not usually performed. EEG studies of patients with absence seizures and their noneffected (no clinical seizures) family members show that these siblings have 3-cps spike and wave pattern but may have no clinical seizures.

Valproic acid (Depakene) or divalproex sodium (Depakote) is the most appropriate drug for absence seizure treatment. Depakote is absorbed in duodenum and not the stomach; this reduces nausea. Liver toxicity and pancreatitis are potential toxic effects; careful laboratory monitoring for these conditions is necessary. This is usually a problem only in patients in whom valproic acid is used with other anticonvulsants. Because sodium valproate has a broad spectrum for seizure control, including major motor type, it is the treatment of choice in absence seizures. Ethosuximide (Zarontin) is the second drug used for absence attacks.

Partial Seizures

Partial seizures are those in which initial clinical disturbance signifies focal unilateral activation of specific anatomical or functional cerebral cortical region. Partial seizures are classified as to whether consciousness is normal (simple) or altered (complex). Partial seizures can spread locally (jacksonian march) and then terminate, or evolve into generalized motor seizure. Partial seizures are characterized by having an initial aura.

Simple Partial Seizures

Simple partial seizures originate from a localized (focal) cortical region to result in motor, somatosensory, autonomic, or psychic symptoms. One type begins with clonic rhythmical flexor movements of the thumb that either stop or spread to contiguous muscle groups such as the wrist, arm, and shoulder, then involve the face and later the leg with initial involvement of hips, knees, ankles, and lastly toes (jacksonian march). In rare instances motor activity remains confined to one group of muscles; this can persist for hours or even years without stopping or spreading (epilepsia partialis continua). If abnormal electrical discharge originates in the frontal region, the seizure begins with adversive (contralateral) deviation of the head, shoulder, and eyes.

Partial somatosensory or special sensory seizures are less common. In one type the patient describes numbness, tingling, or pins-and-needle sensations. Less frequently there are feelings of heat, burning, electricity, or vibration. In these cases abnormal discharge originates in postcentral primary somatosensory cortex. If localized abnormality is in the inferior somatosensory cortex, sensations can be bilateral and involve abnormal visceral sensations in the abdomen and chest. Symptoms of partial special sensory seizures include flashing white lights, a kaleidoscope of colors, or a sensation of darkness moving across the visual field (occipital cortex) or appreciation of sound with buzzing, clicking, or roaring (temporal auditory cortex). Simple partial seizures with neurobehavioral symptoms include language (aphasic) disturbance, memory aberrations, ranging from vivid recall of past experience of déjá vu to faulty recall or jamais vu, and illusions with distortion of size such that objects appear inappropriately large (macropsia) or small (micropsia), affective response (fear or anger), or cognitive effects (forced thinking).

During ictus of simple partial seizure the EEG shows localized spike discharges. In the interictal phase the EEG can show localized spike or slow wave discharge, but *rarely* the EEG can be normal in both ictal and interictal phase. This is because the lesion causing abnormal electrical discharge is located in cortical depths and does not project to the cortical surface. In patients with simple partial seizures complete neurodiagnostic studies—including EEG, CT, MRI, and possibly CSF examination—should be performed because suspicion of underlying focal lesion is high. Diagnostic studies usually demonstrate causal lesions in adult patients, whereas in certain adolescent patients simple partial seizures are benign without an identifiable underlying lesion. Certain metabolic conditions including diabetic nonketotic hyperosmolar coma cause partial seizures in absence of identifiable focal pathologic lesion. Even if diagnostic studies are negative, periodic reassessment is essential because certain lesions are not detected on initial evaluation. Medical treatment of partial seizures can be difficult. No well-controlled clinical studies for this seizure type have demonstrated superiority of one anticonvulsant, but phenytoin or carbamazepine is usually the initial treatment.

Complex Partial Seizures (Temporal Lobe or Psychomotor Seizures)

Complex partial seizures are associated with altered awareness and responsiveness and frequently with stereotyped motor activity (automatisms). The aura can consist of varied behavioral and autonomic sensations, including visceral abdominal sensations (pain, flatulence, nausea, vomiting, and rising or fluttering abdominal sensations), bitter taste in mouth, olfactory hallucinations consisting of unpleasant odors, affective changes with free-floating fear or anger, and structured (auditory or visual) but not command hallucinations.

During the ictal period mental and behavioral responsiveness is altered. The patient suddenly appears dazed, confused, or agitated or can act "crazy."

When the physician speaks to a patient during partial complex seizure, the patient can turn toward the sound and mumble incoherently and nonsensibly. There is no change in body tone; however, stereotyped semipurposeful movements—including picking and repetitive washing or rubbing hands—are observed. During episodes the patient can become agitated and aggressive if restrained. It is unusual for patients to carry out sequential or planned activities during the seizure or the postictal phase. Patients can become incontinent. The seizure usually lasts several minutes and ends gradually, emerging into postictal state, whereas in other cases a complex partial seizure can spread into generalized tonic-clonic seizure.

Ictal EEG findings are variable. Characteristically there are spike discharges that originate from one temporal region and secondarily spread to contralateral hemisphere, or independent spike discharges can originate from both temporal lobes. Postictally there is usually diffuse slowing. In 10% to 30% of cases, the surface electrode EEG shows no ictal pattern change. Interictal EEG frequently shows a spike, spike and wave, or rhythmical slow pattern in the temporal region but can show no abnormality. If a localized discharge originates from the mesial temporal (uncus) region, routine scalp electrodes may show no abnormality and nasopharyngeal, sphenoidal, or special temporal electrodes can be necessary. Complex partial seizures probably do not have a genetic basis. They can begin in childhood or adulthood. The pathological substrate for the complex partial seizures is mesial temporal sclerosis, believed to be related to perinatal hypoxic brain injury. This is especially true when the seizures begin before age 20. In patients with later onset complex partial seizures there is a high incidence of temporal lobe vascular malformations, hamartomas, gliomas, meningiomas, atrophic regions secondary to head trauma or brain infections. CT/MRI can detect these pathological conditions.

Carbamazepine is the drug of choice in controlling complex partial seizures. Phenytoin is the second drug of choice; phenobarbital and primidone are less effective. Newly approved drugs (felbamate, gabapentin, lomotrigine) can make complex partial seizures less of a management problem. If these seizures are refractory to medical therapy, surgical resection of the anterior portion of temporal lobe or corpus callosal sectioning can be necessary for seizure control.

Partial Seizures Evolving to Generalized Tonic-Clonic Seizures

Patients with complex or simple partial seizures can progress to generalized motor seizures. In some instances, the initial seizure portion is not witnessed and the attack can be diagnosed as a generalized motor seizure. An EEG is especially valuable in defining the presence of a localized electrical discharge. If the localized origin is detected, diagnostic evaluation for the underlying cause is mandatory. Treatment should be initiated with either phenytoin, phenobarbital, or carbamazepine.

▪ SEIZURES UNIQUE TO CHILDHOOD

Neonatal Seizures

Neonatal seizures can be difficult to recognize clinically because of their fragmentary nature. They do not have the well-defined stereotyped pattern of other seizure types. Neonatal seizures can simulate normal jitteriness of newborn. Seizures can consist of tonic deviation of head and neck, oral-buccal movements, opisthotonic posturing, or multifocal myoclonic movements. Episodes of apnea without other motor findings are usually not caused by seizures. In equivocal cases the diagnosis is established by abnormal EEG findings. It can be difficult to differentiate jitteriness, benign neonatal sleep activity, or myoclonus from neonatal seizures. There are multiple causes for neonatal seizures. The majority are due to perinatal complications (asphyxia, intracranial hemorrhage, cerebral contusion caused by obstetrical trauma), sepsis, congenital malformations, metabolic disturbances (hypoglycemia, hypocalcemia, hypomagnesemia, biotinidase deficiency, pyridoxine dependency), or drug withdrawal (related to maternal drug addiction).

The prognosis of neonatal seizures depends on the cause. Certain conditions such as benign idiopathic neonatal seizures that occur most commonly on the fifth day of life have a good prognosis; benign familial seizures that occur on the second or third day have favorable outcomes. Pyridoxine deficiency should be suspected if the seizures do not respond to antiepileptic medication. The management goal is to minimize CNS damage. Treatment consists of identifying an underlying cause and controlling seizures with phenobarbital or phenytoin.

Infantile Spasms

Infantile spasms are seizures beginning in children between 3 and 12 months of age. The child may have shown previous neurologic signs or may have been previously normal. Infantile spasms consist of sudden brief flexor spasms of head, neck, trunk, and extremities that cause the child to double up or "jack-knife." Each individual spasm lasts for only seconds; however, they can occur in clusters. The EEG pattern is "hypsarrhythmia" characterized by diffuse, irregular, high-voltage slow waves with interspersed spikes. The West syndrome includes a triad of infantile spasms, mental retardation, and "hypsarrhythmia" EEG pattern.

The prognosis is better if the child was neurologically normal before the attack, if no underlying cause is defined, and if attacks can be rapidly controlled with medication. One fifth of patients with infantile spasms have normal intellectual and behavioral development. CT/MRI should be done because neurocutaneous conditions (tuberous sclerosis) and congenital brain malformations are associated with infantile spasms. These seizures do not respond to conventional anticonvulsants including treatment with valproic acid and clonazepam. The most effective treatments are parenterally administered adrenocorticotropic hormone (ACTH), oral corticosteroids, or clorazepams.

Lennox-Gastaut Syndrome

Some patients develop a seizure disorder characterized by multiple clinical patterns including sudden attacks of altered responsiveness that develop and terminate gradually, sudden akinetic "drop attacks" with the loss of postural tone that cause the patient to fall to the ground, and generalized myoclonus. Attacks usually begin between 2 and 4 years of age. Almost all patients are mentally retarded. EEG shows symmetrical spike and wave pattern usually with frequency of 1.5 to 2.5 cps; this is activated by sleep stage rather than by hyperventilation (as is characteristic of classic absence seizures). Therapy for this disorder has been improved by valproic acid or felbamate.

Juvenile Myoclonic Epilepsy

This is genetically based disorder in which the abnormal gene locus is located in the short arm of chromosome 6. It is classified as generalized epilepsy. The disorder usually begins in adolescence. Symptoms include myoclonic jerks involving shoulders and arms; these characteristically occur on awakening. Initially, myoclonic jerks are not recognized as an epileptic disorder; they can be considered manifestations of anxiety, nervousness, or "tic" disorder. These patients then develop generalized major motor seizures; however, some patients can also have absence seizures. Precipitating events for seizures include alcohol, fatigue, and sleep deprivation. The EEG shows 3.5 to 6 symmetrical polyspike and slow wave discharge. During myoclonic episodes the EEG can show 6 to 16 polyspikes; this can precede the EEG spike and slow wave pattern. Valproic acid is the treatment of choice for this seizure type. This disorder responds well to medication treatment; however lifelong therapy is needed even with good seizure control.

Febrile Seizures

Febrile seizures consist of brief episodes of generalized major motor seizures occurring as the child initially develops febrile response. The child usually has only a brief postictal depression and no focal neurologic deficit, and the interictal EEG (obtained 1 week after the seizure) is normal. The initial seizure usually develops between 6 months and 4 years of age. Three to 5% of children develop seizures as part of febrile illness. In any child who experiences initial seizure and is febrile, the possibility of CNS infection must be excluded by lumbar puncture and CSF analysis. Two thirds of these patients develop recurrent, febrile seizures. Some children also develop nonfebrile seizures. Prognostic factors for development of non-febrile recurrent seizures in these patients include the following:

- Prolonged attack lasting 20 to 30 minutes
- Focal origin of seizures
- Abnormal EEG at least 1 week after the seizure
- No family history of febrile seizures
- Abnormal neurologic development of the child before or after the initial seizure

Fifty to 70% of patients with febrile seizures have a positive family history for this disorder, and the genetic pattern seems to be autosomal dominant. Efficacy of prophylactic treatment of febrile seizures with phenobarbital is controversial. Chronic phenobarbital prophylactic treatment reduces recurrence risk if compliance is maintained. There is no evidence that this decreases subsequent nonfebrile seizures. Treatment with phenobarbital during acute febrile illness is not effective because the period of maximum vulnerability occurs as the temperature rises. Because phenobarbital is associated with sedation and behavioral disturbances in children, the major issue is whether febrile seizures represent a greater potential risk than chronic drug therapy.

▓ DIFFERENTIAL DIAGNOSTIC PROBLEMS

Fit (Seizure) Versus Faint (Syncope)

During syncopal aura the patient can experience lightheadedness, visual blurring, dizziness. This is followed by a loss of consciousness; then the patient falls limply. Certain syncopal patients experience random sporadic myoclonic jerks. In rare syncopal cases, the patient becomes unconscious and assumes a decerebrate (tonic) position followed by random irregular clonic jerks. In convulsive syncope, EEG shows diffuse symmetrical slow wave pattern without spikes. It is important to differentiate convulsive syncope from generalized motor seizure because treating syncope with phenobarbital or diazepam can lead to cardiorespiratory arrest. Following syncopal episodes the patient is dazed for several minutes. Certain seizure features—confusion, focal neurologic deficit—are not seen with syncope.

Epileptic Versus Psychogenic (Nonepileptic)

Emotional factors can precipitate epileptic seizures, but seizures also occur during sleep and when the patient is alone and not being observed. Nonepileptic psychogenic seizures invariably occur in the presence of observers, especially in the setting of emotionally charged situations. There is frequently a history of prior physical or sexual abuse in these patients. In nonepileptic psychogenic seizures onset usually occurs gradually. The aura of nonepileptic seizure can consist of a choking sensation, chest pain, shortness of breath, and palpitations. The patient falls to the ground with writhing, struggling movements and side-to-side head movements. Motor components are not rhythmical in-phase tonic-clonic upper and lower extremity movements but appear as out-of-phase extremity motor activity accompanied by prominent pelvic thrusting and neck movements. There is usually no body rigidity (tonic phase) or abnormal eye movements. During nonepileptic psychogenic seizures patients can bite their lips and injure other people; tongue maceration and incontinence do not occur. There is no epileptic cry, but the patient may talk semicoherently. If restraint is attempted, patients become more violent. Consciousness does not appear to be lost, and the patient may respond to verbal or noxious stimulus. The attack can be aborted by verbal suggestion of the physician. After the psychogenic episode the patient is not post-ictally confused, and there is usually no amnesia, although certain patients cannot accurately report episode details. The patient comes out of the attack *abruptly* without the twilight confusional state that is characteristic of epileptic seizures. Also, clonic jerks stop abruptly rather than gradually slowing; cyanosis, incontinence, and tongue biting are absent, and neurologic signs (abnormal pupillary reactivity, amnesia, Babinski signs) are not seen postepisode. During and immediately after attacks the EEG shows no significant change in psychogenic nonepileptic seizures; this is clearly different from epileptic seizures. In diagnosing psychogenic seizures simultaneous video monitoring and EEG recording has been beneficial. The highest incidence of psychogenic seizures occurs in patients who *also* have epilepsy. If patient is evaluated for "episodes" and is observed to have hysterical seizures, this should not decrease the index of suspicion of epilepsy because of the association between epileptic and psychogenic seizures. It is important to recognize psychogenic nonepileptic seizures *not* caused by abnormal cerebral electrical activity as these do not respond to anticonvulsant medication. These patients are therefore exposed to medication risks without any potential benefit. Provocative testing to induce an "attack" such as using normal saline and the suggestion that this "medication" will induce an attack is helpful; however, ethical considerations of tricking the patient should be considered. Psychogenic seizures represent learned behavior, and appropriate treatment should involve teaching patients more satisfactory psychological coping skills. Psychiatric evaluation is mandatory to identify psychological stressor for psychogenic seizure (prior physical or sexual abuse).

Partial Complex Seizures and Periodic Psychoses

Patients with partial complex seizures become confused and carry out semipurposeful stereotyped repetitive activities. The aura can include hallucinations that are visual or auditory but do not command the patient to action. The patient is amnestic but does not perform purposeful or organized activity. Patients with absence or partial complex status epilepticus may mimic psychoses. EEG should show abnormalities in seizures. Following a seizure, postictal psychiatric disturbances including psychoses may occur. These psychiatric disturbances usually resolve rapidly. Because symptoms are self-limited, antipsychotic medication is rarely necessary. Interictally, patients with partial complex seizures can have psychiatric disturbances including schizophreniform disorders characterized by well-circumscribed psychosis with hallucinations of hyperreligious nature, panic, or anxiety states.

Episodic Confusional States

Episodic confusional states can be transient or prolonged. If occurring suddenly, they can represent partial complex or absence status epilepticus; the EEG would be expected to show continuous abnormal electrical activity if they represent seizure activity. If the confusional episode is caused by drug intoxication, blood and urine toxicology and the EEG would be important to differentiate confusional state not associated with epileptic EEG process, for example, metabolic encephalopathy, from epileptiform process. Transient global amnesia can cause acute confusion with marked impairment of recent memory. These patients can be found wandering and be lost, but they are aware of their identity and address. This condition usually resolves completely in several hours. The EEG is usually normal and does not show epileptic activity.

Simple Partial Seizures or Vascular Episodes (Migraine and Transient Ischemic Attacks)

Simple partial seizures can spread in orderly progression during several seconds or minutes, whereas the focal neurologic (scintillating scotoma, fortification spectra, homonymous hemianopsia, hemiparesis, hemianesthesia, aphasia) phenomena of migraine spread more slowly (10 to 30 minutes). With migraines the onset of neurologic disturbances are usually *followed* by contralateral headache. Syncope can accompany migraines, but altered awareness does not usually occur in patients with migraines. In TIAs focal neurologic deficit develops suddenly with maximal deficit at the onset of attacks. Progression does not occur. There is no altered consciousness, and headache is uncommon.

▨ COMPREHENSIVE MANAGEMENT PROBLEMS

Status Epilepticus

Status epilepticus includes situations in which clinical and EEG expression of seizures occur with continued frequency and the duration of interictal period is decreased. Continuous tonic-clonic motor attacks from which the patient does not completely recover consciousness between individual attacks represent a medical emergency because of the potential risk of permanent neuronal damage resulting from hypoxia, rhabdomyolysis, hyperthermia, autonomic dysfunction, hypoglycemia, lactic acidosis, cardiac arrhythmias, and respiratory depression. The most common cause of status epilepticus is abrupt anticonvulsant medication withdrawal; other causes include brain lesions such as intracerebral hemorrhage, brain neoplasm, and hypoxic-ischemic and traumatic brain injury. The prognosis depends on the nature and extend of the pathologic process. Mortality is 25%; this is lower if the status epilepticus is due to abrupt anticonvulsant medication withdrawal.

Initial management of status epilepticus includes ventilatory support with insertion of an oral airway; this is followed by placement of an endotracheal tube. The patient should be positioned on one side to prevent aspiration. An intravenous pathway is established using large-gauge tubing, and blood is immediately analyzed for glucose, electrolytes (including calcium), liver, and renal function studies. Electrocardiographic monitoring is warranted especially if potentially cardiotoxic medications are used. Insert a Foley urinary catheter for urine output monitoring. It is extremely helpful (but frequently not feasible) to monitor drug treatment with a portable EEG. Initial treatment should include 50 grams of glucose and 200 mg of thiamine administered intravenously after the blood is sampled for laboratory testing.

There are four major anticonvulsant treatment regimens, but no controlled study indicates superiority of one drug. Anticonvulsant medication must be administered intravenously. Diazepam is administered as 5 to 10 mg per minute; this is repeated every 10 to 20 minutes to maximum of 50 to 70 mg. This dosage usually stops seizures within several minutes; however, seizure will recur within 10 to 20 unless a longer-acting anticonvulsant is supplemented (e.g., phenytoin, phenobarbital). Diazepam can cause hypotension, sedation, and respiratory and cardiac depression. Lorazepam (0.01 to 0.05 mg/kg) can be substituted because it has less respiratory depression, no cardiac toxicity, and longer duration of action (4 to 24 hours). The initial dose should be 2 mg per minute; this can be followed by 1 mg every 2 minutes. Phenobarbital is administered in doses of 250 mg over 5-minute intervals. If seizure control is not achieved, this dose is repeated every 15 minutes to a total dose of 20 mg per kg or the EEG shows a burst suppression pattern. Disadvantages of phenobarbital include respiratory depression and excessive sedation. There is synergistic toxicity between diazepam and phenobarbital that can cause cardiovascular toxicity. Phenytoin is administered in doses of 20 mg/kg at a rate not exceeding 50 mg/min. This drug affects the cardiac conduction system, and electrocardiographic monitoring is necessary; it also causes hypotension, and blood pressure monitoring is also necessary. Phenytoin is poorly soluble; it must be given by direct intravenous injection containing normal saline and not mixed with other intravenous fluids. It is alkaline and irritating to veins; direct injection causes pain and has the potential to cause phlebitis. The solvent has recently been changed, and there is now less risk of hypotension and cardiac arrhythmias. Because phenytoin does not depress consciousness, it is possible to follow clinical recovery. Paraldehyde is supplied in ampules that each contain 5 ml. Five ampules are mixed with a solution containing 500 ml of dextrose and water or saline. Because of lipid properties paraldehyde is poorly soluble and droplets are seen in the mixture. It is rapidly administered until seizures stop. This medication causes no acute cardiac toxicity, but unusual effects include metabolic acidosis and pulmonary hemorrhages. Its major disadvantage is that it is difficult to obtain at the present time because limited availability.

If these anticonvulsants are not effective, the anesthesiologist can assist in administering intravenous lidocaine (bolus or infusion technique with initial bolus of 1 to 2 mg/kg administered in 5 minutes). For refractory cases use phenobarbital as an intravenous bolus of 5 mg/kg until the seizures stop or the EEG shows a burst suppression pattern. After this initial bolus use a microdrip maintenance dosage of 1 to 3 mg/kg for 4 hours. If seizures are controlled with this regimen, switch to maintenance phenytoin. For continued refractory seizure use pentobarbital at dose of 12 mg/kg administered at initial dose of 1 to 2 mg/kg per hour. The goal is to obtain complete seizure control and burst-suppression pattern on the EEG. Continue pentobarbital for 24 hours and then decrease dosage after 24 hours. Thiopental (1 gram diluted in 500 ml of normal saline as a microdrip infused at 2 mg per minute until seizures stop and then maintain at 0.5 ml/min for 4 hours) may be used for barbiturate coma, but this has more cardiovascular toxicity than pentobarbital. If necessary, inhalational anesthetic medications (halothane, isoflurane) may be utilized. The role of rectally administered valproic acid has not been determined in status epilepticus.

Other forms of status occur but are not life threatening; however, the possibility of their progressing to generalized major motor status exists. For absence or partial complex status the patient is in a prolonged dazed or unresponsive state. Diagnosis is established by EEG recording. Absence status epilepticus is initially treated with 5 mg of intravenous diazepam; if this is not successful, the dose should be repeated. Partial complex seizure responds to either intravenous diazepam, phenytoin, or phenobarbital. Simple partial seizure usually responds to diazepam, and epilepsia partialis continua is refractory to most medications.

Criteria to Discontinue Anticonvulsant Therapy

Adequate seizure control can be achieved in the majority of patients: generalized major motor, 70% to 80%; absence, 80% to 90%; complex partial, 50% to 60%; simple partial, less than 50%. There are different definitions of "control"; the number of seizures acceptable to the employed patient who needs to drive to work is less than that acceptable to an institutionalized mentally retarded patient. If the goal of therapy is to eliminate all seizures, the patient may be forced to use a higher dose of single drug or multiple drugs with associated risk of drug toxicity.

If the patient is seizure free, the decision to discontinue medication is sometimes reached because patient compliance decreases when patients become asymptomatic. It should be emphasized to the patient that although he or she is seizure free there is a risk that seizures can recur without medication. In this case inconvenience and harm of long-term drug toxicity must be weighed against the potential consequences of seizure recurrence. If the patient is seizure free for 24 months and the interictal EEG has normalized, there is still the possibility of seizure recurrence without medication in 25% to 33% of patients. If seizures recur after medication is discontinued appropriately, they sometimes become more difficult to control. Although this is a general impression, its validity is a highly debated issue. If medication treatment is to be stopped, withdrawal must be gradual and usually requires 2 to 4 months depending on the type and dosage of anticonvulsant medication and prior duration of therapy. Those criteria suggesting the highest probability that seizures will not recur without medication included the following: infrequent seizures before complete control achieved, normal EEG, rapid initial control of seizure, normal neurologic examinations, and normal CT/MRI. Adult patients with simple or complex partial seizures have high recurrence risks. Recurrence is least likely in petit mal seizures when the patient is seizure free for 12 to 24 months and the EEG has normalized. Patients with absence seizures are at significant risk of developing generalized motor seizures; this most frequently occurs at the onset of puberty. Because this represents the period of greatest seizure development vulnerability, cessation of medication for absence attacks should not usually be attempted until the patient is older.

SPECIAL SITUATIONS

Pregnancy

If a patient has long-standing, well-controlled seizure disorder, the risk of precipitating seizures by altering the drug regimen is probably greater than the teratogenic effect of phenytoin, carbamazepine, or phenobarbital; however, many mothers would risk having a seizure in an effort to have healthy child. *All* anticonvulsant drugs cross the placenta, and all have been associated with increased risk of congenital malformations. Most common are orofacial clefts and cardiac abnormalities. Neural tube defects have been reported with valproic acid. There is some evidence that multivitamins containing folate can reduce the risk of major malformations. In high-risk pa-tients alpha-fetoprotein and acetylcholinesterase levels should be obtained as well as ultrasound findings at 16 to 18 weeks of pregnancy. If ultrasound findings are inconclusive for spina bifida or cardiac or limb defects, amniocentesis should be performed.

One third of pregnant women will have an increase in seizure frequency during pregnancy, probably because antiepileptic drug levels frequently fluctuate as a result of changes in protein drug binding and metabolism. During pregnancy, if there is a problem with seizure control, utilize free drug blood levels because of the change in plasma protein binding that occurs in pregnancy. Epileptic patients have higher complication risks during pregnancy and delivery; children born of epileptic mothers have more neonatal complications including growth and developmental problems. If the patient develops a seizure during the first trimester, utilize the most effective antiepileptic drug at lowest effective dose for that seizure type. Poor seizure control is associated with greater risk of adverse events than the potential teratogenic effect of antiepileptic medication. Valproic acid and carbamazepine have increased risk of neural tube defects. Multivitamins with folate may reduce risk of malformations in pregnant women utilizing antiepileptic medication. In the second and third trimesters the major risk is fetal hypoxia during a seizure and respiratory depression and excessive sedation caused by medication (e.g., phenobarbital, primidone). Seizures can develop during pregnancy as manifestations of eclampsia and cortical vein thrombosis. During labor, short acting benzodiazepines are probably the safest and most effective treatment for seizures. Eclampsia with convulsions is initially treated with magnesium sulfate. If this is not effective or causes respiratory depression or weakness, utilize lorazepam or phenytoin.

Drug-Withdrawal Seizures

In our drug-oriented culture drug abuse has become a significant problem. As part of the initial evaluation of a first seizure in any young person, toxicology should be performed. If the seizure is related to drug use and the EEG is abnormal, it is probably not necessary to treat with anticonvulsant medication. There is an exception to this general rule: if a drug-precipitated seizure occurs in a patient with a genetic predisposition for epilepsy, treatment with anticonvulsants would be indicated. The only way to determine this would be to see if subsequent seizures occurred in the drug-free state and then begin antiepileptic medication. In addition, a patient with predisposition for seizures may not develop recurrent seizures if the patient stops using illicit drugs, and prophylactic anticonvulsants may not be needed.

Drug withdrawal seizures are most frequently related to alcohol. These seizures usually occur during or after an episode of heavy alcoholic use and consist of single or multiple short bursts of generalized motor seizures. These attacks are rarely focal, and focal seizures should be evaluated for underlying focal lesions. Acutely it may be necessary to treat with anticonvulsants if seizures are multiple because 5% of patients develop status epilepticus. Although phenytoin has been suggested as a drug to treat acute drug-withdrawal seizures, it is slow to develop therapeutic levels unless an intravenous loading dose is administered. Patients with alcohol-withdrawal seizures should not be treated with chronic anticonvulsant medication because if they begin an alcoholic binge they stop their anticonvulsant medication abruptly and thereby increase risk of drug-withdrawal seizures.

Posttraumatic Seizures

Posttraumatic seizures can be classified by the time of onset that they develop after the seizure (Box 11-3).

BOX 11-3

1 Impact seizures occur immediately after trauma and are most frequent in children. For example, a child is flipped over and strikes his or her head on the gymnasium floor and immediately has a generalized seizure; there is full recovery of neurologic function within 30 minutes, and subsequent examination and EEG are normal. The recurrence rate is low, and anticonvulsants are not usually needed in this situation.

2 Early seizures occur within 7 days of injury and correlate with severity of injury and a prolonged period of impaired consciousness. These can be due to brain hemorrhage and contusional brain injury. Prophylactic treatment with phenytoin can be warranted in those patients who have a high risk of developing seizures (cortical laceration, depressed skull fracture, dural tear, intracerebral hematoma, or contusion) in whom the physiologic derangements caused by the seizure might possibly worsen the patient's clinical condition.

3 Late seizures occur more than 1 week after the trauma. Almost all posttraumatic seizures initially occur within 2 years of trauma. These late seizures can be due to glial scar formation. There is little evidence to support prophylaxis with phenytoin to prevent subsequent occurrence of seizures, and treatment should be withheld until an initial seizure has occurred.

Psychiatric Aspects of Epilepsy

Patients with a well-controlled seizure disorder do not have any characteristic personality or behavioral disturbances. There is no reason why these patients should not lead normal lives with certain simple and practical precautions. In patients with poorly controlled disorders, psychiatric symptomatology can result from social factors that these patients experience or from the results of epileptic cortical hyperexcitability spreading to involve the limbic and septal systems, although these hypotheses are hard to prove. Intelligence in some patients with idiopathic epilepsy is within lower end of intelligence scale, and some require chronic institutionalization. If intelligence is adequate, epileptics should attend regular school unless seizure frequency or sedation from medication makes this impossible. If seizures become frequent, there may be evidence of mental deterioration that is not seen in patients with infrequent seizures.

In patients with partial complex seizures, certain interictal behavioral features have been reported including hypergraphia, hypersexuality, hyperreligiosity, and circumstantiality. In addition, well-circumscribed delusional psychosis with a religious preoccupation is seen in these patients. The relationship of clinical seizures and psychosis is not clear, but some observers have indicated that psychosis becomes more severe when the seizures are well controlled. A tendency toward aggressive but not organized violent or hypersexual behavior is seen in patients with partial complex seizures especially if seizures are poorly controlled.

Social Aspects of Epilepsy

Patients with epilepsy are at risk for bodily injury and should avoid unprotected activities such as climbing, working near electrical machinery, and driving an automobile until control is established. The patients should avoid unprotected water or cycling activities because many epileptic deaths are related to water activities. Despite the potential risk of injury during a seizure, epileptics should attempt to lead a well-regulated but active life. There are no restrictions regarding food; alcohol must be avoided, and patients should not be deprived of sleep.

Patients with epilepsy should adhere to certain restrictions in operating motor vehicles. The law varies for different states, but usually licenses can be obtained when patients have been seizure free for 1 to

2 years. Patients may be required to have a statement verifying the medical condition. It should be noted that patients with epilepsy cannot usually buy automobile insurance through conventional channels and must apply through the Assigned Risk Plan, in which there is pooling of high-risk policies shared equally by all companies. Similar problems are encountered with medical, life, and disability insurance. Because of unjustified and unwarranted prejudice against patients with epilepsy, patients frequently conceal this condition when applying for employment.

Causes of Death in Epileptic Patients

Epileptic patients can suffer sudden, unexplained death. If an epileptic has an attack while driving an automobile, the patient can suffer bodily injury or injure others. During a seizure severe laryngospasm or blockage of the epiglottis by the tongue can cause asphyxia and death. Many deaths are related to water, and epileptic patients can have an attack and drown in a bathtub or in several inches of water.

SUMMARY

The term "seizure" is used to describe a paroxysmal clinical episode usually characterized by an alteration in consciousness and abnormal muscle tone. "Epilepsy" refers to recurrent seizures caused by abnormal cerebral cortical electrical hyperexcitability as manifested by abnormal electrical discharges detected with an EEG. Epilepsy can be generalized as a result of an underlying genetic basis that causes a cerebral dysthymia or be a focal component caused by an underlying structural brain lesion. The diagnosis of epilepsy is established by clinical and EEG criteria, and appropriate treatment should be initiated with antiepileptic medication. Common causes of failure to control epilepsy are patient noncompliance and incorrect diagnosis, for example, pseudoseizure and syncope. It is crucial to control seizures as quickly as possible to prevent brain injury caused by recurrent seizures especially if status epilepticus occurs, but it is also important to use a carefully titrated dosage of antiepileptic medication to minimize systemic and CNS side effects of these medications.

Suggested Readings

Partial Seizures
Curry S, Heathfield KWG, Henson RA: Clinical course and prognosis of temporal lobe epilepsy, *Brain* 94:173, 1971.

Falconer MA, Serafetinides EA, Corsellis JAN: Etiology and pathogenesis of temporal lobe epilepsy, *Arch Neurol* 10:233, 1964.

Theodore WH, Porter RR, Penry JK: Complex partial seizures: clinical characteristics and differential diagnosis, *Neurology* 33:1115, 1983.

Cascino GD: Intractable partial epilepsy: evaulation and treatment, *Mayo Clin Proc* 65:1578, 1990.

Psychogenic Non-Epileptic Seizures
Desai BT, Porter RJ, Penry JK: Psychogenic seizures: a study of 42 attacks in 6 patients, with intensive monitoring, *Arch Neurol* 39:202, 1982.

Lesser RP: Psychogenic seizures, *Neurology* 27:823, 1986.

Epilepsy—General
Elso IS, Penry JK: Epilepsy in adults, *Ann Neurol* 9:3, 1981.

Escueta AV, Treiman DM, Walsh GD: The treatable epilepsies, *N Engl J Med* 308:1508, 1576, 1981.

Gastaut H: Clinical and electroencephalographic classification of epileptic seizures, *Epilepsia* 11:102, 1970.

So EL, Penry JK: Epilepsy in adults *Ann Neurol* 9:3, 1981.

Scheuler ML, Pedley TA: The evaluation and treatment of seizures, *N Engl J Med* 323:1468, 1990.

French J: The long-term therapeutic management of epilepsy, *Ann Intern Med* 120:411, 1994.

Status Epilepticus

Escueta AV, et al: Management of status epilepticus, *N Engl J Med* 306:1337, 1982.

Oxbury JM, Whitty CWM: Causes and consequences of status epilepticus in adults: a study of 86 patients, *Brain* 94:733, 1971.

Walsh GO, Delgado-Escueta AV: Status epilepticus, *Neurol Clin North Am* 11:835, 1993.

Chang CWJ, Bleck TP: Status epilepticus, *Neurol Clin North Am* 13:529, 1995.

Seizures Unique to Childhood

Gomez MR, Kloss DD: Epilepsies of infancy and childhood, *Ann Neurol* 13:113, 1983.

Initial Seizure Management

Hauser WA, et al: Seizure recurrence after a first unprovoked seizure, *N Engl J Med* 307:522, 1982.

Bert AT, Shinnar S: The risk of seizure recurrence following a first unprovoked seizure, *Neurology* 41:965, 1991.

Hopkins A, Garman A, Clarke C: The first seizure in adult life, *Lancet* 1:721, 1988.

Hauser WA: Should people be treated for a first seizure? *Arch Neurol* 43:1287, 1986.

Hauser WA, Rich SS, Annegars JF: Seizure recurrence after a first unprovoked seizure, *Neurology* 40:1163, 1990.

Discontinuing Antiepileptic Medication

Shinnar S, et al: Discontinuing antiepileptic medication in children with epilepsy after two years without seizures, *N Engl J Med* 316:976, 1985.

Callaghan N, Garrett A, Goggin T: Withdrawal of anticonvulsant drugs in patients free of seizures for two years, *N Engl J Med* 318:942, 1988.

Epilepsy and Pregnancy

Yerby MS: Epilepsy and pregnancy, *Neurol Clin North Am* 11:777, 1993.

Antiepileptic Medication

Leppik IE, Graves N, Devinsky O: New antiepileptic medications, *Neurol Clin North Am* 11:923, 1990.

CHAPTER

Head Trauma

12

Head trauma from motor vehicle accidents, industrial mishaps, falls, and physical assault has become a significant part of medical practice. Even though specialized care by a neurosurgeon is required in many cases, the general physician must understand when neurosurgical consultation is required and what should be done until the surgeon arrives. In addition, all physicians must be aware of the sequelae of head trauma and their assessment and management.

In most cases of head trauma, the mechanism of injury is a blunt force to the head that is of sufficient force to cause a concussion. The term *concussion* can be most simply defined as an immediate impairment of neural function secondary to a mechanical impact to the head. The loss of consciousness is the most consistent symptom; however, less commonly there can be impaired vegetative function (respiratory slowing, bradycardia, hypotension) and motor impairment including hypotonia, areflexia, and Babinski signs. There is usually full recovery from a simple uncomplicated concussion, but the patient can have residual amnesia for the events of the injury. The neurodiagnostic studies show no structural pathologic lesions in patients with cerebral concussion.

The severity of the concussion can be defined by the length of posttraumatic amnesia experienced by the patient or by the length of coma (Table 12-1). The length of posttraumatic amnesia, though difficult to assess at times, seems to give the most valid prediction of eventual outcome. The length of unconsciousness is usually easier to determine and therefore often used. Posttraumatic amnesia is measured from the last memory before the trauma to the return of full continuous memory after the trauma. The amnesic period can be divided into two sections: one, the period before the trauma (retrograde amnesia), and two, the period after the trauma (anterograde amnesia). In the more severe cases of head trauma in which the coma period is greater than 24 hours, the assessment of the changing level of consciousness using the Glasgow coma scale (see Chapter 9, Stupor and Coma) is important in predicting eventual outcome. A prognosis based on examination in the first 48 hours is not particularly valid but improves steadily thereafter.

TABLE 12-1 Severity of Concussion Defined by Length of Posttraumatic Amnesia

Severity of Concussion	Length of Amnesia
Slight	0–5 minutes
Mild	5–60 minutes
Moderate	1–24 hours
Severe	1–7 days
Very severe	>7 days

■ PATHOPHYSIOLOGY

A blow to the head causes its injury basically by putting excessive strain on the brain and supporting tissues. The scalp can be lacerated, the skull can be fractured, or a hematoma can form from torn blood vessels. These can occur in the scalp, under the galeal aponeurosis (subgaleal), between the dura and skull (epidural), between the dura and arachnoid (subdural), or in the brain (intracerebral). Contusions (bruises) can occur on the cortical surfaces. Such focal damage can occur at the point of impact or frequently on the opposite pole of the brain along the force line (contrecoup). The contrecoup injury is most frequently seen in deceleration injuries where the moving head strikes a stationary object (e.g., when a patient falls and the head hits the floor). Subarachnoid blood is usually present, and widespread damage can also occur throughout the white matter. These white matter lesions are due to the shearing forces initiated by the brain's rapid acceleration (when the head is struck) or deceleration (when the moving head hits a stationary surface). The major damage to the brain seems to be caused by the rather free rotational and lateral motion of the brain within the skull. This motion allows the brain to move against rough surfaces of the base of the skull and also to twist and distort itself. It is these distortional forces and movement that produces the strain and stretching of axons and vessels.

■ CLINICAL HISTORY AND EXAMINATION

In head trauma cases, it is important to know the exact mechanism of the injury. A blow to the head with a hammer will produce a much different pattern and extent of injury (focal damage to underlying brain) than would a fall from a motorcycle at 45 mph. The latter accident will likely cause injuries to the head, neck, long bones, chest, and so on. Cervical injuries (whiplash) can also cause brain trauma as a result of the rapid acceleration and rotation of the head.

The physician should inquire whether the patient had been drinking or taking illicit or sedative drugs. Such substances can depress the level of consciousness and make the effects of the trauma appear more significant than they actually are. The examiner should ascertain if the patient experienced a period of unconsciousness and, if so, for how long. If the patient is still in a coma on arrival at the emergency department, witnesses or ambulance attendants can be asked whether consciousness was regained after the trauma. Some patients are initially rendered unconscious by a head injury, then slowly awaken to the point of being able to carry on a conversation only to slip into coma again. A history of a lucid interval such as this is crucial when present, for it quite frequently indicates that the patient is rapidly developing a life-threatening epidural hematoma. The lucid interval is not pathognomonic for epidural hematomas and can be seen in cerebral contusion, subdural hematoma, and intracerebral hematoma; however, its presence adds further urgency to evaluation and treatment.

In the alert patient, it is necessary to establish the length of posttraumatic amnesia and to question the patient as to the presence of any neurologic symptoms (e.g., headache, dizziness, confused feeling, and diplopia). Is the patient oriented to place and time? Sometimes the only sign of significant cerebral dysfunction is disorientation.

In the seriously injured patient who is still comatose, the adequacy of the airway and circulation must be assessed immediately. The clinician should auscultate the chest and then establish adequate ventilation. An important word of caution: almost all head trauma involves extension, flexion, or rotational injury to the cervical spine with possible fracture. *Be very careful not to move the neck any more than is absolutely necessary!* An unstable cervical spine can easily damage the spinal cord if moved.

The adequacy of circulation must next be evaluated and shock treated if diagnosed. Another word of caution: shock cannot be due to intracranial bleeding except in young infants. It can be secondary to blood loss from a large scalp laceration, but it is usually due to injuries elsewhere in the body (e.g., spleen, liver, kidney, lungs, thigh muscles). When taking the pulse the examiner should make note of bradycardia. In some patients with a rapidly expanding intracranial lesion the pulse will drop, respiration will slow, and blood pressure often rises. This is called the Cushing reflex.

The head should be examined for obvious signs of trauma. All deep scalp lacerations should be clean and palpated. A fracture line or depression under a laceration indicates that there is a possible communication from the scalp to the intracranial compartment. In such cases the risk of intracranial infection is great. The examiner should look for evidence of basilar skull fracture: blood behind the eardrum, cerebrospinal fluid leaking from either the nose (rhinorrhea) or the ear (otorrhea), or slowly developing ecchymosis around the eyes (raccoon eyes) or over the mastoid process (Battle's sign).

After the patient is stable and has adequate ventilation and circulation, a full neurologic examination should be performed. Special attention should be directed toward the level of consciousness, alterations in mental status, pupillary symmetry and reactivity, and symmetry of reflexes and motor control.

◼ CLINICAL SYNDROMES

There are many clinical management problems presented by patients with head trauma. These problems have two phases: the management of the acute trauma and the appreciation and treatment of the sequelae of the injury.

Concussion

The loss of consciousness is the most consistent defining feature of concussion; however, less commonly there can be impaired vegetative function (respiratory slowing, bradycardia, hypotension), mental confusion, and motor disturbances including weakness, hypotonia, areflexia, and Babinski sign. The period of impaired consciousness rarely lasts longer than 30 minutes, and there is usually full recovery; however, the patient usually remains amnestic for the episode. Because there is full recovery the pathophysiologic substrate of concussion is not clearly known; however, it is probably due to the acute distortion of the brain stem ascending activating system (reticular formation). If a trauma-related abnormality is found on CT or MRI, the disorder is no longer considered to be a simple concussion. It is believed that patients with concussion have suffered a reversible pathophysiologic disturbance. There is impaired brain function (caused by reversible electrical conduction disturbance) without evidence of pathologic injury to brain tissue. It is possible that a mild form of white matter shearing injury has occurred, but it is insufficient to produce abnormal findings of the neurologic examination or brain scan. The patient who has had a simple concussion but is awake on arrival at the emergency department should have full physical and neurologic examinations and probably a plain skull x-ray to check for a linear fracture.

Because neck injury is often associated with head injury, cervical spine roentgenography can be considered. If the skull and cervical spine roentgenograms are negative and neurologic examination including mental status is clear, the patient can usually be discharged to the care of a responsible person, although hospital admission for 24 hours could be justified. If released, the patient should be carefully observed for 24 to 48 hours at home. Any signs of decreased arousability, confused mental status, pupillary changes, or unilateral weakness should prompt immediate return to the hospital for further diagnostic tests, especially a CT scan of the brain.

There is often a question as to which patient is to be admitted. The usual guidelines in considering admission are listed in Box 12-1.

The CT/MRI scan has revolutionized the evaluation of head trauma patients. CT scans can readily identify the presence of most intracranial injuries including hematomas, large contusions, tissue ischemia, mass effect, edema, and hydrocephalus. CT scanning will not demonstrate white matter shearing injuries, which are seen more clearly with MRI.

Contusion

A contusion represents damaged neuronal tissue on the cortical surface, basically a bruise with evidence of tissue necrosis, edema, and extravasated blood. These are most common at superficial cortical regions at the impact point or where the moving brain rubs or comes to a stop along the inner surface

BOX 12-1

1 Patients still unconscious on arrival in the emergency department

2 Patients with positive (focal) neurologic signs

3 Lethargic or confusional patients

4 Patients with evidence of basilar skull fracture on examination

5 Patients with skull fracture on roentgenography

6 Patients with severe headaches

7 Patients with nausea and vomiting

8 Patients under the influence of alcohol or drugs (in such patients, trauma-related alterations in the level of alertness and mentation cannot be accurately assessed)

9 Persons living alone or at a great distance from the hospital

of the skull. They are frequently seen directly underneath depressed skull fractures. The most common locations for contusion are on the inferior surface of the frontal and temporal lobes. With blows to the occipital region there can be an occipital contusion (coup injury) and frontal contusion (contrecoup lesion) as a result of the vacuum phenomenon as the brain accelerates from front to back within the skull. If there is a contusion with actual discontinuity of brain tissue, this is called a brain laceration. Contusions can be multiple and small and can resolve spontaneously; however, larger confluent contusions can form large focal lesions with intracerebral hematomas. These lesions can cause mass effect and result in focal neurologic deficits and impaired consciousness; at times surgical evacuation can be indicated. The diagnosis of cerebral contusion can be established by CT scanning.

Diffuse White Matter Shearing Injury

The brain usually shows no surface cortical contusions; however, hemorrhagic contusions do occur in the white matter, most commonly in the corpus callosum and cerebellar peduncles. There is often intraventricular blood and ventricular dilatation. As the process evolves, the hemorrhage resolves. There can be atrophy of white matter with microscopic evidence of wallerian axonal degeneration. Clinically, these patients with CT evidence of white matter lesions are usually comatose with bilateral motor impairment and Babinski signs. CT scanning can show hemorrhages in the white matter and ventricles; however, MRI is more effective in demonstrating the nonhemorrhagic white matter shearing injuries.

Posttraumatic Increased Intracranial Pressure

In patients who have suffered head injury elevated intracranial pressure can result from structural brain injury (e.g., contusions, hematomas, edema). With increased intracranial pressure there can be reduced brain perfusion. This results in cerebral ischemia and further elevation of intracranial pressure. When intracranial pressure is due to a focal lesion there can be a significant shift of intracranial structures and herniation syndromes. With supratentorial mass lesions there is transtentorial descending herniation with distortion of the midbrain. In some patients severe diffuse brain swelling and edema can occur after trauma in the absence of contusions and hematomas. The mechanism of this diffuse edema is not understood, but it can be a very serious, often fatal, complication of closed head injury. Treatment of increased intracranial pressure includes the following:

- Hyperventilation to reduce PCO_2 and induce cerebral vasoconstriction to reduce blood volume
- Mannitol (1 gm/kg intravenously in adults or 0.25 gm/kg as an initial dose in children)
- Dexamethasone (10 mg intravenously initially and 4 mg every 4 hours)
- Surgical evacuation of the hematoma

Intracranial Hematomas

Small blood vessels in the brain and meninges are often torn when patients sustain a blow to the head. When this occurs, the resultant leakage of blood will form a hematoma that will expand at a rate commensurate with the degree of the vessel tear. The contents of the skull (brain, cerebrospinal fluid, and vessels) have only limited ability to accommodate to the expanding clot, and very soon signs of increased intracranial pressure and herniation develop. In the unconscious patient deterioration because of an expanding clot can be manifest solely by the appearance of decerebrate posturing or sluggish pupils. In the alert patient the first sign of a developing clot is frequently a subtle change in the level of consciousness or mental state. Any deterioration in the patient's neurologic status subsequent to head trauma should alert the physician to the possibility of a developing intracranial clot, and an emergency CT scan should be obtained. Most patients (75%) who become alert after their initial concussion, then subsequently deteriorate and die, have an intracranial hematoma. Failure to recognize an intracranial hematoma is one of the major avoidable factors when patients die after head trauma.

Epidural Hematoma

The epidural hematoma accounts for 15% to 30% of all intracranial clots. These clots develop between the dura and inner table of the skull. Seen more commonly in young patients (10 to 30 years old) the lesion is associated with a linear skull fracture in more than 90% of the cases. The fracture is usually in the temporal or temporoparietal area. In more than half of the cases the fracture crosses the middle meningeal artery groove, and that artery or its companion vein is the major source of the bleeding. In approximately 30% of the cases, however, bleeding can be traced to one of the venous sinuses. Bilateral lesions are distinctly rare, and most epidurals are in the temporoparietal area (70%±).

The hematoma—if of arterial origin—grows very rapidly and can cause deterioration and death within minutes; therefore early recognition is critical. Clinically, 30% to 50% of the patients have a history of a lucid interval after trauma. On the other hand, 15% give no history of an initial loss of consciousness with the trauma.

Early features can be headaches and vomiting, but these findings are not as significant as the appearance of abnormal neurologic signs (e.g., decreased level of consciousness or signs of uncal herniation). Some 60% to 70% of the patients. Seizures are rare. In some patients the pulse may drop, respirations may slow, and blood pressure may rise because of increased intracranial pressure (Cushing reflex). If there are signs and symptoms of raised intracranial pressure, mannitol is administered initially. Dexamethasone is also useful. Corticosteroids can take 6 to 24 hours to be effective, and mannitol or hyperventilation (to cause vasoconstriction) is initially needed in emergency situations.

Prompt surgical evacuation of the clot can be very rewarding if done early enough because 60% of the patients will not have other associated brain damage and recovery can be complete. If treatment is delayed, however, mortality rates are high: 17% when one pupil is dilated and fixed at the time of surgery, almost 50% when both pupils are fixed, and 80% when decerebrate posturing is present.

Subdural Hematoma

The subdural hematoma forms between the dura and the arachnoid. The source of bleeding in chronic subdural hematomas is usually the small veins that bridge the arachnoid space and enter the dural sinuses. Acute subdural hematomas can have mixed arterial and venous bleeding. Subdural hematomas occur commonly in persons 40 years of age and older, particularly in the elderly, in whom mild shrinking of the brain causes stretching of the bridging veins. Documented trauma is implicated in about 50% of cases, but its incidence as a cause decreases with patient age. Bilateral lesions are found in 20% of adult patients but in 50% of pediatric patients. Alcoholics are particularly vulnerable because they are often victims of head trauma and also have blood clotting abnormalities (Figures 12-1 through 12-3). Subdural hematomas in children are often the result of unreported trauma (battering).

Clinical symptomatology is similar to that of epidural hemorrhage in many respects; however, seizures (associated with underlying cerebral contusion or hemorrhage) are more common in subdural hemorrhage, and signs of uncal herniation are less frequent. Skull fracture occurs in less than 50% of cases and is more frequent in the young. Unlike

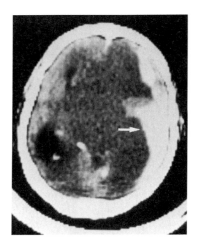

FIGURE 12-1. CT scan (nonenhanced) of a large subdural hematoma.

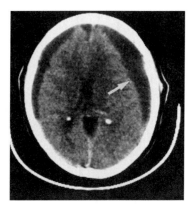

FIGURE 12-2. CT scan demonstrating bilateral hypodense subdural hematomas. The one on the right (*arrow*) is chronic; note lens shape. The one on the left is subacute; note how it follows the contour of the convexity.

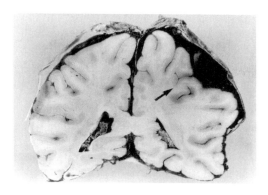

FIGURE 12-3. Pathologic specimen corresponding to the scan in Figure 12-2.

patients with epidural hematoma, in whom the fracture is almost always on the side of the clot, 50% of patients with subdural hematomas have the fracture on the opposite side. A subdural hematoma can be an acute, a subacute, or a chronic lesion; each has its own clinical and prognostic significance.

Acute. An acute lesion develops in less than 3 days, is usually related to severe trauma, and is therefore often associated with intracerebral and epidural clots. This lesion is more common in young patients; frequently the patient does not regain consciousness from the trauma, and a lucid interval is present in less than 30% of the patients. If surgery is performed in the first 4 hours mortality is low, but if surgical treatment is delayed mortality may be high. The prognosis is very closely related to the condition of the patient at the time of surgery. The hematoma can be anywhere in the cranial vault and is often associated with a contused and lacerated brain. Acute subdural hematomas can also occur in the rupture of berry aneurysms or in blood dyscrasias.

Subacute. Lesions can develop in 3 days to 3 weeks, and deterioration can be due as much to swelling of the underlying hemisphere as to the enlargement of the hematoma collection itself; hemiparesis is present in 50% of the patients contralateral to the hematoma, but in 25% it is ipsilateral. Mortality is 25%.

Chronic. A lesion can manifest 3 weeks or more after trauma. Researchers disagree as to pathophysiologic mechanism governing the gradual increase in size of these lesions, but intermittent rebleeding is probably the major factor. Accumulation of fluid caused by an osmotic gradient in the subdural membrane has also been postulated but seems less likely to be the mechanism. Clinically the chronic subdural hematoma can appear as personality or other mental change, signs of focal neurologic dysfunction, increased intracranial pressure, or focal seizures. The diagnosis is established by CT/MRI; angiography, which used to be the definitive diagnostic study, is rarely needed. A fluctuating level of consciousness can occur but is not a prominent feature. Surgery is required, and the mortality rate is 15%. Some hematomas are not diagnosed clinically and can resorb spontaneously or become calcified or even ossified; detection is often made on a scan done for an unrelated condition.

Intracerebral Hemorrhage

By definition intracerebral hemorrhages represent collections of blood of more than 5 ml. They are most commonly found in either the temporal or frontal lobes, although occasionally they can be present in the occipital lobe or cerebellum. These lesions are usually associated with severe trauma and clinically appear as expanding mass lesions with significant focal neurologic deficit (Figure 12-4). Traumatic intracerebral hemorrhage usually occurs in superficial locations. It

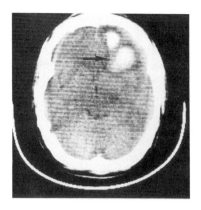

FIGURE 12-4. Traumatic intracerebral hematoma in the right frontal lobe (*arrow*).

is important to differentiate traumatic intracerebral hemorrhage from other types of nontraumatic intracerebral hemorrhage (e.g., hypertension, amyloid angiopathy, rupture angioma, aneurysm) that resulted in a neurologic deficit (e.g., seizure, hemiplegia) and that may have *caused* the patient to sustain head trauma either by a fall or auto accident.

Basilar Skull Fracture or Fractures across Paranasal Sinuses

Any fracture that crosses a paranasal sinus or results in a dural tear of the cribriform plate (causing cerebrospinal fluid rhinorrhea) or temporal bone (causing otorrhea) produces a communication between the subarachnoid space and the environment. The possibility of meningitis occurring in this situation is very real and demands special observation and treatment.

Basilar fractures are difficult to diagnose by roentgenography (less than 50% on routine skull films), so they must be inferred from clinical signs. Special base-of-skull tomograms can help identify these fractures. If the fracture is through a sinus or cribiform plate, air can often be seen intracranially on either the skull film or, even more reliably, CT scan. Cerebrospinal fluid can sometimes be seen in the paranasal sinuses. Chronic cerebrospinal fluid rhinorrhea can usually be accurately diagnosed and the location of the leak identified by introducing a radioactive isotope into the cerebrospinal fluid and performing a nuclide cisternogram. Water-soluble contrast material can also be used and CT scanning employed to identify the site of the leak.

Treatment of a cerebrospinal fluid leak consists of bed rest for 7 to 10 days. The use of prophylactic antibiotics is controversial. If antibiotics are used, they should be continued at least 1 week after the leak closes spontaneously or is closed surgically. Unfortunately meningitis can develop many months or even years after the trauma and even with adequate treatment can recur. Most cerebrospinal fluid leaks stop spontaneously in the first week; this is particularly true of otorrhea. If the leak does not spontaneously seal within 10 days, surgical exploration is necessary. If the fracture and fistula involve the frontal or sphenoidal sinus, the likelihood of spontaneous healing is less, necessitating surgical intervention sooner.

Basilar fracture can also damage facial or acoustic nerves, so assessment of cranial nerve function is necessary in each case.

Depressed Skull Fractures

A skull fracture is considered to be *compound* if there is a scalp laceration. If the dura is torn, this is a *penetrating* injury. Depressed fractures can result from motor vehicle (including motorcycle) accidents or from the head being struck by objects (work-related injuries, assault attacks), or they can be caused by missile injuries. Diagnosis of the fracture is established by a skull roentgenogram, and evidence of an underlying focal contusion is established by CT/MRI scanning. The major complication of depressed fracture is meningitis. Treatment of a depressed fracture consists of surgical debridement, elevation of the fracture, repair of the dura (if it has been torn), and antibiotics.

Sequelae of Head Injury

The most significant sequelae occur in the cases of severe injury, but there are some very important problems that can occur after mild trauma. In general, recovery from any head trauma is better in young patients. Improvement proceeds slowly over many weeks or months.

Diffuse Damage (Posttraumatic Encephalopathy)

The most severe form of diffuse damage is the chronic vegetative state in which the patient has multiple neurologic abnormalities and is so severely damaged that, even though the eyes are open, meaningful contact with the environment is minimal or nonexistent. All grades of recovery occur in diffuse damage, and varying degrees of neurologic impairment are demonstrated. In general the prognosis is directly related to the length of posttraumatic amnesia or coma and inversely related to the age of the patient.

One common sequela of blunt head trauma that is often not fully appreciated until the major motor disabilities have cleared is the behavioral effect of bilateral frontal and temporal damage. Because of the contour of the inner surface of the skull, the orbital (inferomedial) surface of the frontal lobes and the medial temporal lobes are often contused or otherwise damaged during the injury. In moderate concussions other neurologic deficits can be mild. The results of frontal or temporal trauma are twofold. From the temporal damage there develops a recent memory or new learning deficit. This is usually subtle and reversible in slight or mild concussion but can be a significant problem in more severe injuries. Such a deficit can greatly hinder job performance, particularly if the patient must learn a new vocation after the accident. The memory problem can improve slowly over years, but improvement is most rapid in the first 12 months after the trauma. Frontal lesions can cause a very distressing change in personality or temperament. This is characterized by a lack of motivation, apathy, at times euphoric disinterest, a lack of social restraint, and a distressing lack of goal direction. Pursuant to these and other intellectual deficits it is suggested that all patients who suffer significant head trauma should have a full neuropsychologic evaluation before returning to work or entering a vocational rehabilitation program.

Focal Damage

Focal contusions or hematomas will often leave residual focal neurologic deficits (e.g., aphasia, hemiplegia, hemiparesis, visual field defect).

Hydrocephalus

After trauma there is occasionally sufficient blood or fibrous adhesions in the subarachnoid space at the base of the brain to obstruct the flow of cerebrospinal fluid. In such instances a communicating hydrocephalus can develop. This diagnostic possibility should always be considered in any patients with head trauma in whom deterioration occurs. This can be during the acute phase (mostly from blood) or many weeks or months later. The clinical signs in these cases will be gait unsteadiness, incontinence, behavioral changes often simulating a frontal lobe syndrome, or intermittent confusion.

Cranial Nerve Abnormalities

The cranial nerves are anchored to the skull as they exit through the various foramina; because of this they are often damaged when the skull is fractured or the brain is thrown about during acceleration/deceleration injury. The effects injury can have on the first, second, sixth, seventh, and eighth cranial systems are listed in Box 12-2.

 BOX 12-2

1 *First (olfactory).* This is the most commonly damaged nerve, especially with basilar skull fractures. In patients with cerebrospinal fluid rhinorrhea, anosmia (loss of sense of smell) is extremely common. Recovery is slow and related to the severity of the trauma. In general less than 50% of the patients recover full function. On occasion there is recovery for some odors and not others, and sometimes the sense of smell is distorted. To some persons anosmia is a minor inconvenience, but to others it can be a major disability, for instance, for a restaurant chef or wine producer.

2 *Second (optic).* Direct injury to either the second cranial nerve or chiasm occurs. Often the resultant loss of vision is transient.

3 *Sixth (abducens).* This is the most commonly affected nerve of the extraocular muscles.

4 *Seventh (facial).* With fracture through the temporal bone, the seventh nerve is often interrupted acutely. In some patients without fracture, delayed (usually 2 to 3 days) facial paralysis can manifest.

5 *Eighth (acoustic).* In basilar fractures in which otorrhea or hematotympanum is present, hearing can be affected as well as vestibular function.

Seizures and Electroencephalographic Changes

After acute head injury the EEG can show slowing of background rhythm, suppression of voltage, or paroxysms (bursts) of slow activity. This is also true in a high percentage of patients with severe whiplash. The incidence of such abnormalities is highest in children. As acute effects of the injury dissipate (2 to 3 weeks) the EEG will either return to normal or show evidence of focal residual damage or dysfunction. Focal slowing is the most common finding, but focal or even generalized epileptic activity is occasionally seen. If an EEG is to be ordered at all, it is best to obtain it in the recovery phase rather than acutely. One problem with interpreting EEG findings is the high degree of both false-positive and false-negative recordings (more than 15%). The most important information to be gained from the EEG is the probability of a patient developing posttraumatic epilepsy. If the EEG show abnormal bursts, the patient has a 20% to 25% chance of developing seizures and therefore should be treated with anticonvulsants. This is particularly true if there is any family history of epilepsy.

There is a definite risk of developing a chronic, recurring seizure disorder after significant head traumas. The four factors listed in Box 12-3 significantly raise the probability of developing posttraumatic epilepsy.

In simple concussions in which there is only a fleeting loss of consciousness, the probability of developing a seizure disorder is no greater than that in the general population.

Seizures can first appear many years after an accident, and prophylactic treatment does not seem to be efficacious in preventing their appearance. Most posttraumatic seizures are focal and are more difficult to

BOX 12-3

1 Depressed fractures particularly with dural tear have a very
   high incidence of seizures (>50%)

2 Penetrating wounds or grossly destructive lesions have high
   incidence (>50%)

3 Amnesia (>24 hours)

4 Time after injury that the first seizure occurs:
   a Immediate (little chance of chronic seizures)
   b First week (33%)
   c First to eighth week (70%)

treat than idiopathic epilepsy. Posttraumatic epilepsy
is a chronic disorder, with only a 40% cure rate after
5 years.

Posttraumatic Syndrome

Posttraumatic syndrome is the most common and
probably most complex sequela of head trauma. The
basic elements of the syndromes are headache, dizziness, difficulty concentrating, and a host of vague
behavioral symptoms such as anxiety, depression, and
nervous instability. This syndrome is curiously more
common in trivial or slight trauma than it is in serious
injury. It is logical that some of these symptoms
should occur after an acute injury because a blow to
the head will have a number of organic effects such
as the following: injury to the soft tissues of the skull
or meninges will cause headache; labyrinthine dysfunction has been well documented to explain the
dizziness, and trauma to the ascending activating system as well as limbic system and cortex will lead to
difficulty with concentration, memory, and emotional
stability.

The syndrome usually lasts a few weeks to a few months. The symptoms gradually disappear but can be exacerbated by strenuous physical exercise, emotional stress, or the use of alcohol. Patients in laboring jobs or highly stressful jobs should be warned that symptoms might recur when they return to work. Employers must also know this and be sympathetic. Rest and symptomatic treatment are usually all that is required.

A major problem arises when the symptoms do not abate in a reasonable length of time. Such patients often become depressed and angry, which are factors that can cause the symptoms to increase. Because many head injuries occur in vehicle or work-related accidents, the problems of fault and compensation arise. When a person feels that someone also is to blame for his or her injury, anger and desire for recompense can consciously or unconsciously perpetuate the symptoms. It has been repeatedly shown that head injuries incurred during sporting events have a much lower incidence of posttraumatic symptomatology than injuries in which fault is an issue. Many, but not necessarily all, of the patients with symptoms lasting more than 6 to 12 months probably have considerable psychologic, legal, financial, or other social factors responsible for the perpetuation of their symptoms. The physician should maintain a sympathetic interest in helping the patient over the posttraumatic period but must also be aware of these other often significant factors. Simple symptomatic treatment is best. Narcotic medications should not be given for more than a few weeks after the accident, except in rare cases.

In some patients trauma to the scalp and branches of the external carotid artery produces migrainelike headaches. These headaches should be treated in the same fashion as other migraines, but the success of treatment is not as satisfactory.

■ SUMMARY

Head trauma is a common medical problem. Most head injuries are mild, but some patients develop serious complications such as intracranial hematomas (e.g., subdural or epidural). Neurosurgical consultation is the most important aspect of the management of significant head trauma, but the evaluation and management of mild head trauma can be adequately handled by any physician. CT scanning has been a great comfort in screening head trauma patients but is not necessary in all cases. The posttraumatic syndrome is one of the complex problems from head injury; this condition is usually managed by the primary care physician.

Suggested Readings

Head Injury—Evaluation

Feiring EH, editor: *Brock's injuries of the brain and spinal cord,* New York, 1974, Springer.

Jennett B, Teasdale G: *Management of head injuries,* Philadelphia, 1981, FA Davis.

Levin HS, Benton AL, Grossman RG: *Neurobehavioral consequences of closed head injury,* New York, 1982, Oxford University Press.

Teasdale GM: Head injury, *J Neurol Neurosurg Psychiatry* 58:526, 1995.

Vinken PJ, Bruyn GW, editors: *Handbook of clinical neurology: injuries of the brain and skull,* parts I and II, vols 23 and 24, Amsterdam, 1976,1977, Elsevier-North Holland.

Vinken PJ, Bruyn GW, Klawans HL, et al, editors: *Handbook of clinical neurology,* vol 57, Revised Series 13, Amsterdam, 1990, Elsevier Science.

Walker AE, Caveness WF, Critchley M, editors: *The late effects of head injury,* Springfield, Ill, 1969, Charles C Thomas.

White RJ, Likavec MJ: The diagnosis and initial management of head injury, *N Engl J Med* 327:1507, 1992.

Posttraumatic Seizures

Annegers JF: Seizures after head trauma, *Neurology* 30: 683, 1980.

Temkin NR, Dikmen SS, Wilensky AJ: A randomized double blind study of phenytoin for the prevention of posttraumatic seizures, *N Engl J Med* 323:497, 1990.

Traumatic Brain Hemorrhage

Gutman MB, Moulton RJ, Sullivan I: Risk factors predicting operable intracranial hematomas in head injury, *J Neurosurg* 77:9, 1992.

Markwalker TM: Chronic subdural hematomas: a review, *J Neurosurg* 54:637, 1981.

C H A P T E R

Neurologic Disorders of Childhood

13

Neurologic evaluation of children is important because 25% of hospitalized children have some type of neurologic disease. The neurologic evaluation of a child begins with a complete and accurate history from the parents or guardian of the child. Hospital birth records and perinatal information are essential. Developmental events should be compared with standard tables (e.g., Denver Developmental Screening Test). In older children records of performance in school or day-care centers can provide information concerning intellectual and emotional characteristics of the child. Other prior medical problems or a family history of neurologic disease can give a clue to the ongoing neurologic process.

To understand the disease processes and the pathogenesis of pediatric neurologic diseases, the reader should be familiar with normal development of the brain as is described in embryology textbooks. The cerebrum that begins as a smooth round structure evolves into a complex convoluted bihemispheric structure through a well-organized and predictable pattern. At the same time the neurons proliferate and differentiate and are organized through proliferation and enlargement of synaptic connections. Growth of the brain continues after birth, and, although myelination occurs mainly in the first year of life and is almost completed by the second year, it continues until the third decade of life.

The neurologic examination of children varies according to patient age. In infants, observation of the patient on the lap of a parent or guardian is least threatening and reveals the patient's spontaneous activities. The ability to grasp objects from the floor or from above the head and transfer them from hand to hand demonstrates motor function and coordination. Using small objects for this test facilitates evaluation of vision. Hearing can be tested by snapping fingers, shaking keys, or creating a loud noise to startle the infant. Head control can be evaluated by simple observation or by pulling the patient to a sitting position by his or her hands to reveal head lag. Sensation can be tested by pinching or tickling the skin surfaces of extremities and trunk. In addition to testing the stretch reflexes, one should test infants with the following maneuvers to obtain certain postures and movements that can indicate whether there are abnormalities of motor function: The *Moro reflex* is elicited by making a loud noise, sudden withdrawal of head support, and slapping the bed or examining table. The resulting startle response consists of an elevation, abduction, and clasping of the arms. This reflex disappears at 4 or 5 months of age. The *tonic neck reflex* is elicited by passively turning the head to either side. The response consists of extension of the limbs on the side the head is rotated toward and flexion of the limbs on the opposite side. This reflex should disappear after 6 months, and a normal child usually breaks the response in 15 to 30 seconds. The *parachute response* is elicited by holding the infant at the trunk and then dropping the infant forward with the head downward. The normal 7-month-old infant will thrust the arms forward for support or protection. The *Landau maneuver* is elicited by suspending the infant in a prone horizontal position. An infant who is older than 6 months will respond by extending the neck and trunk. The presence or absence of these reflexes indicate the degree of maturation of the nervous system and will give an indication of focal deficits when the response is asymmetrical or of more defuse neurologic deficit in a symmetrically absent response. No neurologic examination is complete without measuring the patient's head circumference to detect microcephaly or macrocephaly and visualizing eye grounds to look for cherry-red spots and splinter hemorrhages. Hepatosplenomegaly can indicate some type of storage disease. The following questions about a child with neurologic disease need to be answered:

- Is the disease process acute or chronic?
- Is the disease static or progressive ?
- If it is static, when did it happen?
- Is it a primary nervous system process or part of a systemic disease ?
- If it is a primary disease process, is it confined to the central nervous system, the peripheral nervous system, or both ?
- If it is a CNS process, does it affect cortex, white matter, or both ?

These questions may not have an answer in every case, but asking the questions helps the examiner arrive at a diagnosis.

DISORDERS OF MOTOR EXECUTION

Children who have disorders of motor execution are clumsy and show poor performance of sequential motor acts but with preservation of motility and no alterations of muscle strength, tone, or posture. These motor deficits have been called, incorrectly in the past, "soft neurologic signs." In most of these children there are associated learning disorders and hyperactive behavior. The presence of these disorders can cause long-term educational and social disadvantages. The physician needs also to remember that in a few cases these findings can be the early manifestations of more serious and progressive neurologic disorders. *Dyspraxia* is the inability to perform sequential motor tasks in the presence of good motor strength, sensation, and cooperation. In children with dyspraxia, motor milestones have usually been normal, but the children have difficulty buttoning, zippering, and tying shoes and using combs, toothbrushes, and scissors. The best single office test that is most likely abnormal for manual dyspraxia is the finger-to-nose test. When the examiner asks the child to touch the tip of his nose with his index finger, the child is able to touch his nose with his finger, but then he may use the other hand's finger to touch the examiner's finger. Although this test is very reliable, a battery of tests are needed to make a definite diagnosis. Failure of other imitation tasks can also help in the diagnosis. In dyspraxia of speech buccalfacial gesturing is not imitated by the patient and can affect speech (dilapidated speech). The cause of the pure dyspraxia is unknown, but dyspraxia can be part of a more severe neurologic disorder. *Clumsiness* is a disorder of speed and dexterity of movements in children who have normal strength and muscle tone. In the preschool years parents of clumsy children can think that their children are lazy, slow, or uncooperative. In the early school grades in which the demands are more motor than intellectual, the children usually do poorly. This disorder frequently produces low self-esteem and, later, depression in some of the children. Teachers need to know about the diagnosis to be able to understand, tolerate, and help these children. *Adventitious movements* appear early in childhood and are frequently associated with clumsiness. There are mainly three types of adventitious movements: choreas, tremors, and synkinesis. *Choreas* are more easily detected when the children stand with the legs slightly apart, the arms pronated and extended, and the wrists dorsiflexed. Once in this position, rapid asymmetrical movements of the fingers can appear, and in severe cases there are associated facial and arm movements. The acute onset of chorea in school-age children may alert the physician to a rheumatic or collagen vascular disease etiology. In severely retarded children on neuroleptics, abnormal movements suggest drug induced dyskinesia. *Tremor* is a rhythmic distal involuntary oscillatory movement that can appear at rest or be aggravated by movements (intention tremor). A cerebellar lesion needs to be excluded. If the tremor is severe, medication should be used. *Synkinesis* is an involuntary movement that occurs during voluntary action such as opening of the mouth when the child opens his eyes and the other way around or the presence of mirror image movements. Mirror movements are more frequently seen in association with agenesis of the corpus callosum. No treatment is available for this condition.

CEREBRAL PALSY

Cerebral palsy is a clinical description of a heterogeneous group of disorders that affect control of movement or posture (motor dysfunction). The symptoms appear early in life, can change in the first two years (hypotonia can turn into spasticity or dyskinesias), are of a fixed nature, and are caused by a nonprogressive brain lesion or dysfunction. In 55% to 60% of the cases, the cause cannot be established. *Cerebral palsy does not mean mental retardation and is not always an outcome of difficult labor*. In spite of spasticity, Babinski signs are not constant features. Associated features include seizures, language disorders, dystonia, ataxia, speech impairments, and occasionally mental retardation. The classification of cerebral palsy is based on clinical features and includes the following:

- *Spastic diplegia*. Bilateral spasticity that is worse in the legs, with scissors posturing and gait. It is commonly associated with prematurity. Associated features can include seizures and a variable degree of mental impairment.
- *Spastic quadriplegia*. Severe bilateral spasticity that is worse in the legs, with few voluntary movements, pseudobulbar palsy, frequent aspiration, and commonly severe intellectual impairment. Seizures and optic atrophy can be seen.
- *Spastic hemiplegia*. Unilateral spastic hemiparesis is present at birth but is not usually recognized until sometime in the first 2 years of life. The paresis can be associated with athetotic posturing or other abnormal movements. Although seizures are frequent, mental impairment is less severe.
- *Spastic double hemiplegia*. Bilateral spasticity that is worse in the arms. Mental retardation and seizures are frequent.

- *Extrapyramidal cerebral palsy.* Diffuse hypotonia occurs at birth and changes into progressive choreoathetosis in the first 2 years of life. Dysarthric speech is frequent and can be associated with drooling as a result of impaired swallowing. Seizures and mental impairment are rare.

- *Mixed forms of cerebral palsy.* These are manifested by combinations of spasticity with abnormal movements.

Treatment of cerebral palsy needs to be individualized for every patient according to the patient's needs. The treatment should be directed toward early and intensive physical therapy, bracing when indicated, and, in selected patients, surgical intervention for release of contractures or elongation of Achilles tendons. For most CP patients learning some way of communication is more important than ambulation. Muscle relaxants including diazepam, dantrolene sodium, and baclofen can help temporarily in some of the spastic types.

MENTAL RETARDATION

Intelligence has been defined as the capacity to obtain new knowledge and solve problems. It consists of a series of special and natural abilities: to have curiosity, observe, comprehend, think, and remember and use these qualities in a rational way during social interactions. Intelligence can be modified by schooling and training but is predominantly innate. Intelligence has been measured by different tests designed to measure special abilities and to predict scholastic achievement. Mental retardation is an "incomplete or insufficient general development of mental capacities" as defined by the World Health Organization. Adams and Victor differentiate two groups of mental retardation: the *severely impaired* (IQ less than 20), or pathologic mentally retarded and the *less severely impaired* (IQ is 45 to 70), or subcultural, physiologic, or familial mentally retarded. The severely impaired patients often have neurologic impairment and are more frequently males; most need to be institutionalized. The less severely impaired show no neurologic impairment, are frequently females, and do not require institutionalization; the parents and siblings are often subnormal. The brains of the less severely impaired look normal with conventional histologic techniques, but a sparsity of dendritic arborizations and abnormal dendritic spines have been found with Golgi-Cox preparations, suggesting a synaptic transmission problem. Management should be directed toward the planning of the patient's special education and training to achieve independent living when possible.

AUTISM

Autism is a heterogeneous syndrome characterized by development of excellent motor skills and retentive memory but failure to use language for communication (lack of speech, abnormal speech content, or prosody), profound withdrawal from contact with people, and an obsessive desire to preserve sameness (Kanner). Autistic children frequently show repetitive stereotyped movements (whirling or rocking) and demonstrate selectivity of attention such as ignoring noises or painful stimuli yet concentrating on spinning objects or self-induced sounds. They ignore other persons' feelings or existence and make no eye contact. Imitation is poor, and they show abnormal social play. In most cases there is no family history of the same syndrome. A good number of neurologic disorders, including those caused by prenatal infections, perinatal anoxia or trauma, or metabolic or chromosomal abnormalities, can have the same clinical phenotype, but none provide clues as to the cause of autism. The screening of these disorders depends on the clinical information obtained by the physician. In autistic cases that show no other neurologic deficit, neuropathologic studies have described subtle cytoarchitectonic abnormalities in the temporal lobes, neostriatum, and thalamus suggestive of a dopaminergic disturbance. However, a definite cause is still elusive. The EEG is frequently normal, and the imaging studies can show nonspecific subtle abnormalities. The prognosis is usually poor with only one third of the cases developing some form of speech (communication). Treatment consists of behavior modification and the use of some antipsychotic medications. Fenflurazine, a serotonin-depleting agent, has shown mixed results. There is poor response to CNS stimulants.

▨ HYPERACTIVITY-ATTENTION DEFICIT DISORDER

The normal level of activity varies considerably among children from the time of birth. Some normal children are very placid, and others are extremely active. Activity is normally accentuated when a child begins to run and walk. Males are generally more active than females, and cerebral defects can accentuate hyperactivity. Hyperactive behavior can become apparent when a child cannot stay in one position for more than a few seconds; is very inattentive, distractible, or impulsive; and is unable to maintain adequate concentration in school and often other situations. This problem is occasionally seen as the sole impediment to adequate school performance, and teachers may demand a medical consultation. To make a diagnosis of hyperactivity in a child, the physician needs to obtain information from different sources, including the child's teachers, and the diagnosis should be made after observation for at least 12 months. Parental marital problems and parental depression, anxiety, and substance abuse need to be investigated. The cause of the disorder is not known but resembles the postencephalitic syndrome. Some cases are familial. Some patients can show "soft neurologic signs" but not more than what is seen in the normal pediatric population. Imaging studies have revealed asymmetry in the anterior part the cerebral hemispheres. The prognosis is variable, but nearly half of the patients improve around adolescence. However, as a group the patients have a higher incidence of truancy, alcohol abuse, and juvenile delinquency. The treatment should be individualized and should include counseling for the patient and the family, adjustments in the school programs, and use of stimulants when needed. Three medications are most frequently used. Methylphenidate (Ritalin) takes 30 minutes to work, and its action lasts 4 to 6 hours; thus, the patients need to take one 5 mg tablet in the morning and one at noon. Some patients need a third dose in the afternoon. The undesirable side effects include anorexia, insomnia, headache, abdominal pain, and hypertension. A 20 mg sustained-release tablet can be used for one dose a day in the mornings. Dextroamphetamine (Dexedrine) has a longer half-life than Ritalin and can be used in patients who are unresponsive to Ritalin. Pemoline (Cylert) is the third choice of medication. It has a 12-hour half-life, but the medication needs several days or weeks to reach the maximum effect.

DEVELOPMENTAL DYSLEXIA

Developmental dyslexia, or congenital word blindness, is a specific visuoperceptual defect of reading in an otherwise intelligent person. Children with this disorder have extraordinary difficulty identifying printed words and also have difficulty spelling and writing despite the ability to recognized individual letters. However, dyslexics are able to recognize the meaning of diagrams, objects, and pictures. There are several levels of reading performance, from minor faulty letter sound associations to an almost complete inability to read. The disorder is highly familial, and left-handedness is statistically higher in patients and relatives. Hyperactivity and attention deficit disorders are frequently associated with dyslexia. Neuropathologic studies have revealed cytoarchitectonic dysplasias in the perisylvian regions of the left hemisphere. The significance of these changes is undetermined. Imaging studies can detect subtle changes in the same regions. Treatment should be started after a complete evaluation of the deficit is made and should emphasize the needs of the child, including phonetics and using better learning strategies. Most dyslexic children finish high school, and most live independent successful lives. Some variations of disorders of higher cortical functions include *dysphasia, dysgraphia,* and *dyscalculia.* These disorders also are most likely associated with other brain pathology, can be identified by special neuropsychologic testing, and should be treated accordingly.

▨ EPILEPSIES

The epilepsies have been reviewed in Chapter 11. Only the most frequent types that may be seen by primary care doctors will be emphasized here.

Febrile Seizures

Febrile seizures occur at the onset of an acute febrile illness in a child who is usually between 3 months and 5 years of age and who most likely has a family history of febrile seizures. The seizure occurs early in the illness when the temperature is rising rapidly. The most frequent seizure is the generalized tonic-clonic type, but other types of seizures can occur including focal motor seizures and seizures manifested by staring, stiffening of the limbs, or just limpness. The febrile illness is usually a tonsillitis, upper respiratory infection, or otitis media. Recurrence after the first febrile seizure occurs in one third of the patients. The younger the patient is when a febrile seizure occurs, the more likely it is that there will be a recurrence. The risk factors for later epilepsy include developmental abnormality or neurologic deficit before the seizure, a family history of epilepsy in one parent, a history of a febrile seizure that was focal or that lasted more than 15 minutes, and an abnormal EEG. The differential diagnosis includes bacterial or viral meningitis or encephalitis, epidural or subdural empyema, hypernatremic dehydration, septic embolization, Reye's syndrome, and any other infection. Management consists of controlling the seizure by lowering the patient's temperature and treating the seizure with anticonvulsants. The cause of the fever needs to be investigated and treated. Treatment with anticonvulsants has not been shown to prevent the development of epilepsy. Parents of children with the first seizure need to be reassured and counseled regarding the favorable prognosis in most of the patients.

Benign Rolandic Epilepsy

Benign Rolandic epilepsy is an important form of autosomal dominant childhood epilepsy that remits spontaneously. The seizures occur more frequently between the ages of 5 and 10 (range 2 to 12) and are characterized by a single nocturnal generalized seizure of focal onset and diurnal focal motor seizures. The nocturnal seizure starts with brief twitches of the mouth with salivation and gurgling sounds followed by generalization of the seizure. Unfortunately most parents see only the generalized part. The daytime seizures are focal in onset. In most cases there is no loss of consciousness and no amnesia or postictal confusion. The seizure starts in the face and is associated with speech arrest, salivation, and guttural sound. Involvement of the arm and leg on the same side can occur. There are no automatisms, hallucinations, or auras associated with the seizures. The seizures are sporadic, and the interictal neurologic examination is normal. The interictal EEG shows high-amplitude spikes followed by slow waves that can be seen isolated or in groups and that originate in the midtemporal and Rolandic (central) region. The EEG pattern is seen in 50% of patients' close relatives, but only 12% of the people with this EEG abnormality develop seizures. When this sterotype seizure occurs along with the EEG pattern, the use of costly imaging studies should be avoided. Treatment may not be necessary after the first or even the second seizure. Monotherapy with phenytoin or carbamazepine easily controls the seizure.

Lennox-Gastaut Syndrome

This syndrome is characterized by medically intractable recurrent seizures of various types that frequently begin in the first 6 years of life (rarely after 10), are frequently associated with severe mental retardation, and show a slow spike-wave or slow spike-wave discharges on the EEG during a portion of the awake state. The type of seizure varies. *Tonic* contractions of muscle groups occur commonly during sleep and are associated with impaired consciousness that lasts from a few seconds to 1 minute. *Atonic* (astatic) seizures are also known as drop attacks. There is no warning, and they are sudden in onset and are associated with loss of tone and momentary loss of consciousness. There is no postictal confusion. Facial injuries can occur because most children fall forward. Myoclonic jerks frequently precede the atonic seizure. Nocturnal generalized tonic-clonic seizures occur in 60% to 70% of the patients. Seizure frequency is variable from day to day in the same child. Seizures occur more frequently during inactivity or drowsiness and can be as frequent as 50 or more per day. The prognosis of this syndrome is poor, and the response to anticonvulsants is dismal. Most patients need polytherapy. Treatment should be individualized for each patient.

Infantile Spasms

Infantile spasms are also known as salaam seizures, flexion spasms, massive spasms, jack-knife seizures, massive myoclonic jerks, and infantile myoclonic seizures. All these terms describe the type of seizure that is seen in these infants, which varies from brief head nods to violent flexion of the trunk and limbs. The minor forms can be misdiagnosed as colics or other medical problems. The onset of the seizures is confined to the first 2 years of life. The seizures usually occur in clusters, during sleep or after awakening. The EEG is highly abnormal and frequently shows diffuse high-voltage random slow waves and multifocal spikes, called hypsarrythmia. Infantile spasms can occur without a clear cause (idiopathic) or can be found in infants with severe hypoxia, congenital malformations, congenital infections, neonatal intracranial hemorrhage, and metabolic disorders such as phenylketonuria.

Tuberous sclerosis is frequently associated with infantile spasms. The prognosis is poor for most patients but is worse in those with associated neurologic disease. In the idiopathic cases the patients are left with significant neurologic impairment. The treatment consists of adrenocorticotropic hormone (ACTH) or corticosteroids. Clonzepam and valproic acid have also been used with moderate success.

Benign Juvenile Myoclonic Epilepsy of Janz

This disorder is characterized by the presence of mild myoclonic jerks (see myoclonic epilepsy, p. 337) that affect predominantly the neck and upper limbs in a patient who is alert. The jerks are more frequent in the mornings and are aggravated by sleep deprivation. Some patients can have absence or generalized tonic-clonic seizures. The seizures affect predominantly males with an onset in the second decade (age 8 to 24) and a family history of the disorder. The EEG is characterized by 3.5 to 6 Hz spike-wave or multiple spike-wave complexes. The seizures are easily controlled with long-term use of valproic acid.

▧ MALFORMATIONS OF THE CENTRAL NERVOUS SYSTEM

Most major deviations from normal embryonic development of the brain occur early in the first trimester of embryonic life and can be produced by a variety of genetic, infectious, metabolic, toxic, and irradiation insults. Although the nature of the insult may be obscure, the time of the insult can be determined. This group accounts for 75% of fetal deaths and 30% to 40% of deaths during the first year of life. Surviving children can have intellectual impairment or various somatic anomalies.

Spina Bifida

Spina bifida, myelomeningocele, and myelodysplasia are failures of closure of the vertebral arches with variable involvement of the spinal cord and meninges. These defects are more frequently found in the lumbar areas. *Spina bifida occulta* is not accompanied by protrusions of meningeal or spinal cord elements. Symptoms are absent or appear late in life. It can be associated with dimples of overlying skin, dermal sinuses, lipomas, diastematomyelia (division of spinal cord by fibrous tissue, cartilage, or bony spicules), or syringomyelia. The defects can be detected only by x-rays or imaging studies of the spine. *Meningomyelocele* is evident at birth, is most frequently found in the lumbosacral region, and can rupture during birth causing leakage of cerebrospinal fluid. Neurologic deficits vary according to the level of the lesion and consist of weak legs with inverted feet held in equinovarus position, depressed stretch reflexes, sensory loss (in the feet and saddle or perirectal region), and sphincteric disturbances. In 90% of patients with lumbar meningomyelocele, there is an associated Chiari type II malformation usually with hydrocephalus. The exact cause of the defect is not known, but in families with one affected child there is a 10% chance of another child having a similar defect. Treatment consists of immediate surgical closure of the defect. Folic acid, 4 mg a day, supplementation in subsequent pregnancy decreases incidence of neural tube defects in women who have given birth to affected infants. Folic acid, 0.4 mg, is recommended to decrease incidence of birth defects in all pregnancies.

Chiari Type I Malformations

Chiari type I malformation consists of cerebellar tonsillar displacement through the foramen magnum down into the cervical spine but without brain stem displacement. The malformation is usually asymptomatic until later in life, when brain stem and upper cervical cord symptoms of a progressive nature can occur as a result of adhesions between the cerebellum, lower brain stem, and spinal cord. MRI is used to diagnose the lesion. Treatment consists of surgical decompression through a laminectomy and occipital craniectomy.

Chiari Type II Malformation

This malformation consists of elongation of the pons, medulla, and fourth ventricle and downward displacement of the brain stem along with the cerebellar tonsils through the foramen magnum into the cervical spinal canal (Figure 13-1).Very frequently there is an association of other malformations such as aqueductal stenosis, microgyria, gray matter heterotopia, and syringomyelia. The malformation should be suspected in all newborns who have meningomyelocele and are born with or develop hydrocephalus early after birth. The diagnosis is confirmed by MRI. Treatment consists of relief of hydrocephalus.

Dandy-Walker Syndrome

This syndrome consists of a cyst dilatation of the fourth ventricle, hypoplasia of the cerebellum, and hydrocephalus (Figure 13-2). Frequently there are other anomalies such as agenesis of the corpus callosum, facial clefts, and cardiac abnormalities. The expanded posterior fossa produces upward displacement of the tentorium along with the torcular and lateral venous sinuses. The large posterior fossa causes dolichocephaly. CT scanning and MRI confirm the presence of the lesion.

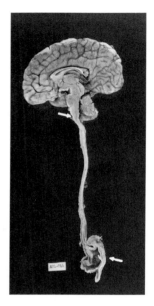

FIGURE 13-1. Sagittal section of brain and spinal cord showing meningomyelocele (*lower arrow*) and Chiari type II malformation. *Upper arrow* shows level of foramen magnum. Note hydrocephalus.

■ NEUROCUTANEOUS SYNDROMES

Neurocutaneous syndromes are genetically determined disorders that affect the CNS, skin, and other viscera. They can be present at birth or appear later in life.

Neurofibromatosis is an autosomal-dominant inherited disease with marked variability of expression and a slight preponderance in males. There are two different syndromes. Neurofibromatosis type I is the most frequently found syndrome and is linked to chromosome 17(17q11.2). Neurofibromatosis type II is linked to chromosome 22(22q11-q12).

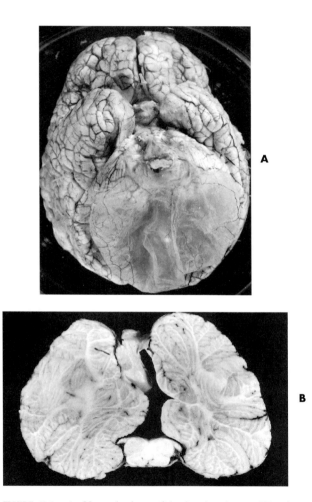

A

B

FIGURE 13-2. **A,** Ventral view of brain showing a dilated fourth ventricle covered by a membrane. **B,** Same specimen as **A.** Note the defect of the cerebellar vermis and the attachment of the membrane.

Neurofibromatosis Type I

This is a clinically and genetically heterogeneous syndrome with almost 100% penetrance and a high rate of spontaneous mutations. The diagnosis of neurofibromatosis has to be based on finding two of the following features: family history of neurofibromatosis type I, café au lait spots, neurofibromas, axillary or inguinal freckling, optic glioma, Iris (Lisch) nodules, or one of the distinctive osseous lesions (thoracic scoliosis, anterolateral bowing of the tibias, pseudoarthrosis, sphenoid wing dysplasia). Age is an important factor in the appearance of some of these lesions. Café au lait spots are better recognized after the first year of life, the Lisch nodules are seen in all affected patients only after age 20, and neurofibromas grow with age. These last three findings are seen in all adult patients with neurofibromatosis type I. Five café au lait spots measuring more than 5 mm in diameter before puberty and six measuring more than 15 mm after puberty are required to suggest or confirm the diagnosis. The location in the sun-protected areas and the trauma- or rubbing-inducing factor are very characteristic of these freckles. The tumors can occur distally, can be cutaneous or subcutaneous, and are usually localized or nodular (neurofibromas) or can be diffuse or less localized (plexiform neurofibromas). Proximal tumors are usually schwannomas. Acoustic neuromas do not occur in this type of neurofibromatosis. The symptoms associated with these tumors include neuropathic pain and esthetic problems. The CNS problems in neurofibromatosis I can include developmental delays, mental retardation, seizures, loss of vision, and headaches. Some of the CNS symptoms are caused by brain or blood vessel dysplasia. CNS tumors include multiple meningiomas and optic nerve and brain stem gliomas. Spinal cord lesions include syringomyelia, hydromyelia, and compressive myelopathies caused by tumors or bone deformities. Imaging studies are helpful in diagnosing these conditions. The treatment consists predominantly of symptomatic management of the lesion by different specialists, including neurosurgeons and orthopedic doctors. Excision of symptomatic intracranial tumors is mandatory. Mental retardation and seizures should be treated accordingly.

Neurofibromatosis Type II

Also known as bilateral acoustic neuroma or central neurofibromatosis, this condition is a genetically distinct entity from neurofibromatosis type I. Acoustic neuromas, usually bilateral and seen before the age of 30, are always present. Café au lait spots, posterior lens opacities, absence of Lisch nodules, and a family history of the disease are confirmatory of neurofibromatosis type II. Other CNS tumors including meningiomas and gliomas (except for optic verve gliomas) are more frequent than in type I. Mental retardation, seizures, and macrocephaly do not occur. Clinical symptoms of acoustic neuromas consist of tinnitus, deafness, headaches, and brain-stem dysfunction. Syringomyelia and hydromyelia may occur. MRI studies confirm the diagnosis and can detect small resectable acoustic tumors before they produce permanent deafness. Genetic counseling is very important.

Tuberous Sclerosis

Tuberous sclerosis is inherited as an autosomal dominant disease with markedly variable expression, high penetrance, and a high spontaneous mutation rate. The disease is also genetically heterogeneous and has been linked to chromosome 9(9q34) in 35% of the families and to chromosome 11(11q21-23) in other families. The diagnosis is based on finding one of the characteristic malformations such as the focal cortical dysplasias (tubers), subependymal nodules, giant cell subependymal tumors, retinal astrocytic hamartomas, facial angiofibroma (misnamed adenoma sebaceum) or ungual fibromas. The diagnosis can also be based on finding several less specific lesions, such as cardiac rhabdomyomas, renal angioleimyolipomas, pulmonary angiomyolipomas, or rectal polyps. The clinical neurologic manifestations include a high frequency of seizures that vary from infantile spasms in infancy to posterior focal (partial) seizures before 2 years of age to temporal and frontal seizures later on. Mental retardation is found in half of the patients of all ages. All mentally retarded patients with tuberous sclerosis have seizures, but one third of the tuberous sclerosis patients have seizures without mental retardation. Visceral lesions include involvement of the kidneys and the heart. The renal lesions include multiple cysts or angiomyolipomas. The cardiac rhabdomyomas are usually asymptomatic. Benign rectal polyps and vascular dysplasia have also been described. Treatment consists of control of the seizures with the appropriate anticonvulsant medication, surgical resection of intraventricular tumors when hydrocephalus develops, and resection of renal and other visceral lesions when indicated.

Sturge-Weber Syndrome (Encephalotrigeminal Angiomatosis)

Sturge-Weber syndrome does not have a well-defined inheritance pattern. Although most cases are sporadic, a few are autosomal recessive or autosomal dominant. The disease is characterized by dysplasia of mature capillaries in the distribution of the first division of the trigeminal verve, ipsilateral occipitoparietal leptomeningeal angiomatosis with degeneration and calcification of the underlying cortex as a result of ischemia, contralateral hemiplegia, and contralateral focal or generalized seizures. Glaucoma in the eye ipsilateral to the vascular lesions can be present. Aspirin and other antithrombotic agents prevent important neurologic sequelae. Anticonvulsant therapy controls the seizures. Hemispherectomy has been performed for many intractable seizures.

▪ DEGENERATIVE AND METABOLIC DISEASES

Degenerative diseases comprise a group of rare neurologic disorders, usually inherited and frequently progressive, that can appear early after birth or later in life with severe developmental neurologic regression. Metabolic diseases must be suspected when these criteria are associated with recurrent unexplained ataxia or spasticity, recurrent episodes of altered consciousness or unexplained vomiting, unexplained acidosis, or mental retardation in the absence of major congenital anomalies. The confirmation of the diagnosis should be made by detection of abnormal substances or their metabolites in the urine or blood and titration of specific enzymes in urine, blood or more accurately from tissue culture of fibroblasts obtained through a skin biopsy. In some of the metabolic disorders in which the exact enzymatic defect has not yet been found but accumulation of abnormal metabolites is deposited in the tissue, biopsy of peripheral nerve, muscle, bone marrow, or brain tissue nay be necessary and should be done where adequate facilities are available. Although treatment is available for only a few of these disorders, an exact diagnosis is important for genetic counseling and prognosis. Bone marrow transplantation has been sucessful in a few cases when done early in the course of the disease. Intrauterine diagnosis by amniocentesis may be possible in pregnancies at risk for certain of these disorders and can be helpful in deciding whether to terminate the pregnancy. Only a treatable and preventable disorder will be described here.

Hepatic Encephalopathy and Reye's Syndrome

Reye's syndrome is an acute encephalopathy of childhood of undetermined cause. The disease is preceded by a viral illness, especially influenza B and varicella. Frequently the affected children have received aspirin, phenothiazines, or trimethobenzamide (Tigan). The disease is characterized by vomiting followed by delirium, lethargy, coma, and seizures. During coma the child can develop decorticate or decerebrate posture or opisthotonos, the pupils dilate, and breathing becomes irregular. Biochemical alterations consist of early hypoglycemia, especially in younger patients, and hyperammonemia, abnormal liver enzymes without elevation of bilirubin, and elevated serum levels of free and short-chain fatty acids. Striking intracranial hypertension produced by severe cerebral edema produces the change in sensorium and eventually results in death. Mortality correlates with the level of consciousness at admission to the hospital. Fatty degeneration of the liver, kidneys, and heart without cell necrosis is a constant feature in postmortem studies. Recovery in nonfatal cases occurs in 2 or 3 days.

Treatment consists of intravenous administration of hypertonic glucose solutions in the early stages that may prevent progression of the disease. Control of temperature, early monitoring of intracranial pressure, and reduction of intracranial pressure by hyperventilation and use of mannitol is important. Early correction of metabolic derangements and control of intracranial pressure can lead to recovery in most patients.

▦ SUMMARY

The neurologic evaluation of a child is different from that of an adult, and in a good number of cases it requires the expertise of a pediatric neurologist. Only the most frequent pediatric neurologic problems are reviewed here. The history need to be obtained from the parents or guardian of the child. The hospital records may need to be obtained to review the perinatal history and the birth events. In older children records of performance in school or day-care centers are important to learn about the emotional and intellectual characteristics of the child. Important reasons for pediatric consultation of the neurologist are disorders of motor execution such as dyspraxia, clumsiness, and adventitious movements as well as attention deficit disorders, which are discussed in this chapter. There are important differences between cerebral palsy and mental retardation that are important for the primary care physician to know. There are also special types of seizures, some of them begign, that need to be differentiated from the more malignant types seen in the pediatric population. Finally, the most frequent neurocutaneous syndromes are delineated here.

Suggested Readings

Suggested Readings—General

Adams RD, Victor M: *Principles of neurology,* ed 5, New York, 1993, McGraw-Hill.

David RB: *Pediatric neurology for the clinician,* Norwalk, Conn, 1992, Appleton & Lange.

Schaefer GS, Bodensteiner JB: Evaluation of the child with idiopathic mental retardation, *Pediatr Clin North Am* 39:929, 1992.

Swaiman KF, Wright FS: *The practice of pediatric neurology,* ed 2, St Louis, 1982, Mosby.

Volpe JJ: *Neurology of the newborn,* ed 2, Philadelphia, 1987, WB Saunders.

Birth Injuries

Allen WC: The intraventricular hemorrhage complex of lesions: cerebrovascular injury in the preterm infant, *Neurol Clin North Am* 8:529, 1990.

Freeman JM, Nelson KB: Intrapartum asphyxia and cerebral palsy, *Pediatrics* 84:240, 1988.

Developmental Abnormalities

Dunsker SB, Brown D: Craniovertebral anomalies, *Clin Neurosurg* 27:430, 1980.

Loesser JD, Albord EC: Agenesis of corpus callosum, *Brain* 91:553, 1968.

Sawaya R, McLaurin RL: Dandy-Walker syndrome, *J Neurosurg* 55:89, 1981.

Hydrocephalus

DeMeyer W: Megalencephaly, *Pediatr Neurol* 2:321, 1986.

Naidich TP, Schott LH, Baron RL: Computed tomography in the evaluation of hydrocephalus, *Radiol Clin North Am* 20:143, 1982.

Neurocutaneous Syndromes

Riccardi VM, Von Recklinghausen: neurofibromatosis, *N Engl J Med* 305:617, 1981.

Roach ES: Encephalofacial angiomatosis, *Pediatr Clin North Am* 39:606, 1992.

Roach ES: Neurocutaneous syndromes, *Pediatr Clin North Am* 39:600, 1991.

Roach ES: Tuberous sclerosis, *Pediatr Clin North Am* 39:591, 1991.

Metabolic Diseases

DiMauro S, Moraes CT: Mitrochondrial encephalomyopathies, *Arch Neurol* 50:1197, 1993.

Kolodny EH, Cable WJL: Inborn errors of metabolism, *Ann Neurol* 11:221, 1982.

Naidu S, Moser HW: Peroxisomal disorders, *Neurol Clin North Am* 8:507, 1990.

Hypotonic Infant

Rabe EF: The hypotonic infant, *J Pediatr* 64:222, 1964.

Dubowitz V: *The floppy infant*. London, 1969, Spastics International Medical Publications.

Neurobehavioral Disorders (Organic Brain Syndromes)

14

The neurobehavioral disorders are a group of conditions in which brain damage or dysfunction produces primarily intellectual (cognitive) and behavioral change rather than motor or sensory abnormalities. The behavior change can be in intellectual functions, such as the memory failure in dementia, or emotional, as is seen in the personality change accompanying frontal lobe lesions. In widespread diseases such as dementia and delirium, many aspects of behavior will be affected, whereas with focal lesions from strokes or tumors more restricted abnormalities such as inadequate verbal comprehension may be all that is demonstrated on examination. These syndromes are encountered in everyday medical practice and can usually be diagnosed with a careful history, a brief mental status examination, and some basic knowledge of the clinical syndromes.

▣ EVALUATION

The clinical evaluation of the patient with a behavioral change requires a history and a mental status examination that are tailored to elicit specific organic symptoms and signs. The history should be taken from both the patient and someone who knows the patient well because the patient is frequently unable to give an accurate history of the illness. In the history of the current illness it is important to ask exactly how the patient's behavior has changed and over what period of time. From the patient with behavioral change in whom organic brain disease is suspected, specific historical information should be obtained as outlined in Box 14-1.

Specific Review of Systems for Organic Behavior Change

During the review of systems for organic behavior change several changes must be observed (Box 14-2).

After a careful history a screening mental status examination such as that outlined in Chapter 1 should be performed. Neurologic and physical examinations are also necessary. In dementia and delirium the neurologic examination is frequently normal, but the elicitation of localizing neurologic signs suggests that a focal lesion is responsible for the behavior change. Such signs as papilledema or stiff neck also suggest specific intracranial disease (e.g., mass lesion, intracranial hypertension, or meningitis). The physical examination can also reveal the cause of the behavior change (e.g., pulmonary failure, hypothyroidism, Addison's disease, and extremely high blood pressure). Unfortunately, it is impossible to discuss every neurologic or medical disease in which behavior change can be the main or an accompanying symptom; therefore only some of the more common organic syndromes will be presented here.

BOX 14-1   Pertinent General History

1   *Age.* Behavioral change in the elderly is most likely organic.

2   *Education and vocation.* This information establishes the level of expectation on the mental status examination.

3   *Handedness.* Knowledge of handedness is important in assessing the laterality of a focal lesion in aphasic patients.

4   *Review of medical history.* Endocrine, vascular, renal, hepatic, pulmonary, and many other medical diseases can affect the brain and therefore behavior.

5   *Review of neurologic history.* Strokes, head trauma, seizures, and parkinsonism are all important causes of brain disease that can affect behavior.

6   *Family history.* There are many familial forms of dementia: Huntington's disease, Alzheimer's disease, Pick's disease and others.

7   *Medications.* Many medications or combinations of medicine can produce delirium and sometimes a dementia-like state.

8   *Alcohol or drug abuse.*

9   *Toxic exposure.* Insect sprays, hydrocarbon vapors, and other toxins can affect the brain.

10 *Psychiatric history.* Depression is well known to masquerade as dementia in the elderly. Any significant psychiatric illness will effect cognitive functioning and raise the possibility of brain disease or dysfunction.

ACUTE CONFUSIONAL STATE (DELIRIUM)

An acute confusional state (variously labeled delirium, metabolic encephalopathy, or acute brain failure) is as the name implies—a rapidly developing mental change in which the patient looks and acts confused. More specifically the clinical picture is one of altered and fluctuating alertness, incoherent or

BOX 14-2

1 Memory difficulty
2 General loss of intellectual ability
3 Word-finding problems in speech
4 Geographic disorientation (e.g., getting lost)
5 Personality change
6 Inattention or difficulty concentrating
7 Bizarre behavior (e.g., nocturnal wandering, improperly clothed)
8 Lethargy or excessive sleepiness

clouded mental processes, marked inattentiveness, and usually a change in activity level featuring either agitation or lethargy. In addition, hallucinations, most often visual or tactile (e.g., spiders crawling on the skin); emotional changes such as suspiciousness, irritability, euphoria, or violence; indistinct speech; and autonomic changes such as dilated pupils, tachycardia, and diaphoresis can be present. The course of the condition is typically rapid in onset (hours to days) with considerable fluctuation in symptoms during the day and a distinct propensity for nocturnal exacerbations. If the cause is not determined and proper treatment instituted, the mental state will deteriorate, and the patient will become stuporous and comatose and can eventually die.

The causes are many and closely parallel those of stupor and coma. Predisposing factors include increasing age, early dementia, previous brain damage, and a previous history of delirium. The cause of a confusional state is almost always medical or neurologic rather than psychiatric (e.g., mania, schizophrenia);

therefore the physician's first obligation is to review the patient's medical status with particular attention to medications. Older people are especially sensitive to medications and can become confusional on even small doses of standard prescription drugs. Common offenders are psychotropics, antiparkinsonism drugs, diuretics, sedatives, strong analgesics, and of course alcohol and illicit drugs. Frequently it is the combination of drugs that produces the problem.

The next area to consider is systemic illness. Some of the most common are generalized metabolic dysfunction; organ failure (e.g., cardiac, renal, pulmonary, or hapatic); sepsis; marked hypertension; endocrine disease; or electrolyte disturbances. Neurologic disease such as increased intracranial pressure, brain tumor, meningitis, or acute cerebral infarction (particularly in the frontal lobe or inferior parietal region of the non-dominant hemisphere) can also cause the syndrome. In many cases, however, it is a combination of factors that is involved. Nowhere is this more true than in the post-operative patient, in whom medications, electrolyte fluctuations, fever, and the primary disease itself all combine to produce an abnormal metabolic milieu for the brain. Alcohol withdrawal, which can itself produce a classic delirium, can also be a factor in any patient who stops drinking on entrance to the hospital. Sleep loss is another very important factor that is well known for its capacity to produce and perpetuate confusional behavior.

The evaluation of the confusional patient is similar to that for coma and involves a complete history, physical examination, and neurologic examination, after which blood counts, chemical screens, and drug screens are obtained. The remaining evaluation is largely dictated by what is found at this point. A spinal tap or a CT scan of the brain is indicated if primary neurologic disease is suspected or the patient does not respond to medical management within 24 to 48 hours, but these tests are usually not necessary for routine cases.

▣ DEMENTIA

Dementia is a very common clinical entity in which there is a progressive deterioration in intellectual and social adaptive functions; there is usually associated behavior and personality change. Although previously divided into presenile and senile varieties, this distinction seems to be unjustified; the dementing illnesses seen before age 65 appear identical to those seen thereafter. Not included within the dementia category are the patients with intellectual loss secondary to head trauma, encephalitis, or other acute lesions. These are not progressive conditions and are more conveniently classified as encephalopathies.

It is now realized that some dementia can be reversed. In general it is the younger patients (40s or 50s) who will prove to have the reversible conditions; nevertheless a full evaluation should be made in all demented persons.

Alzheimer's Disease/Senile Dementia

Alzheimer's disease is by far the most common dementia, probably constituting more than two thirds of all dementia cases. Its onset is insidious, and its course is long (10 years average with some patients living 15 to 20 years). Initial symptoms are usually a subtle personality change and recent memory difficulty. The personality change is usually characterized by apathy, lack of interest, hypochondriasis, and often an accentuation of previous personality traits. If examined carefully, the patients can also show difficulty with abstract reasoning on proverb interpretation, constructional impairment on drawings, and subtle word finding difficulty. There are no gait, motor, coordination, or reflex abnormalities in the early stage. As the disease progresses, aphasia, agnosia, apraxia, and inattention occur along with marked worsening of memory and other intellectual functions. The patients, however, remain alert and can be somewhat hyperactive. The standard neurologic examination is almost always normal except that a snout reflex can occasionally be elicited. Treatment is largely directed toward control of associated agitation, depression, or anxiety. There can be some improvement with oral anticholinesterase drugs, although the success of such agents has been far less satisfying than has been the experience with dopamine in parkinsonism.

Vascular Dementia (Arteriosclerotic Dementia)

Cerebrovascular disease can produce a progressive dementia, but the prevalence of the disorder has been overestimated in the past. Approximately 15% to 35% of all demented patients have a vascular dementia, and another 10% to 15% have what is now called a mixed dementia: Alzheimer's dementia plus brain damage from strokes that contribute to the cognitive decline. The clinical picture is usually one of stepwise deterioration, with multiple acute exacerbations and a gradual accretion of positive neurologic findings such as pseudobulbar paralysis, labile affect, reflex asymmetries, and aphasia. Memory function is usually quite good, which is uncommon in Alzheimer's disease.

There are several mechanisms by which cerebrovascular disease can result in dementia. In hypertensive patients multiple small lacunar infarcts throughout the brain, though more prevalent in the white matter and basal ganglia, produce the most common form of vascular dementia—multiinfarct dementia (50%±). A second type of vascular dementia is produced by multiple emboli to the cortex of the brain. These emboli can be of cardiac origin or from lesions in the major vessels leading to the brain. A third mechanism is chronic fluctuating hypoxia. Patients with hypotension, poor cardiac output, or severe stenosis of the major cerebral vessels will experience decreased cerebral blood flow especially when standing. This hypoxia leads to confusion and can eventually produce ischemia to the brain such that cells in the temporal lobes can be damaged (the memory circuits) and areas of demyelination can be seen in the hemispheric white matter.

CT and MRI scans will demonstrate these areas of infarction and demyelination very well. Caution must be exercised when interpreting these scans, however, because many of these findings, usually to a lesser degree, can be seen in patients with Alzheimer's disease and even in some normal elderly individuals.

Treatment of vascular dementia depends on the cause, control of hypertension, prevention of cerebral emboli, or raising blood pressure in those patients with significant hypotension.

Pick's Lobar Atrophy

Pick's lobar atrophy is a cause of dementia in which the cerebral atrophy is localized to the frontal and temporal lobes. The atrophy is frequently asymmetric with the left hemisphere more commonly affected than the right. In patients with primary frontal atrophy there is a decline in personal appearance and social appropriateness. The frontal patients also are withdrawn, talk less, and eventually become mute. If temporal atrophy is more prominent, memory loss and language problems will predominate the clinical picture. Usually the clinical picture in Pick's disease is sufficiently different from Alzheimer's disease that the clinical diagnosis can be made. The focal atrophy on CT or MRI scan further increases the accuracy of the diagnosis (Figure 14-1). This contrasts with the pathologic findings in Alzheimer's disease in which the cerebral atrophy is more diffuse. Clinical symptomatology is consistent with that expected for the frontal-temporal predilection.

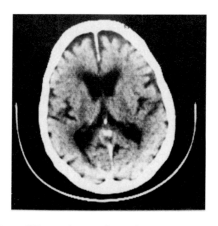

FIGURE 14-1. CT scan in a patient with Alzheimer's disease. Cortical atrophy is prominent, and the ventricles are enlarged. This ventricular enlargement, often called hydrocephalus ex vacuo, is secondary to atrophy and not pressure. A word of caution about the interpretation of atrophy seen on the CT scan: Many normal elderly persons will demonstrate cerebral atrophy; therefore the diagnosis of dementia must be made on clinical grounds and not from the CT scan. Conversely some patients with unequivocal clinical evidence of Alzheimer's type dementia will have a normal-appearing CT scan.

Alcoholic Dementia

Chronic alcoholism produces dementia as well as some of the more well-known alcoholic behavioral syndromes of delirium tremens and Wernicke-Korsakoff syndrome. The dementia is usually mild and is characterized by mild memory loss and apathy. Any alcoholic patient with severe memory loss probably has Alzheimer's disease plus the effects of alcohol. The exception is when the memory loss was sudden and occurred after a period of confusion (Wernicke-Korsakoff syndrome).

Mass Lesions

Neoplasms, abscesses, subdural hematomas, or any other mass lesion can produce a gradual deterioration in mental capacities. The clinical picture, however, almost always shows focal neurologic findings, an altered level of consciousness, seizures, papilledema, or focal behavioral change such as aphasia and frontal lobe symptoms. Certain neoplasms can cause tissue infiltration and not mass effect. In these cases the patient can develop progressive dementia without other neurologic signs.

Hydrocephalus

In adults the condition called "normal pressure hydrocephalus" (NPH) has been identified as a correctable cause of dementia. Communicating hydrocephalus (often with normal intracranial pressure) can produce a rather characteristic clinical picture of which mental deterioration is one feature. More prominent and usually appearing first, however, are a very unsteady gait and urinary incontinence. The gait disorder is called gait apraxia, and it is characterized by a magnetic quality in which the patient does not pick the feet off the ground. The mental change that follows can be intermittent confusion, memory difficulty, frontal lobe personality change, or psychiatric symptoms.

The pathogenesis of this syndrome is due to impairment of the reabsorptive surface of the arachnoid villi in the subarachnoid spaces. This leads to progressive ventricular dilatation but with normal intraventricular and lumbar cerebrospinal fluid pressures. Computed tomography shows dilatation of all ventricles without enlarged subarachnoid spaces. (Figure 14-2) The most valuable test for both diagnosing and predicting the response of shunting is a spinal puncture with removal of 25 or 30 ml of spinal fluid. If the opening pressure is greater than 110 mm H_2O and the removal of fluid produces a significant improvement in the patient's clinical symptoms, then the diagnosis is established, and shunting is highly likely to greatly improve the patient's mental as well as physical symptoms.

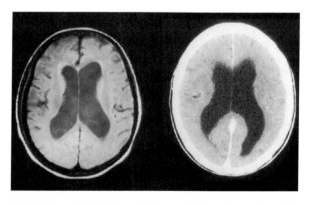

FIGURE 14-2. MRI (*left*) and CT scan (*right*) of a patient with communicating hydrocephalus. Note the enlarged ventricles and small cortical sulci for the patient's age (75 years old).

Other Causes of Dementia

The effects of the other causes of dementia can be either potentially reversible, degenerative irreversible, or infectious irreversible. Box 14-3 lists the diseases that can be reversible or irreversible.

The evaluation of a patient with dementia should include the following:

- CT scan (see Figures 14-1 and 14-2) or MRI scan
- Complete blood cell count
- Chemical profile
- Thyroid studies
- Vitamin B_{12} and folate levels
- VDRL test
- Urine screen for drugs and toxins (if indicated)
- Lumbar puncture with cerebrospinal fluid analysis (if serum VDRL and FTA are abnormal or if meningitis is suspected)

Electroencephalography is sometimes useful particularly if Creutzfeldt-Jakob disease is suspected. Lumbar puncture is not required in every patient, although it should be considered if the diagnosis is not established by the other workup. Neuropsychologic evaluation can be useful when the diagnosis is in doubt or if the mental competency level needs to be evaluated.

Two words of warning need to be issued concerning the evaluation of dementia. The first is that the CT scan can show atrophy in normal elderly persons and no atrophy in patients with significant Alzheimer's disease. The second point is that depression can often mimic dementia. The depressed patient often has apathy and memory complaints, so the physician must be very cautious making a diagnosis of dementia in a depressed patient. Most dementia is irreversible and untreatable, whereas depression is

BOX 14-3

Potentially Reversible

1 Chronic meningitis *(Cryptococcus,* fungus, *Mycobacterium tuberculosis)*

2 Myxedema

3 Vitamin B_{12} deficiency

4 Pituitary or parathyroid disease

5 Wilson's disease

6 Meningovascular syphilis

Degenerative Irreversible

1 Pick's disease

2 Huntington's disease

3 Parkinsonism

Infectious Irreversible

1 Creutzfeldt-Jakob disease

2 General paresis

3 Acquired immune deficiency syndrome (AIDS)

4 Viral (herpes simplex, arbovirus)

quite the opposite; the implication of an erroneous diagnosis cannot be overstressed.

A full neuropsychologic test battery and psychiatric consultation are often necessary to make the correct diagnosis in complex cases. Depressed or anxious patients can perform poorly on mental status testing yet return to normal functioning when their emotional problem is treated. Such patients are diagnosed as having a pseudodementia or dementia of depression. Such conditions usually appear rather suddenly after an emotional crisis and show fluctuating and inconsistent findings from a history and mental status examinations.

NEUROBEHAVIORAL SYNDROMES SECONDARY TO FOCAL LESIONS

Aphasia

Aphasia is a language disturbance that is secondary to brain damage. Improper syntax, word choice, and imperfect comprehension are the principal features. The demonstration of aphasia is unequivocal evidence of brain dysfunction and most frequently indicates left-hemisphere involvement. Almost all right-handed persons have their speech in the left hemisphere; but left-handed persons, particularly those with a family history of left handedness, frequently have bilateral speech representation. In rare cases right-handed individuals are right-hemisphere dominant for language.

The evaluation of language includes listening to spontaneous speech and evaluating comprehensive, repetition, and naming of objects. In the acute aphasia following a stroke the patient can also show confusional behavior, so it is often difficult to assess aphasia fully early in its evolution.

Global aphasia. Global aphasia is caused by a large lesion involving the entire middle cerebral artery territory. Spontaneous speech consists only of explicatives or stereotyped sounds. Comprehension, repetition, naming, reading, and writing are similarly profoundly affected. Hemiparesis and hemianesthesia are usually present.

Mixed aphasia. Many patients exhibit some problems in all language functions without any single function being relatively spared or impaired. This is not surprising, particularly in vascular disease in which there is such a great variation in patterns of ischemia and infarction.

Broca's aphasia. This type of aphasia is usually produced by a lesion in the frontal lobe that involves Broca's region 44 and surrounding tissue. The patients have markedly reduced spontaneous speech and dysarthria. They produce only a few single words and do so with great effort. Usually the words are highly meaningful nouns or verbs. Because temporal and parietal lobes are spared, comprehension is near normal. Repetition is impaired to the same degree as spontaneous speech, and naming errors are common. The patients are usually hemiparetic. Reading for comprehension is good, but writing is impaired.

Wernicke's aphasia. Wernicke's classic aphasic syndrome is caused by a lesion in the posterior temporal area and contiguous parietal lobe. The patient's spontaneous speech is fluent, circumlocutory, surprisingly devoid of content, and paraphasic. Comprehension is severely impaired, as is repetition. Naming is paraphasic. No hemiparesis is present, but a visual field defect is sometimes observed. The patient may be considered to have a primary psychiatric disorder on initial examination because the most prominent feature of the syndrome is bizarre language output. That the patient has had a stoke or other focal lesion is overlooked because of the lack of classic motor signs usually associated with those conditions.

Conduction aphasia. Conduction aphasia is an uncommon but interesting type of aphasia in which spontaneous speech, comprehension, and naming are quite good (paraphasia is often present), yet repetition is severely impaired. The lesion causing this syndrome is in the posterior sylvian fissure region and extends into the deep white matter in that area.

Transcortical aphasia. Transcortical aphasia is an unusual yet not uncommon aphasia. It is the direct linguistic opposite of conduction aphasia. In these patients repetition is excellent, whereas spontaneous speech, comprehension, and naming are nil or severely involved. The lesion causing this interesting syndrome is a border zone infarction caused by carotid stenosis, hypoxia from decreased perfusion, or carbon monoxide poisoning. The lesion has the appearance of a backwards "C" and involves the border zone cortex between the anterior and middle cerebral arteries anteriorly and the middle and posterior cerebral arteries posteriorly. If the lesion is predominantly anterior, comprehension can be good and speech production absent (transcortical motor aphasia); conversely, if the lesion is posterior, speech can be present (albeit aphasic), but comprehension is poor (transcortical sensory aphasia).

Anomic aphasia. Some patients develop an aphasic syndrome in which the ability to name objects is the only significant defect. Speech is fluent yet halting as the patient searches for specific nouns or verbs. Comprehension and repetition are good, but naming is very poor and often grossly paraphasic. There is no specific lesion localization for this syndrome, but inferior temporal lobe or parietal lobe lesions are the most common.

Frontal Lobe Syndrome

In patients with destruction of the frontal lobes, a rather characteristic behavioral syndrome occurs. Patients develop apathy and lose motivation and goal direction. They do not initiate activities unless encouraged by others, including washing and dressing themselves. They are often euphoric and indifferent, at times to the point of inappropriate jocularity or childishness. Irritability that is short-lived, perseveration, and a tendency to act inappropriately in social situations are also frequently present. They have difficulty sustaining attention, and they cannot make mental shifts in their thinking (perseveration). In some cases depressive symptoms are prominent. Causes include tumors (glioma, metastatic, meningioma, and pituitary adenoma), hydrocephalus, Pick's disease, alcoholic dementia, general paresis, head trauma, and Huntington's disease. To develop the syndrome bilateral damage must be present. The prognosis for normal social integration and productive employment is unfortunately not good after significant frontal damage even when intellectual functions are spared.

Organic Amnesia

Amnesia, as the term is used in neurology, refers to a defect in recent memory or, more properly, in the ability to learn new material. Learning requires the limbic structures of the hippocampi, mammillary bodies, dorsal medial thalami, and perhaps other limbic structures. When brain disease specifically damages these structures *bilaterally,* a severe organic amnesia or recent memory deficit results. There are several common causes: thiamine deficiency in the Wernicke-Korsakoff's syndrome (mammillary bodies and dorsal medial thalami), herpes encephalitis (hippocampi), head trauma (hippocampi), bilateral temporal lobe strokes, and a transient form called transient global amnesia. In these cases the patients constantly repeat the same questions and usually appear rather confused during the attack. In Alzheimer's and senile dementia it is the hippocampi and the cholinergic neurons in the basilar nuclei that are involved earliest and most severely. In Korsakoff's syndrome, usually seen in alcoholics, the amnesia is usually the only significantly abnormal cognitive function; IQ and other functions can be normal. In other conditions mentioned above the cortical involvement is more widespread, and other mental status changes can be demonstrated. In psychiatric amnesia (dissociative or fugue states) the patient blocks out periods of time, yet during that time (during which the patient later claims not to remember) the patient is able to learn adequately if tested. Behavior during that time is frequently normal and not noticed to be abnormal by others. In organic amnesia recent memory is impaired, but remote memory is spared.

Parietal Lobe Syndromes

Damage to the parietal lobes produces a host of interesting signs, many of which can easily be overlooked on cursory examination. Box 14-4 outlines the signs that can be seen on the parietal lobes.

▉ EVALUATION

Any person showing evidence of a focal lesion on higher cortical function testing should be evaluated in the same fashion as one would be if the patient had any other focal neurologic deficit (electroencephalography, CT/MRI scanning, and angiography).

▉ SUMMARY

The neurobehavioral disorders, previously called organic brain syndromes, represent the myriad ways in which the patient's behavior can be changed by physical disease affecting the brain. Sudden events will produce the global changes described as acute confusion, a global behavioral abnormality that usually produces an altered level of alertness. If a focal

1 Signs that can be seen with lesions in either parietal lobe
   a Drawing and other constructional tasks are frequently impaired; lesions of the right parietal give more dramatic abnormalities, however (constructional apraxia)
   b Right-left disorientation
   c Finger agnosia (inability to recognize fingers and their relative position on the hand)
   d Calculation errors (dyscalculia). In left parietal lesion this can be a loss of basic arithmetic processes, whereas with right lesions calculation failure is usually on the basis of spatial errors (inability to keep numbers in their proper alignment).
   e Contralateral astereognosis or graphesthesia (inability to integrate sensory stimuli for identification of objects placed in the hand or writing on the skin).

2 Left parietal lesions
   a Reading and writing problems. With lesions in the inferior parietal lobule (angular and supramarginal gyri, areas 39 and 40) there is a defect in the translation of verbal language into written language. The resultant syndrome is called an alexia with agraphia; the syndrome is often accompanied by an anomic aphasia.
   b Gerstmann syndrome. On rare occasions left superior parietal lesions produce this syndrome in which a combination of finger agnosia, right-left orientation, dyscalculia, and dysgraphia is present. Constructional impairment apraxia is also present but is not part of the original syndrome.
   c Ideomotor apraxia. This fascinating inability to carry out rather complex motor acts such as flipping a coin, drinking through a straw, or using a hammer is often seen with parietal lesions, usually the left. Left frontal lesions can also produce apraxia.

3 Right parietal lesions
   a Unilateral neglect. Lesions in the right parietal lobe frequently produce an interesting condition in which the patient neglects both the left side of the body and the left side of the environment. The patient may shave only the right side of his face, completely ignore people to the left, and fail to use the left arm even though it has normal strength. Occasionally, the patient will frankly deny having any defect at all. This syndrome is occasionally seen with left-hemisphere lesions but not with the frequency that it is seen with right lesions.
   b Geographic disorientation. Patients often lose their orientation in their environment and can even get lost in their own houses.

lesion has been the cause of the change, then there will also be evidence of a specific cognitive loss that is dependent on the location of the lesion. The slowly developing changes represent a dementia syndrome whose cause can usually be determined with a full medical and neurologic evaluation.

Suggested Readings

Dementia—General

Clarfield AM: The reversible dementias: do they reverse? *Ann Intern Med* 109:476, 1988.

Cummings JL, Benson DF: *Dementia: a clinical approach,* Boston, 1983, Butterworths.

Le May M: CT changes in dementing diseases: a review, *Am J Neuroradiol* 7:841, 1986.

Mesulam MM: *Principles of behavioral neurology,* Philadelphia, 1985, FA Davis.

Strub RL, Black FW: *Behavioral neurology: a clinical approach,* ed 2, Philadelphia, 1988, FA Davis.

Stuss DT, Benson DF: *The frontal lobes,* New York, 1986, Raven Press.

Whitehouse PJ, The concept of subcortical and cortical dementia, *Ann Neurol* 19:1, 1986.

Whitehouse, PJ, editor: *Dementia,* Philadelphia, 1993, FA Davis.

Vascular Causes of Dementia

Babikian V, Ropper AH: Binswanger disease, *Stroke* 18:2, 1987.

Caplan LR: Binswanger disease, *Neurology* 45:626, 1995.

Hachinski VC, Lassen NA, Marshal J: Multi-infarct dementia, *Lancet* 2:207, 1974.

Alzheimer and Pick Disease

Katzman R: Alzheimer's disease, *N Engl J Med* 314:964, 1986.

Knapp NJ, Knopman DS, Solomon PR: A 30-week randomized controlled trial of high-dose tacrine in patients with Alzheimer disease, *JAMA* 27:985, 1994.

Mendez MF, Selwood A, Mastri AR: Pick disease versus Alzheimer disease, *Neurology* 43:289, 1993.

Normal Pressure Hydrocephalus

Huckman MS: Normal pressure hydrocephalus: evaluation of diagnostic and prognostic tests, *Am J Neuroradiol* 2:385, 1981.

Vannestc JA: Three decades of normal pressure hydrocephalus, *J Neurol Neurosurg Psychiatry* 57:1021, 1994.

Huntington Disease

Martin JB, Gusella JF: Huntington's disease: pathogenesis and management, *N Engl J Med* 315:1267, 1986.

Infectious Causes of Dementia

Lipton SA, Gendelman HE: Dementia associated with acquired immunodeficiency syndrome, *N Engl J Med* 332:934, 1995.

Marra CM: Syphilis and human immunodeficiency virus infection, *Sem Neurol* 12:43, 1992.

Simon RP: Neurosyphilis, *Arch Neurol* 42:606, 1985.

Confusional States and Delirium

Lipowski ZJ: *Delirium,* Springfield, Ill, 1980, Charles C Thomas.

Aphasia

Absher JR, Benson DF: Disconnection syndromes, *Neurology* 43:862, 1993.

Benton AL: Gerstmann syndrome, *Arch Neurol* 49:445, 1992.

Damasio AR: Aphasia. *N Engl J Med* 326:531, 1992.

Levine DN, Calvinio R, Rinn WE: The pathogenesis of anosognosia for hemiplegia, *Neurology* 41:1770, 1991.

CHAPTER

Neoplasms of the Nervous System

15

A neoplasm is an abnormal mass (tumor) of tissue produced by a disturbance of cell growth caused by an autonomous proliferation of cells. The lack of lymphatics and the paucity of connective tissue in the central nervous system (CNS) modifies the spreading and cell growth of these lesions. The site of the lesion (medulla versus frontal lobe) and the rapidity of growth are more important than the traditional distinction between histologically benign and malignant neoplasms.

CNS tumors can originate within the intracranial cavity if they are found above the foramen magnum or within the spinal canal if they are found below the foramen magnum. The distinction between *intracranial* and *intraspinal* is important because they differ in their clinical manifestations, frequency, and prognosis. More than 50% of intracranial tumors are histologically malignant and surgically not feasibly resectable, whereas more than 50% of intraspinal tumors are histologically benign and surgically resectable.

Unfortunately, 85% of CNS tumors originate above the foramen magnum.

INTRACRANIAL TUMORS

Primary intracranial tumors can arise in the brain tissue itself (intraparenchymal or intraaxial), most of them being gliomas, or they can originate in tissues outside the brain tissue (extraparenchymal or extraaxial) such as the meninges (meningiomas), cranial nerves (schwannomas), pituitary gland (adenomas), or bony structures (osteomas, sarcomas). *Secondary* tumors originate in other organs and can reach the CNS by direct extension (nasopharynx) or by the bloodstream (hematogenous metatases).

The incidence of CNS tumors seen in a given hospital differs greatly and depends on whether the hospital has a neurosurgical service, the type of facilities, and the availability of specialists (neurosurgeons, neuroncologists). Autopsy figures vary according to the thoroughness with which the brain is examined. Also, the incidence of tumors has changed with time. An increase in the incidence of brain tumors is the result of prolonged longevity. An increase in brain metastasis is the result of improvement in the treatment of primary systemic tumors and longer survival of cancer patients. Primary CNS lymphomas have increased because of the high frequency in human immunodeficiency virus–infected patients. It is possible for intracranial tumors to be asymptomatic and be found incidentally at autopsy. In adult admissions to general hospitals metastatic tumors are probably the most common intracranial neoplasm, followed by the gliomas. Both groups combined make up 60% of all intracranial neoplasms. Meningioma is the third most frequent tumor (13% to 18%), followed by the schwannomas (8%) of

the acoustic nerve. The incidence of pituitary adenomas varies in the different surveys (3% to 12%), but
they are the fourth most frequent intracranial tumors
in adults. Pinealomas and midline embryologic nest
tumors (teratomas and craniopharyngiomas) are rare
tumors of childhood, whereas medulloblastomas/
primitive neuroectodermal tumors (PNT) and gliomas
are frequent childhood tumors. The distribution of
intracranial gliomas shows a preponderance of 2:1 in
males, whereas meningiomas occur 2:1 in females.

Age is an important factor for the type and localization of intracranial tumors. The CNS is the second
most common site of primary tumors in children. In
this age-group 70% of intracranial tumors are infratentorial (posterior fossa). Early in childhood (first
decade) cerebellar medulloblastomas/PNTs are the
most frequent tumors followed by cerebellar astrocytomas. Brain stem gliomas are seen in adolescents,
whereas ependymomas of the fourth ventricle are usually seen in children and young adults. The supratentorial tumors in childhood include the craniopharyngiomas and the pinealomas followed by astrocytomas.

Tumors in adults are chiefly supratentorial (70%)
and include metastasis and glioblastoma multiforme
followed by the meningiomas and pituitary adenomas
and other gliomas. The infratentorial (posterior fossa)
tumors in adults include the acoustic neuromas
(schwannomas) and cerebellar hemangioblastomas
followed by gliomas, meningiomas, and other rare
tumors (Table 15-1).

The accuracy of the histologic diagnosis and the
safety of diagnostic brain biopsies have improved
with the combination of better imaging resolution,
immunocytopathology, and stereotactic needle biopsies. Close cooperation and communication between

TABLE 15-1 Intracranial Neoplasms

Children	Posterior fossa, 70% (infratentorial)	Infancy: medulloblastoma, midline cerebellum Childhood: cerebellar astrocytoma, cerebellar hemisphere Adolescence: brain stem, glioma Children and young adults: ependymomas fourth ventricle
	Anterior and middle fossa, 30% (supratentorial)	Craniopharyngioma: suprasellar Pinealomas: pineal region, third ventricle Glioma: optic nerve, thalamus
Adults	Anterior and middle fossa, 70% (supratentorial)	Glioblastoma multiforme Metastatic Meningioma Pituitary adenomas Other gliomas
	Posterior fossa, 30% (infratentorial)	Cranial nerve schwannomas Cerebellar hemangioblastomas Meningiomas, metastatic

neurosurgeons, radiologists, and pathologists optimize the use and accuracy of needle biopsies for brain tumors. The intraoperative use of the microscope, technological surgical advances, and presurgical embolization of highly vascular tumors have improved the postoperative outcome.

Symptomatology

Intracranial neoplasms cause signs and symptoms by their general or local brain effects. General effects are due to space occupation by the tumor, obstruction of cerebrospinal fluid (CSF) flow, and edema of adjacent cerebral tissue. These effects produce *increased intracranial pressure* and manifest clinically by *headache, vomiting, and papilledema.* Intracranial hypertension is not always present in CNS tumors and correlates better with the rapidity of tumor growth or obstruction of CSF pathways rather than with the presence or size of the tumor. Benign, slowly growing tumors such as meningiomas, pituitary adenomas, or slowly growing infiltrating gliomas give signs of increased intracranial pressure very late in their course. The *headache* of tumor is frequently intermittent, usually worse in the morning hours, with a tendency toward increasing frequency and severity. It is aggravated by straining, coughing, and change in posture and can be localized to the site of the tumor but is usually generalized. *Nausea* and *vomiting* are rare features and more frequently noted in patients with cerebellar tumors. *Papilledema,* when present, is good evidence of increased intracranial pressure.

The local effects can be *irritative* and produce focal or generalized seizures. Onset of seizures in nonalcoholic or nondrug abusers older than 30 years of age suggests intracranial neoplasm. Seizures can occur in both intraaxial or extraaxial *hemispheric* neoplasms. Seizures are rare in childhood neoplasms. Effects of *destruction* are loss of function (focal weakness) at the level of the lesion and liberation of lower centers (spasticity and hyperreflexia). Frequently the onset of symptoms is slow and the clinical course progressive. Bleeding into the substance of a necrotic tumor such as a metastatic tumor or a glioblastoma, however, can appear as a sudden catastrophic illness (strokelike onset), particularly if tumors have grown "silently" in areas such as the frontal or temporal lobes. Certain rapidly growing malignant tumors such as glioblastoma multiforme or metastasis can evolve clinically in a few days.

◼ NEOPLASMS OF CHILDHOOD

Infratentorial Tumors

Medulloblastomas and Primitive Neuroectodermal Tumors

Medulloblastomas, also known as primitive neuroectodermal tumors (PNT), are highly malignant, rapidly growing tumors derived from nests of small undifferentiated cells located in the cerebellum. They are predominantly found in infants and young children and arise in the vermis of the cerebellum. As they grow, these tumors occupy the fourth ventricle. In older patients the tumor arises laterally in the cerebellar hemispheres (circumscribed desmoplastic medulloblastomas/PNT). Seeding by tumor cells in the subarachnoid space of the spinal cord and cerebral hemispheres is frequent. Clinical signs are those due to cerebellar lesions and are primarily truncal ataxia and early signs of increased intracranial pressure because of obstructive hydrocephalus. Palliative treatment consists of radical surgical removal of the tumor followed by maximal radiation therapy because of the radiosensitivity of the tumor. Chemotherapy can be helpful for recurrent tumors. Some therapeutic protocols have reported a 50% to 60% incidence of long-term, disease-free survival.

Cystic Cerebellar Astrocytomas

Most cerebellar astrocytomas are cystic, slowly growing, benign, well-differentiated tumors derived from astrocytes. They are found predominantly in children (first decade). They usually arise laterally in either one of the cerebellar hemispheres. Frequently they are large cystic lesions containing a mural nodule and protein-rich fluid. Clinical findings are those of homolateral appendicular (limb) ataxia and head tilting to the same side as the lesion. Signs of increased intracranial pressure are caused by compression of the fourth ventricle. Treatment consists of drainage of the cyst with resection of the mural nodule. Radiation therapy is not usually indicated. The prognosis is usually good, with long survivals even after partial resections.

Brain Stem Gliomas

Brain stem gliomas are tumors arising from astrocytes, usually in the pons, with a variable degree of cell differentiation. Most are fibrillary or diffuse in type, but glioblastomas or glioblastomatous degeneration can occur. The higher the location in the brain stem the more undifferentiated the tumor is likely to be. These tumors are found predominantly in late childhood (peak age 8 years) and adolescence and manifest clinically as slowly progressive long pyramidal tract signs and multiple cranial nerve involvement. Papilledema and other signs of intracranial hypertension are very late because of the infiltrative growth up and down the brain stem axis. These neoplasms usually originate in the midpons. They can grow upward into the midbrain and thalamus or downward into the medulla or can extend exophytically into the cerebellopontine angle cisterns. Survival is short in children who have cranial nerve palsies, patients who have a hypodense tumor on noncontrast CT, or patients with tumors that involve the entire brain stem on CT. Biopsy and partial resection can be done in exophytic tumors. Surgical drainage of cysts found on imaging studies helps some patients. Radiation therapy can prolong survival in some patients. The full extent of these lesions is seen with MRI.

Ependymomas

Ependymonas are benign, slowly growing, well-circumscribed intraventricular tumors derived from ependymal cells. The fourth ventricle is the most common site (70%), but ependymomas can be found anywhere in the ventricular system. When localized in the fourth ventricle, they are most common in the first two decades of life. Because the tumor tends to grow into the ventricular cavity, clinical symptoms are late. Changes in the mental status and frontal lobe signs are due to progressive hydrocephalus, as are signs of intracranial hypertension. Although histologically benign, they are difficult to resect completely because of their location. Partial surgical resection, shunting, and irradiation are palliative treatments. Malignant transformation can occasionally be seen in recurrent tumors.

Supratentorial Tumors

Supratentorial tumors in children are rare. The most frequent supratentorial tumors are craniopharyngioma and pinealoma. Also, solid, diffuse, well-differentiated astrocytoma can be seen. Gliomas (astrocytomas) of the optic nerves and hypothalamus are seen more frequently in patients with neurofibromatosis. Gliomas (astrocytomas) can also arise in the thalamic region or cerebral hemispheres in children and young adults.

Craniopharyngiomas

Craniopharyngiomas (adamantinomatous type) originate from squamous cell nests believed to be remnants of Rathke's pouch or from metaplastic cells from the adenohypophysis. One of the most frequent supratentorial tumors of childhood, a craniopharyngioma is a benign, slowly growing lesion that calcifies and adheres to surrounding neural tissue. Parasellar in location, it is usually suprachiasmatic, producing compression of the hypothalamus and chiasm (Figure 15-1). Clinical manifestations are those of visual field defects (bitemporal or other defects caused by chiasmal compression) and hypothalamic syndrome (short stature, failure to thrive, delay in sexual development, diabetes insipidus). Suprasellar calcifications can be detected on plain skull roentgenography, and they are well delineated by CT and magnetic resonance imaging (MRI) scanning (see Figure 15-1). Because of their location and the fact that they can adhere to neural tissue, total surgical removal without removing adjacent brain tissue is usually impossible. Craniopharyngioma (papillary type) has another peak of prevalence around the fourth and fifth decades. Calcification in this age-group is less frequent. Symptoms are visual defects caused by chiasmal compression or endocrine deficiencies caused by hypothalamic compression.

Pineal Tumors

The most frequent form of tumor in the pineal region and third ventricle is the *germinoma* (atypical teratoma). This is a malignant and infiltrative tumor derived from primitive germ cells identical to those seen in the gonads. Because the tumor grows within the third ventricle, tumor cells frequently seed into the ventricular system and the subarachnoid spaces. The tumor can originate within the pineal gland (true pinealoma) or in the parasellar area (ectopic pinealoma). It predominantly affects young adolescent males (12 years). Symptoms in pineal area tumors consist of compression of the quadrigeminal plate and posterior commissure, giving origin to Parinaud's syndrome (vertical, mainly upward gaze palsy, pupillary

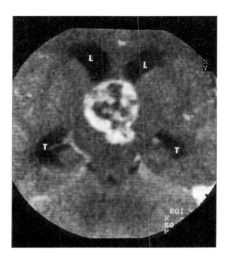

FIGURE 15-1.   CT scan of brain with contrast showing a midline suprasellar (area of third ventricle) multicystic calcified craniopharyngioma.

irregularity with nonreactivity to light) and compression of the aqueduct producing hydrocephalus. Diabetes insipidus, visual field defects, and hypothalamic pituitary failure can be seen in lesions situated in the anterior third ventricle. These are the most radiosensitive CNS tumors. Radiation therapy should include the entire CNS axis because of the frequent CSF seeding. Survivals of more than 20 years after radiation therapy have been reported. Other rare pineal tumors are the *teratomas*. These tumors are usually benign with a range of well-differentiated tissue elements derived from three germ layers. Although they are benign tumors histologically, they are difficult to resect completely. Other tumors of the pineal parenchyma are the *pineocytoma* and the *pineoblastoma/PNT,* which are quite rare lesions.

Thalamic astrocytomas are seen between 1 month to 18 years of age (mean 7.7 years) and usually show signs of increased intracranial pressure or hemiparesis. Survival rates vary according to the degree of differentiation of the tumor. *Optic nerve* and *chiasmal gliomas* are pilocytic or anaplastic astrocytomas seen in children (mean age 6 years) that cause visual loss and endocrine symptoms. CT/MRI scanning guides the diagnosis and neurosurgical treatment, establishing the best site for biopsy or ventricular shunting. Radiation therapy can be indicated in some cases.

NEOPLASMS OF ADULTHOOD

Most of adult neoplasms (70%) are supratentorial. The two most frequent tumors are the metastatic type and glioblastoma multiforme followed by the meningiomas, pituitary adenomas, and other gliomas. Glioblastomas and brain metastasis are very close in rate of frequency, and together they constitute 60% of adult brain tumors. There are predominantly two posterior fossa neoplasms seen in adults: schwannoma of the cranial nerve and cerebellar hemangioblastoma. Clivus meningiomas, chordomas, and epidermoid cysts are rare posterior fossa lesions.

Supratentorial Tumors
Metastatic Tumors

Intracranial metastases are increasing in frequency because of longer survival of patients with other visceral primary tumors and more effective treatment of systemic metastasis. Eighty-one percent of metastases are cerebral, 16% are cerebellar, and only 3% are found in the brain stem. Neurologic symptoms can be the first manifestation of some systemic neoplasms, most commonly lung cancer. Signs of increased intracranial pressure, seizures, dementia, or focal motor or sensory deficit are seen (Figure 15-2). Symptomatology is usually progressive, but acute onset (strokelike) can be seen in some tumors that bleed (Figure 15-3). A triphasic clinical course (sudden onset, stabilization sometimes with improvement, followed by worsening) can be seen in metastatic neoplasms or with glioblastoma multiforme. The most frequent primary sources are lung tumors in both sexes followed by breast tumors in females. Both tumors are followed in frequency by melanoma and colon tumors. Multiple brain lesions are frequent and are likely to be associated with lung cancer and melanomas. Colon, breast, and renal cell (clear cell) tumors have a tendency to produce solitary lesions. Diagnosis of a solitary lesion is important because of its resectability if found in a surgically accessible (superficial) brain area. Most hemispheric lesions are found in arterial border zones, predominantly in the parietal lobe. Although most lesions are intra-parenchymal nodules, the dura can be infiltrated and thickened in a hemorrhagic subdural seeding. Also, diffuse infiltration of the meninges (*meningeal carcinomatosis*) is predominantly seen with gastrointestinal and breast adenocarcinomas. Vasogenic edema surrounding metastases is a constant feature. The edema is frequently severe and can cause cerebral herniations but responds dramatically to corticosteroid therapy. Irradiation therapy and corticosteroids are palliative measures for both intracranial and intraspinal metastases. Chemotherapy is useful in some patients.

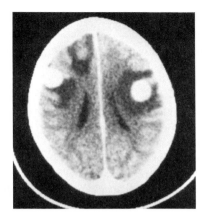

FIGURE 15-2. CT scan with enhancement showing multiple bilateral round metastases surrounded by edema (low-density areas).

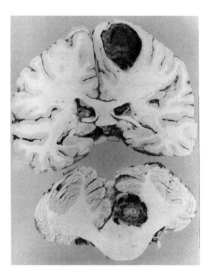

FIGURE 15-3. Brain and cerebellum showing well-circumscribed metastatic lesions with hemorrhage.

Glioblastoma Multiforme

Glioblastoma multiforme is a highly malignant, rapidly growing tumor of glial cell origin that usually arises *de novo* but occasionally can start as an astrocytoma or oligodendroglioma. It is the most frequent primary tumor in adults and is found mainly in the frontal and temporal lobes but can arise in any part of the CNS including the brain stem (Figure 15-4). It predominantly affects males in the fourth and fifth decade, but it can be found in young patients. Symptoms are usually progressive but of short duration, and, when discovered, the tumors are usually large. Because the lesions are highly necrotic and vascular, they have a tendency to bleed and in some cases can appear as an apoplectic episode (strokelike onset), which primarily occurs in patients with tumors in the frontal or temporal lobes. Rarely, glioblastoma can appear as a seizure disorder only. The initial diagnostic studies can be negative; however, subsequently seizures worsen or a neurologic deficit develops, and repeated studies show a large neoplasm. Even after radical resection, radiation therapy, and chemotherapy, mortality is still high, with neurologic deterioration and death occurring within 2 years. Treatment protocols have prolonged survivals only a few months.

Meningiomas

Meningiomas are benign, slowly growing, extraaxial tumors derived from arachnoidal cells, chiefly those in the arachnoidal villi, hence their tendency to arise along venous sinuses. They are the third most common tumor seen in adults, and most occur in females (2:1). The most frequent site is in the parrasagittal region, with some of them arising from the falx cerebri

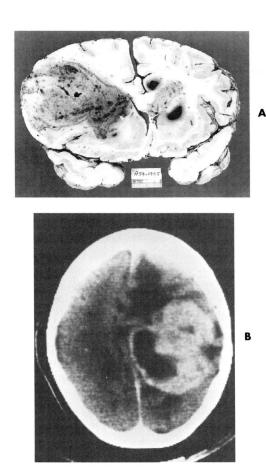

FIGURE 15-4. A, Coronal section of a brain showing a glioblastoma multiforme. Note infiltration of the tumor across the corpus callosum and areas of hemorrhagic necrosis. **B,** CT scan with enhancement showing a glioblastoma multiforme surrounded by edema (*lucent area*).

(Figure 15-5). Other sites are the sphenoid ridge and tuberculum sella; more unusual locations are the tentorium cerebelli, foramen magnum, clivus, and within the ventricular system. When seen in the clivus, they can compress the brain stem. The neoplasm grows outside, displacing and compressing, rather than infiltrating, nervous tissue. The neurologic findings, when present, depend on the site of the tumor. Headache, focal or generalized seizures, dementia, and progressive ocular and motor deficits can be the clinical signs. Papilledema is not a frequent finding because the tumors grow slowly. CT scanning demonstrates a sharply marginated, homogeneously enhanced lesion. Hemorrhages and calcifications within the tumor are rare. Angiography demonstrates the tumor's blood supply. MRI delineates the tumor clearly. Treatment consists of surgical resection, which is not always successful because of the tumor's location in an inaccessible area or its vicinity or infiltration into the venous sinuses. The tumor can recur if it is not completely resected. Because most of the tumors are highly vascularized and their circulation is derived from the dural vessels, enlargement of the vascular marking and hyperostosis caused by reaction to infiltration by the tumor on the adjacent skull can be seen on plain skull roentgenograms. Preoperative embolization of the tumor facilitates its resectability.

Pituitary tumors

Most pituitary neoplasms arise from the glandular (anterior lobe) portion of the gland, hence the name pituitary adenoma. Available techniques measure increased serum hormone levels in the presence of functional tumors. Certain small lesions can be demonstrated with imaging studies. When a pituitary biopsy is done it is possible to demonstrate hormone granules

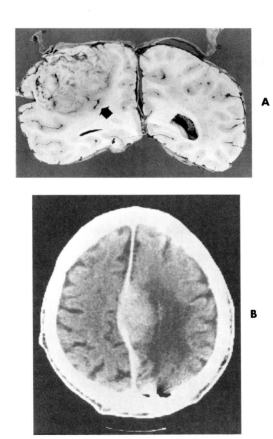

FIGURE 15-5. **A,** Coronal section of brain showing a convexity meningioma. Upper arrow shows displaced cortex and surrounding edema. Ventricle is compressed on same side. Lower arrow shows hippocampal herniation. **B,** CT scan with enhancement showing a parasagittal meningioma surrounded by edema (*lucent area*).

within the tumor cells by immunocytochemical staining (immunoperoxidase). Pituitary adenomas are classified according to hormonal secretions and cytoplasmic granules stained by immunocytochemistry. These lesions include the prolactin cell adenoma (prolactinoma), growth hormone cell adenoma, mixed prolactin and growth hormone adenoma, corticotropic cell adenoma, and acidophilic stem cell adenoma. Forty-one percent of the adenomas are prolactinomas, 19.5% are growth hormone producing, and 16.7% are adrenocorticotropic hormone (ACTH) producing. Nonsecreting hormone neoplasms (null cell or oncocytomas) are rare. Prolactinomas can appear as amenorrhea, galactorrhea, and infertility in young females; in males they can cause impotence. The serum prolactin levels are usually elevated. CT scanning shows a normal size sella and a small hypodense lesion in a slightly enlarged or normal gland (microadenoma). MRI scanning is more sensitive in detecting these small tumors. Prolactinomas can also grow to erode and enlarge the sella and can compress the optic chiasm, producing bitemporal superior quadrantanopias or hemianopsia. (Macroadenomas are larger than 10 mm in size). As the tumor enlarges, symptoms of panhypopituitarism can appear. Bleeding within the tumor (pituitary apoplexy) can produce an acute onset of blindness and signs of subarachnoid hemorrhage. The tumor can also extend laterally into the cavernous sinus or grow down into the sphenoidal sinus to cause CSF rhinorrhea. The adenoma can be resected transsphenoidally (microadenomas) or by bifrontal craniotomy. Bromocriptine can reduce the prolactin level and tumor size. Adenomas are also radiosensitive tumors. The growth hormone-secreting tumors appear in adults as enlargement of hands, feet, jaws, and frontal bones (acromegaly) or as gigantism in children. Endocrinologic studies show elevated serum growth hormone levels. The tumor can be circumscribed (microadenoma) or grow above the sella. Surgical resection is always necessary. ACTH-secretin adenomas are usually small (microadenomas) and appear as Cushing's disease, manifested by "moon faces," hirsutism, hypertension, osteoporosis, "buffalo hump," and diabetes mellitus. Endocrinologic studies confirm the presence of hypercortisolism in serum. The most frequent cause of Cushing's syndrome is iatrogenic use of corticosteroid, but it also can be produced by primary adrenal disease. Transphenoidal microsurgical exploration is the procedure of choice in ACTH-producing pituitary microadenoma.

Other Supratentorial Tumors

Other less common supratentorial tumors include oligodendrogliomas, astrocytomas, and lymphomas (microgliomas). Oligodendrogliomas are rare tumors derived from oligodendroglial cells. They are predominantly seen in adults, frequently in the frontal lobes of the cerebral hemispheres. Frequently they are calcified (28%) and can also bleed. Papilledema, paresis, and seizures are frequent symptoms. Astrocytomas can also be found in adults and are usually low-grade infiltrative tumors. Gemistocytic astrocytomas are seen in the temporal lobe of young adults and have a tendency to become anaplastic astrocytomas. Primary CNS lymphomas (microgliomas) or reticulum cell sarcomas of the brain are tumors derived from B lymphocytes. They are frequently multicentric and are reported most frequently in patients on immunosuppressive therapy. The diagnosis requires brain biopsy and is of importance because the tumor may respond to a combination of radiation and chemotherapy. Primary CNS lymphoma is the most frequent CNS tumor in patients with acquired immune deficiency syndrome (AIDS) and in these patients carries a poor prognosis regardless of therapy. Meningeal lymphomatous infiltration produces multiple cranial nerve involvement.

Infratentorial Tumors

There are two main tumors in adults that originate in the posterior fossa structures: the schwannoma of cranial nerves and the cerebellar hemangioblastoma.

Schwannoma of Cranial Nerves

Schwannomas are benign, slowly growing tumors found in peripheral nerves, usually sensory roots, and are derived from Schwann cells and fibroblasts. They frequently arise from the intracanalicular portion of the eighth nerve, frequently the vestibular branch (acoustic neuroma), but can also originate from the fifth or seventh nerve. Bilateral tumors of this type are found in patients with von Recklinghausen's disease. The earliest clinical symptom is hearing loss, especially speech discrimination, followed by symptoms caused by compression of structures in the pontocerebellar angle with homolateral cerebellar dysfunction, facial weakness or facial sensory deficit, and long tract signs if the tumor has compressed the pons. Treatment consists of resection of the lesion. Other tumors occupying the cerebellopontine angle area include meningiomas, chordomas (arising from the clivus), and epidermoid cysts (cholesteatomas).

Cerebellar Hemangioblastoma

Cerebellar hemangioblastoma is a benign, slowly growing tumor composed of a mixture of endothelial cells and stromal (foam) cells of obscure origin. The tumors are usually cystic with a mural nodule but can be solid hemorrhagic lesions found in one of the cerebellar hemispheres. They are found in young and middle-aged adults. In approximately 20% of the cases the tumor is familial (Lindau's disease) and can be associated with tumors in the spinal cord, retinal angiomas, pancreatic and hepatic cysts, and renal tumors (von Hippel-Lindau disease). Clinical symptoms are those of a cerebellar deficit associated with polycythemia as a result of release of erythropoietin by the tumor or one of its precursors. Signs of increased intracranial pressure may be evident because of displacement of the fourth ventricle. CT/MRI studies differentiate these lesions from other neoplasms, except from cystic cerebellar astrocytomas. Treatment consists of surgical resection.

Chordoma is a rare posterior fossa, destructive, slowly growing tumor of notochordal origin seen predominantly in young adult males that arises in the clivus area and can compress the brain stem. Chordomas are also seen in the lumbosacral spine.

Intraspinal Tumors

Intraspinal tumors can best be understood if they are related to the dura. Imaging studies (CT/MRI) have improved the diagnostic accuracy. The most common intraspinal tumors are the extradural (epidural) tumors, which are very frequently metastatic to vertebral bone and produce signs because of compression of nerve roots or the spinal cord. A combination of high dose steroids and radiotherapy is the best therapeutic approach. Most of the intradural tumors are primary (Figure 15-6). The intradural tumors can arise within the spinal cord tissue (intramedullary), most of them being gliomas, or they can originate outside the cord in the nerve roots (schwannomas) or the arachnoid (meningiomas). Meningiomas, schwannomas, and ependymomas are in most cases surgically resectable. The level at which the tumor originates is also important because most of the cervical tumors are astrocytomas, most thoracic tumors are meningiomas, most lumbar area tumors are schwannomas, and most sacral and filum terminale tumors are ependymomas. The most frequent spinal tumor is the extradural metastatic tumor. The most frequent intramedullary tumor is the ependymoma.

Colloid Cyst

This epithelial cyst predominantly appears in the anterior third ventricle and can produce intermittent hydrocephalus by blocking the foramina of Monro. The main symptom is intermittent headache occurring over a period of several years, sometimes relieved by changing the position of the head. Sudden death is frequent and is a result of herniation of the lateral ventricle through the tentorial opening. The treatment consists of surgical resection or CT/MRI-guided aspiration of the cyst.

Epidermoid and Dermoid Cysts

These cysts, also known as pearly tumors, are not true neoplasms. They grow by desquamation of keratine from the well differentiated squamous epithelium that lines the inner portion of the cyst's wall. The dermoid cyst also contains adnexal appendages. These lesions are predominantly found in the posterior fossa in the cerebellopontine angle, the parapontine region or within the fourth ventricle. The clinical features are those of compression of the cerebellum or brain stem. CT/MRI shows a very low density lesion and occasional peripheral calcification. The treatment consists of surgical resection of the lesion.

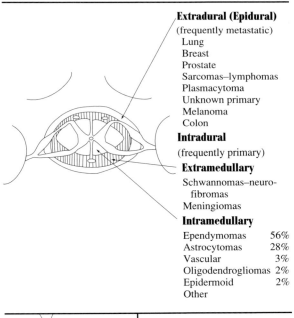

Extradural (Epidural)

(frequently metastatic)
Lung
Breast
Prostate
Sarcomas–lymphomas
Plasmacytoma
Unknown primary
Melanoma
Colon

Intradural

(frequently primary)

Extramedullary

Schwannomas–neuro-
   fibromas
Meningiomas

Intramedullary

Ependymomas	56%
Astrocytomas	28%
Vascular	3%
Oligodendrogliomas	2%
Epidermoid	2%
Other	

C	Astrocytomas
T	Meningiomas
L	Schwannomas
E	Ependymomas

**Incidence of Primary
   Intraspinal Tumors**

Schwannomas	29.0%
Meningiomas	25.5%
Gliomas	22.0%
Sarcomas	11.9%
Vascular	6.2%
Other	

FIGURE 15-6.   Intraspinal tumors.

Paraneoplastic Syndromes (Remote Effects of Cancer on the Nervous System)

There is a group of neurologic disorders that occur in patients with a carcinoma, but that are not due to direct infiltration of the nervous system by neoplastic cells. Every one of these conditions can appear before the malignancy, during its course, or at a time when the malignancy is thought to be in remission. These disorders are characterized pathologically by destruction of central or ganglionic neurons and by perivascular lymphocytic cuffs in affected regions. The histopathologic findings, the presence of antineuronal antibodies in the CSF and serum of affected patients, the synthesis of specific antibodies within the CNS, the detection of intraneuronal IgG within these patient's brains, and the response to immunosuppressive therapies suggest an autoimmune cause. Commercially available determination of Hu and Yo paraneoplastic autoantibodies can confirm the autoimmune cause for the neurologic symptoms associated with the syndromes. Box 15-1 shows neurologic syndromes, which can occur singly or in combination.

▒ SUMMARY

Neoplasms of the nervous system are abnormal masses produced by a disturbance of cell growth caused by an autonomous proliferation of cells. Neoplasms can be primary if they arise from intracranial and intraspinal tissues or secondary if they originate outside the brain and spine and invade the CNS (metastasis). Primary tumors can originate from the brain parenchyma (gliomas) or from the meninges (meningiomas), the pineal gland (pinealomas), or the pituitary gland (pituitary adenomas). Age, sex, and

BOX 15-1

1 *Cerebellar degeneration.* This represents a pancerebellar disturbance with gait and truncal ataxia occurring along with ataxia of the arm and legs. The patients can also be dysarthric and have horizontal nystagmus. This disorder is most commonly associated with lung and ovarian carcinoma and lymphoma. The cerebellar dysfunction does not usually improve despite tumor removal, but clinical improvement has been reported after successful tumor treatment. Antibodies to the Yo antigen are the most common paraneoplastic antibodies to Purkinje cells found in these patients.

2 *Peripheral neuropathy and sensory neuronopathy.* Subacute or chronic mixed sensorimotor neuropathy is the most frequent type of neuropathy associated with neoplasia. The neuropathy is usually seen in adult males and appears as distal numbness, dysesthesias, and paresthesias. It is most common with carcinoma of the lung, but it can be associated with cancer of the gastrointestinal system and with multiple myeloma. It is important to remember that sensorimotor neuropathies are also a common complication of certain antineoplastic drugs (e.g., vincristine, cisplatin). The sensory neuronopathy consists of paresthesias, pain, and unsteadiness (especially in a dark environment) and severe sensory ataxia associated with small cell bronchogenic carcinoma. The pathologic features, which explain the clinical findings in sensory neuronopathies, are degenerative changes in the dorsal root ganglia with secondary changes ascending into the posterior columns of the spinal cord. Several tests to detect autoantibodies (SGPG, MAG, and Hu) are commercially available to identify the cause of the patient's neuropathy.

3 *Subacute necrotizing myelopathy.* This rare condition is characterized by a rapidly progressive necrotizing myelopathy. Initial symptoms are paresthesias and weakness in the feet which rapidly spread to the legs, trunk, and arms. These patients have loss of bladder and bowel function and develop paraplegia with bilateral Babinski signs. Pathologic findings are necrotic lesions in both the gray and white matter of the spinal cord. Diagnostic tests, including imaging studies, are necessary to differentiate this remote effect from spinal epidural metastases.

4 *Encephalomyelitis.* This condition has usually been associated with oat-cell bronchogenic carcinoma. This inflamma-

Continued.

BOX 15-1—cont'd

tory disorder can affect all levels of the neural axis (cerebral hemispheres, brain stem, spinal cord) with predominant involvement of the gray matter. Pathologically there is destruction of neurons, microglial proliferation, and perivascular lymphocytic cuffing. If the cerebral hemispheres are involved, there is a tendency for the limbic system (i.e. *limbic encephalitis*). These patients show neurobehavioral abnormalities (confusion, memory loss, anxiety, depression, hallucinations). The CSF shows sterile lymphocytic pleocytosis (without neoplastic cells) and an elevated protein content.

5 *Motor neuron disease.* A form of motor neuron disease associated with neoplasia has been recognized; however, there is only one reported case in which the symptoms of amyotrophic lateral sclerosis remitted following the successful treatment of the neoplasia. Both motor neuron disease and carcinoma cause weight loss, weakness, muscle wasting, and cachexia and occur most commonly in patients older than 50 years old, so the association may be more apparent than real. Not all patients with symptoms of motor neuron disease require a complete search for an occult neoplasm.

6 *Dermatomyositis.* When seen in adults, particularly in males, this can be associated with an occult neoplasm.

7 *Eaton-Lambert myasthenic syndrome.* This is characteristically seen in adults, predominantly males. The fatigue caused by this syndrome rarely affects the eye muscles and is associated with areflexia that returns after exercising the tested muscle. Patients may also complain of a metallic taste in the mouth.

8 *Progressive multifocal leukoencephalopathy.* This is a viral infection produced by the JC virus. It was first described in patients with systemic lymphomas and is seen predominantly in immunosuppressed patients. It is now an infection frequently seen in AIDS patients.

location of the tumor are important factors in the diagnosis of these lesions. Most tumors in children are infratentorial, meningiomas are more frequent in females and rare in children, and glioblastomas are more frequent in adult males. Systemic cancer can affect the CNS and PNSS by producing not only metastasis but also paraneoplastic syndromes due to autoimmune phenomena. New developments in imaging techniques have improved detection and improved complete delineation of these lesions. Innovations and refinements in surgical procedures have improved the surgical treatment of some of these tumors.

Suggested Readings

General

Black PM: Brain tumors, *N Engl J Med* 324:1471, 1991.

Burger PC, Scheithauer BW: *Tumors of the central nervous system, series 3*, Washington, DC, 1993, Armed Forces Institute of Pathology.

Burger PC, Scheithauer BW, Vogel FS: *Surgical pathology of the nervous system and its coverings,* ed 3, New York, 1991, Churchill Livingstone.

Gjerris F: Clinical aspects and long-term prognosis of intracranial tumors in infancy and childhood, *Dev Med Child Neurol* 18:145, 1976.

Leibel SA, Sheline GE: Radiation therapy for neoplasms of the brain, *J Neurosurg* 66:1, 1987.

Lyons MK, Meyer FB: Cerebral fluid: physiology and the management of increased intracranial pressure, *Mayo Clin Proc* 65:684, 1990.

Pollack IF: Brain tumors in children, *N Engl J Med* 330: 1500, 1994.

Weisberg LA: Intracranial neoplasms, *Neurol Clin North Am* 2:695, 1984.

Acoustic Neuromas

Harner SG, Laws ER: Clinical findings in patients with acoustic neurinoma, *Mayo Clin Proc* 58:721, 1983.

Hart RG, Gardner DP: Acoustic tumors: atypical features and recent diagnostic tests, *Neurology* 33:211, 1983.

Gliomas

Albright AL, et al: Prognostic factors in pediatric brain stem gliomas, *J Neurosurg* 65:751, 1986.

Bernstein M, et al: Thalamic tumors in children: long-term follow-up and treatment guidelines, *J Neurosurg* 61:649, 1984.

Fletcher WA, Imes RK, Hoyt WF: Chiasmal gliomas: appearance and long-term changes demonstrated by computerized tomography, *J Neurosurg* 65:154, 1986.

Mork SJ, et al: Oligodendrogliomas: incidence and biological behavior in a defined population, *J Neurosurg* 63:881, 1985.

Stroink AR, et al: Diagnosis and management of pediatric brain stem gliomas, *J Neurosurg* 65:745, 1986.

Lymphoma

Hochberg FH, Miller DC: Primary CNS lymphoma, *J Neurosurg* 68:835, 1988.

Meningiomas

Black PM: Meningiomas, *Neurosurgery* 32:643, 1993.

Quest DD: Meningiomas: an update, *Neurosurgery* 3:219, 1978.

Metastases

Clouston PD: The spectrum of neurologic disease in patients with systemic cancer, *Ann Neurol* 31:268, 1992.

Greenberg HS, Kim JH, Posner JB: Epidural spinal cord compression from metastic tumor: results with a new treatment protocol, *Ann Neurol* 8:361, 1980.

Patchell RA, Posner JB: Neurological complications of systemic cancer, *Neurol Clin North Am* 3:729, 1985.

Weiss L, Gilbert HH, Posner JB: Brain metastasis, New York, 1980, GK Hall.

Pituitary Neoplasms

Ciric I: Pituitary tumors, *Neurol Clin North Am* 3:751, 1985.

Klibanski A, Zervas NT: Diagnosis and treatment of hormone secreting pituitary tumors, *N Engl J Med* 324:822, 1991.

Scheithauer BW, et al: Pathology of invasive pituitary tumors with special reference to functional classification, *J Neurosurg* 65:733, 1986.

Wilson CB: A decade of pituitary microsurgery, *J Neurosurg* 61:814, 1984.

Pineal Neoplasms

Bruce JN, Stein BM: Pineal tumors, *Neurosurg Clin North Am* 1:123, 1990.

Jooma R, Kendall G: Diagnosis and management of pineal tumors, *J Neurosurg* 58:654, 1983.

Spinal Cord Neoplasms

Bryne TN: Spinal cord compression from epidural metastasis, *N Engl J Med* 327:614, 1992.

Slooff JL, Kernohan JW, MacCarty CS: *Primary intramedullary tumors of the spinal cord and filum terminale,* Philadelphia, 1964, WB Saunders.

CHAPTER

Diseases of the Peripheral Nerves and Motor Neurons

16

▣ PERIPHERAL NEUROPATHIES

The peripheral nervous system (PNS) includes all structures related to the Schwann cells from the pia-arachnoid membrane to the nerve endings. The first (olfactory) and second (optic) cranial nerves are not considered peripheral nerves. These nerves are extensions of the central nervous system (CNS) and contain oligodendroglia instead of Schwann cells. All of the other cranial nerves, the spinal motor and sensory nerves, and peripheral components of the autonomic nervous system are included in the PNS.

Disorders that affect the peripheral nerves can affect one or more components of the nerve fiber. Disorders that predominantly affect the myelin are known as *demyelinating neuropathies.* When the disease process affects the distal portion of the axons with preservation of the parent cell bodies in a dying-back manner, it is known as an *axonopathy.* Disorders that affect the cell bodies in the dorsal root ganglia and their axons are known as *neuronopathies.*

To understand the pathophysiology of peripheral nerve disease, the physician must be familiar with the anatomy of nerves, roots, and plexuses and the distribution and function of the different nerves (see Chapter 1).

▨ SYMPTOMS AND SIGNS

Symptoms and signs vary according to the nerves affected but can be motor, sensory, or autonomic or a combination of any or all three.

Motor Findings

The weakness or paralysis in neuropathies is usually hypotonic in type and is associated with atrophy that develops over days, weeks, or years. The weakness can develop *acutely* in external compression of a superficial nerve ("Saturday night" or "crossed leg" paralysis), when penetrating trauma injures a nerve, or when vascular occlusion causes infarction of nerves as in diabetic femoral neuropathy or ophthalmoplegia (third cranial nerve) or in vasculitides such as in polyarteritis nodosa. A *subacute* onset of weakness takes less than 4 weeks as is usually seen in infectious polyneuropathies. The weakness in *chronic* neuropathies progresses slowly over a month to several years. The patients show distal wasting of muscles. Chronic neuropathies are usually due to hereditary or toxic-metabolic causes. Pes cavus, hammer toes, and kyphoscoliosis are associated with chronic hereditary neuropathies. The weakness in mononeuropathies is localized to the muscles innervated by the affected nerve. The weakness in polyneuropathies frequently begins distally in the feet and hands and progresses in an ascending symmetrical fashion to involve the legs and arms and sometimes the facial, bulbar, and respiratory muscles. Proximal muscle weakness in neuropathies suggests a radicular involvement. *Fasciculations* are a rare occurrence in neuropathies and, when present, suggest distal motor axonal involvement. *Myokymia* or undulating worm-like rhythmic movements of muscle is rarely seen in neuropathies except in radiation-induced neuropathy, where it is common. Muscle *cramps* can occur in uremic neuropathy.

Sensory disturbances appear in two different ways. *Positive* sensory symptoms occur when aberrant sensation occurs in the absence of normal stimulation. *Negative* symptoms occur when adequate stimuli fail to produce a sensory response.

Postive sensory symptoms: A sensation *numbness* or tingling (*paresthesia*) in the hands or feet over the distribution of one or more nerves is a frequent complaint in sensory neuropathies and can be the first sign of nerve involvement. Some patients experience a peculiar unpleasant sensation of tingling in the feet that occurs mainly during the night and that can be temporarily relieved by movement of the affected limb, the so-called restless legs syndrome. Ischemic pain of peripheral vascular disease, which has to be differentiated from this, occurs during activity rather than at rest and improves with rest rather than with exercise. Paresthesias are characteristic of acquired neuropathies, whereas numbness is seen in congenital neuropathies. *Dysesthesia,* or unpleasant feeling triggered by any ordinary stimuli, is usually evident after partial nerve injury or during recovery from some neuropathies. A burning sensation, *hyperesthesia,* or an exaggerated normal feeling, *hyperpathia,* is felt when the stimulus is moving rather than when stationary pressure is applied. Dysesthesias, hyperesthesias, and hyperpathias can occur in diabetic and alcoholic neuropathies and in some of the neuropathies associated with malignancies (multiple myeloma). Terms frequently used in reference to abnormal sensation in some peripheral neuropathies are *neuralgia,* which implies stabbing or throbbing pain in the course or distribution of a nerve as is found in tic douloureux or herpetic neuritis, and *causalgia,* which implies burning, persistent pain that radiates distally along an injured nerve trunk. When causalgic pain is associated with autonomic dysfunction, such as abnormal sweating, trophic changes, or edema, it is known as reflex sympathetic dystrophy.

Negative sensory symptoms: Sensory loss can be an early sign and occasionally the only sign of peripheral neuropathy; however, it frequently is associated with motor disturbances. Sensory loss can be limited to one nerve trunk as in herpetic neuritis or, more frequently, can be bilateral, symmetrical, and distal in a stocking or glove distribution as is seen in most polyneuropathies. There are several different patterns of sensory loss: (1) Loss of all modalities of sensation in a distal distribution with gradual return of sensation is usually produced by conduction blocks caused by demyelination. (2) Loss of touch-pressure, vibratory, and position sense with preservation of pain and temperature, so-called sensory ataxia, is seen in tabes dorsalis, but also is seen in some diabetic neuropathies and Friedreich's ataxia. This type of sensory deficit is due to large fiber loss. (3) Selective loss of pain and temperature with preservation of touch-pressure and other modalities is seen in leprosy and some hereditary sensory neuropathies. This type of sensory deficit is due to loss of small myelinated sensory fibers. (4) A pure sensory syndrome with positive (dysesthesia) and negative (hypesthesia) phenomena and associated with sensory ataxia is seen in neuronopathies and is due to damage to nerve cell bodies in the dorsal root ganglia.

Autonomic Findings

Orthostatic hypotension without change in the pulse rate is probably the most important and in some cases the earliest abnormality in some autonomic neuropathies. Painless nocturnal diarrhea, heat intolerance, and localized excessive sweating in unaffected areas with anhidrosis in affected areas may be the complaint of some patients. Other symptoms of autonomic dysfunction include bladder (atonic) dysfunction manifested by difficulty voiding, sexual impotence, retrograde ejaculation, decreased tearing, and pupillary abnormalities. Autonomic involvement is seen predominantly in diabetic and amyloid neuropathies.

Muscle Stretch Reflexes

Stretch reflexes are decreased (hyporeflexic) early in most demyelinating neuropathies and abolished (absent or areflexic) in established neuropathies. Preservation of stretch reflexes can be seen in axonal neuropathies. The presence of Babinski signs should alert the physician to a central disease process or a more diffuse process involving peripheral nerves and corticospinal tracts as is noted in subacute combined degeneration or Friedreich's ataxia.

Nerve Enlargement: Observation and Palpation

Inspection and palpation of the nerves is an essential part of the examination when the diagnosis of peripheral neuropathy is being considered. Enlarged nerves are easier to detect in slender patients. When superficial nerves are enlarged they can even be seen through the skin. The physician should observe and palpate for nerve enlargement along the course of the great auricular nerve in the posterolateral surface of the neck and the superficial peroneal nerve over the anterior aspect of the ankle or the dorsal aspect of the feet. Palpation of enlarged nerves needs to be done in the supraclavicular area for the supraclavicular nerves, above the elbow for the ulnar nerve, and at the lateral aspect of the neck of the fibula for the common peroneal nerve.

LABORATORY TESTS

The diagnosis of peripheral neuropathy can be confirmed by *electrophysiologic studies.* Nerve conduction studies define the distribution and extent of the neuropathy and differentiate between an axonal and demyelinating process. They also can differentiate between an acquired demyelinating neuropathy and a hereditary neuropathy. The presence of multifocal conduction blocks indicates an acquired demyelinating neuropathy, whereas hereditary neuropathies show uniform slowing of conduction velocities. Nerve conduction studies can localize the level of the lesion in compressive (entrapment) neuropathies. *Laboratory* investigation should include a complete blood cell count, erythrocyte sedimentation rate, fasting blood glucose, serum protein and plasma immunoelectrophoresis, liver function tests, chest roentgenograms, thyroid function tests, and serum vitamin B_{12} and folate levels. Cryoglobulins, urinary porphyrins, and heavy metals should be ordered in selected cases. Ganglioside-monosialic acid antibodies are detected in some patients with multifocal neuropathies and lower motor neuron disease. Myelin-associated glycoprotein and sulfate-3-glucuronyl paragloboside are detected in some patients with inflammatory neuropathies. Commercially available motor and sensory neuropathy panels are already available. Deoxyribonucleic acid analyses for the CMT1A duplication and for peripheral neuropathy with liability to pressure palsies are commercially available. *Cerebrospinal fluid* (CSF) protein is elevated in some neuropathies, most frequently in Guillain-Barré syndrome and chronic inflammatory demyelinating polyneuropathy. Finally nerve biopsy can be helpful in the diagnosis of neuropathies caused by vasculitis (polyarteritis nodosa), autoimmunity, infections, and amyloid neuropathies; it should be done only where special competence and facilities are available.

▦ APPROACH TO THE PATIENT WITH A SUSPECTED NEUROPATHY

Many different disease processes can affect peripheral nerves; however, the clinical features are uniform and stereotyped. When confronted with peripheral nerve diseases the following questions should be answered:

Evolution

Is it an acute (a few hours or days), subacute (less than 4 weeks), or chronic (more than a month) process?

Is it a recurrent or chronic relapsing disease?

Distribution

It is an isolated lesion of one nerve (*mononeuropathy*), or are multiple isolated scattered individual nerves affected (*multiple mononeuropathy*)?

Is it a symmetrical bilateral involvement of nerves (*polyneuropathy*)? If so, are the spinal roots also involved (*polyradiculoneuropathy*)?

What nerve is affected? Is it a peripheral or cranial nerve (*cranial neuropathy*)?

Is an entire plexus or part of the plexus involved (*plexitis or plexopathy*)?

Are the distal or proximal parts of the nerve involved?

Modality

Is the nerve involved motor in type (pure *motor neuropathy*)?

Is it a sensory nerve (pure *sensory neuropathy*)?

Are the autonomic nerves involved (*autonomic neuropathy*)?

Is there a combination of different types of nerves involved (*mixed neuropathy*)?

Electrophysiology and Pathology

Is the neuropathy caused by damage of the myelin (*demyelination*)? Is it segmental? Or diffuse?

Is it due to axonal damage (*axonal neuropathy*)?

Is it both axonal and demyelinating?

Is it due to nerve cell damage of the dorsal root ganglion (*neuronopathy*)?

Is it the neuropathy due to nerve fiber ischemia? (*vasculitis*)?

Is it due to chronic autoimmune inflammatory phenomena (*chronic inflammatory demyelinating polyneuropathy*)?

Has a focal portion of the nerve been injured, causing a compressive or entrapment neuropathy?

By the time you have answered most of the questions listed above, you should have an idea of the type of neuropathy and the cause of the nerve lesion.

Etiology

Is there evidence of systemic disease that can provide a clue as to the disease cause (e.g., diabetes, uremia, connective tissue disorder, cancer, alcoholism)?

Has the patient been exposed to neurotoxic agents?

Is there a family history of the same disease? If so, who is or has been affected? (Obtaining a pedigree of the family will determine the possible inheritance pattern.)

▣ CLINICAL SYNDROMES

Of the disease processes that affect peripheral nerves, only the most common problems and those that typify a group of similar disorders are discussed here.

Neuropathies Caused by Compression and Entrapment

Neuropathies can be produced by local injury of superficial nerves (compression) or during passage of the nerve through a narrow anatomical site (entrapment). The compression can be external (outside the skin) or internal such as that caused by hematoma, inflammation, or scarring. Predisposing factors in both compression and entrapment include pregnancy, hypothyroidism, acromegaly, and rheumatoid arthritis. Increased susceptibility to compression of nerves occurs in malnutrition, diabetes, alcoholism, renal failure, and genetic defects. In certain compressive neuropathies the onset can be abrupt; the patient wakes up after a deep sleep induced by heavy alcohol ingestion or heavy sedation by drugs and has so-called Saturday night palsy or paralysis, which is produced by compression of the radial nerve against the humerus. In most compressive neuropathies the onset is more insidious and is produced by repeated minor (sometimes occupational) trauma. The main symptoms are variable degrees of weakness in the innervated muscles and paresthesias confined to the cutaneous distribution of the nerve. Pain is poorly localized and can be felt in areas away from the compression site. Sensory examination is important followed by palpation of the nerve to look for nerve thickening and percussion of the nerve to look for local pain or paresthesias (Tinel's sign). Only the most frequent and important neuropathies will be mentioned here. Electrophysiologic studies are very important to confirm the diagnosis, to localize the site of compression, and for prognostic information.

Carpal Tunnel Syndrome

Carpal tunnel syndrome is produced by compression of the median nerve as it passes beneath the transverse carpal ligament at the wrist. It is the most common entrapment neuropathy and usually causes nocturnal bouts of pain and paresthesias in the wrist and hand that can radiate proximally into the forearm, elbow, and at times to the shoulder. Distally the discomfort radiates into the palmar aspect of the thumb, index finger, and middle finger. Patients may complain of sensory impairment involving the entire hand; however, detailed sensory testing usually shows decreased sensation on the palmar surface of the hand involving the first three fingers and the radial side of the ring finger with normal sensation on the ulnar side of the ring finger. Weakness of the opponens pollicis and abductor pollicis brevis may be seen later. Thenar atrophy is a late sign. The signs and symptoms are aggravated by kneading, typing, or any activity involving flexion and extension of the wrist. This condition is very common in typists, carpenters, and plumbers; these occupations involve repetitive pressure on the median nerve at the wrist. Percussion of the median nerve at the wrist can produce painful discomfort radiating to the hand (Tinel's sign). Treatment consists of wrist immobilization in a neutral position in early cases, local injection with cortico-steroids and anesthetics in mild cases, or surgical decompression after failure of conservative treatment or in advanced disease.

Ulnar Entrapment

The ulnar nerve can be compressed at the elbow, at the axilla, or at the wrist and hand. The condylar groove or the cubital tunnel at the elbow is the most frequent site for ulnar entrapment. Predisposing factors for compression include elbow deformities from previous fractures, arthritis, and soft tissue tumors. Numbness and tingling of the fourth and fifth fingers and the medial border of the palm are frequent complaints. Weakness can be absent, or else an insidious progressive wasting of hand muscles can develop without sensory symptoms. Treatment consists of padding the elbow, nonsteroidal antiinflammatory agents, or surgical transposition of the nerve.

Radial Nerve Injury

The radial nerve can be compressed or entrapped in the axilla. This injury commonly results from incorrect or prolonged use of a crutch or compression of the axilla during intoxicated sleep. Radial nerve injury at this level can cause weakness of the triceps, wrist extensors, brachioradialis, and finger extensors. The most frequent compressive site is at the humerus as the nerve courses around the bone. Compression at this level can occur during sleep (Saturday night palsy) or during general anesthesia. This compression causes weakness of extension of the forearm and "wristdrop" with an inability to extend the wrist but with preservation of the triceps muscle. Because the hand cannot be placed in the position of function, there appears to be marked weakness of the hand. This apparent weakness is eliminated by placing the wrist in a splint with the hand in the neutral position of function. The sensory loss of radial nerve injury is limited to a small area adjacent to the dorsum of the thumb. Most patients will recover with time and with avoidance of further compression. Treatment includes placing the wrist in a splint to allow use of the hand. Surgical exploration is indicated when there is continuous worsening of the symptoms.

Common Peroneal Nerve Palsy

Common peroneal nerve palsy is produced by compression of the nerve as it passes around the head and neck of the fibula. Pressure is usually produced during sleep or anesthesia, by casts or obstetrical stirrups, by tight high boots, by squatting, or by habitual leg crossing while seated. Symptoms consist of footdrop as result of the inability to dorsiflex the foot and toes and numbness on the lateral aspect of the leg and dorsum of the foot. Treatment consists of physical therapy and foot braces (ankle-foot orthosis) and removal of the compressive agent.

Lateral Femoral Cutaneous Nerve Compression

The lateral femoral nerve innervates the anterolateral thigh from the pelvic crest to the knee. The nerve passes underneath the inguinal ligament. Compression of this nerve can result from abdominal or pelvic surgery or can be caused by wearing tight garments around the hip region. This nerve is commonly damaged in patients who are obese or who have diabetes mellitus. Because this is a superficial purely sensory nerve, symptoms include numbness, paresthesia, or dysesthesia over the lateral thigh with no motor weakness. This syndrome is called *meralgia paresthetica*.

Femoral Nerve Injury

The femoral nerve is derived from the second through fourth lumbar roots. The nerve can be injured in the abdomen (e.g., caused by neoplasm, hemorrhage, or abscess) or as it exits from the pelvic region. Motor symptoms include weakness of the psoas and quadriceps muscles such that there is weakness of hip flexion and impaired leg extension. The anterior thigh can appear wasted as result of quadriceps atrophy. The knee jerk is diminished. Sensory impairment involves the anteromedial thigh. For patients with femoral neuropathy computed tomography (CT) scanning of the abdomen and pelvis should be performed to exclude a mass compressing the femoral nerve. If these tests are negative, diabetes mellitus must be excluded as the cause of the femoral neuropathy.

Sciatic Nerve Injury

The sciatic nerve is derived from the fourth and fifth lumbar and first and second sacral roots. Sciatic nerve involvement affects both the peroneal and the posterior tibial nerve branches. This nerve supplies the hamstring muscle and all muscles below the knee (including dorsiflexion and plantar flexion and eversion and inversion of the foot). The sensory distribution involves the posterior thigh, posterior and lateral leg, and the entire foot. In complete sciatic nerve injuries the knee cannot be flexed and the entire foot is paralyzed. If there is gluteal muscle weakness and sensory impairment in the saddle (buttock) region, this indicates involvement of the sciatic nerve at the lumbosacral plexus in the pelvis. The sciatic nerve can be injured by abdominal and pelvic fractures, poorly administered (intramuscular) injections into the buttock region, by tumors. It is important to differentiate a lumbosacral plexopathy or herniated disk with radiculopathy from a sciatic nerve injury.

Posterior Tibial Nerve Injury

The posterior tibial nerve is a branch of the sciatic nerve. It passes from the popliteal fossa down the leg and through the tarsal tunnel (located along the medial calcaneus at the ankle). The motor branch of this nerve supplies plantar flexion and inversion of the foot as well as all intrinsic foot muscles except the extensor digitorum brevis. The sensory supply is the plantar (sole) foot surface. The posterior tibial nerve can be compressed at the tarsal tunnel to cause pain and dysesthesias over the sole of the foot. It is important to consider tarsal tunnel syndrome with posterior tibial nerve entrapment in the differential diagnostic consideration of foot pain.

◾ NEUROPATHIES ASSOCIATED WITH SYSTEMIC DISEASES

Diabetic Neuropathy

Clinical signs and symptoms of neuropathy are seen in approximately 20% of diabetic patients, but electrophysiologic studies done in asymptomatic diabetics demonstrate a higher percentage of subclinical involvement. Rarely, the neuropathy can be the initial sign of diabetes. Symptoms of neuropathy in childhood diabetics are rare. There are different patterns of presentation: symmetric polyneuropathies, focal and multifocal neuropathies, and mixed forms.

Symmetric polyneuropathies: Distal, symmetrical, sensory polyneuropathy of insidious onset is the most common form. Symptoms usually start with paresthesias of the feet and legs in a typical length related pattern. The hands are rarely affected. The anterior midline of the abdomen (truncal neuropathy) is affected in severe cases. Burning paresthesias of the feet that are worse during the night can be seen. Leg weakness is rare. Areflexia of the Achilles tendon is a constant feature. There is loss of pain and touch in a stocking-glove distribution. Acute painful neuropathy can occur and is preceded by a rapid and profound weight loss. It is most frequently seen in males and can be associated with impotence. The symptoms subside with adequate control of the diabetes and weight gain. In some patients there is predominance of loss of vibratory, position, and deep pain sensation with neuropathic arthropathy and unreactive pupils resembling tabes dorsalis (diabetic pseudotabes). Transient painful paresthesias can be described by some diabetic patients following treatment with insulin (treatment induced neuropathy). The symptoms improve with continuous control of the diabetes. Symmetric mild distal weakness can be associated with sensory neuropathies. Proximal symmetric lower limb motor neuropathy, also known as diabetic amyotrophy, can occur. It is insidious in onset and is associated with poorly defined pain.

Autonomic neuropathy: Autonomic involvement increases the risk of death in diabetic patients. Autonomic dysfunction includes pupillary abnormalities that are frequent and consist of miosis, diminished light reflex, and absence of pupillary dilation in the dark as a result of sympathetic denervation. Tachycardia and postural hypotension can also occur. Painless nocturnal diarrhea or diarrhea after meals is the most frequent gastrointestinal autonomic dysfunction. Impotence correlates with the presence of neuropathy. Bladder atony with overflow incontinence and large residual of volume after micturition indicate parasympathetic denervation.

Focal and multifocal neuropathies: Acute, painful mononeuropathies caused by nerve ischemia occur in diabetes and include mainly femoral mononeuropathy and diabetic ophthalmoplegia. In femoral mononeuropathy the patient develops severe pain in the distribution of the femoral nerve (thigh) accompanied by weakness and atrophy of quadriceps muscle with patellar areflexia. In diabetic ophthalmoplegia the third nerve is the most commonly affected but with no pupillary involvement. The pupillary sparing seen in diabetic third nerve involvement differentiates it from compression of the third nerve by intracranial carotid artery aneurysms. The sixth cranial nerve is less frequently affected. Other presentations of diabetic nerve disease include multiple, painful, asymmetric, usually motor neuropathy (multiple mononeuropathy). The treatment of diabetic neuropathies consists of strict control of the diabetes and maintenance of an ideal body weight. However, autonomic neuropathy and distal sensory neuropathy are more resistant to therapy. Vitamin supplementation and aldolase reductase inhibitors have produced no improvement of the symptoms. Amitriptyline (Elavil) or nortriptyline (Pamelor), 75 to 100 mg at bedtime, frequently relieves the pain in patients with sensory neuropathies, but phenytoin, carbamazepine, or valproic acid, either individually or in combination, can be used.

Uremic Polyneuropathy

Uremic polyneuropathy occurs more frequently in males and has an insidious onset, usually correlating with renal failure. The clinical manifestations are those of dysesthesias, cramps, and restless legs syndrome. The neuropathy is a distal symmetric mixed sensory motor neuropathy that predominantly affects the legs. Some improvement of the neuropathy can occur after dialysis, but only renal transplantation results in sustained improvement.

Alcoholic Neuropathy

Alcoholic neuropathy is most likely the result of dietary deficiency rather than a direct neurotoxic effect of alcohol and is only part of a multisystemic involvement. Alcoholic neuropathy is slowly progressive and manifests predominantly with distal sensory dysesthesias of the feet. The patients describe the pain as burning or stabbing. Hands involvement is late and less severe. Variable weakness and muscle atrophy also occur. Loss of stretch reflexes and autonomic skin changes are frequent. Associated myopathy with or without myoglobinuria can be evident. Autonomic involvement with hypothermia and postural hypotension is also frequent. Treatment consists of dietary improvement, abstinence from alcohol, and vitamin supplements (especially thiamine and other B vitamins).

Amyloid Neuropathy

Peripheral nerves can be involved in primary systemic amyloidosis and rarely in secondary (chronic infection) amyloidosis. The most frequent form of amyloid neuropathy occurs in a familial form known as foot disease or Andrade's disease. It usually starts in young adulthood and progresses slowly for 10 to 15 years. The neuropathy is usually sensory and frequently has the features of pseudo syringomyelia (sensory dissociation). Autonomic involvement is very frequent with predominant gastrointestinal problems (diarrhea). Cardiac arrhythmias, vitreous opacity, and renal involvement along with a positive family history are characteristic of this disorder. Amyloid deposits can be demonstrated in nerve or rectal biopsies.

Monoclonal Gammopahties

A gammopathy is a disorder in which there is an abnormal proliferation of lymphoid cells producing immunoglobulins. In monoclonal gammopathies a single clone of plasma cells in the bone marrow produces immunoglobulin consisting of two heavy polypeptide chains of the same class and subclass and two light polypeptide chains of the same type. The monoclonal proteins are classified according to their type of heavy chain. IgG, IgA, and IgM monoclonal gammopathies are sometimes associated with neuropathies. Neuropathies in monoclonal gammopathies are most likely associated with sclerotic myeloma, multiple myeloma, amyloidosis, macroglobulinemia, or lymphoma. Neuropathies associated with monoclonal gammopathy are rare and, when present, are more frequent in males older than 50. They are usually mixed sensory-motor and are seen predominantly distal in the legs. They respond to treatment of the underlying process. If these diseases have been excluded, the patient is classified as having a monoclonal gammopathy of undetermined significance (MGUS) with an associated neuropathy. However, most patients with MGUS do not have any clinical evidence of a peripheral neuropathy. The significance of MGUS, also known as "benign," is not clear and is controversial. Antibodies that are active in MGUS associated with peripheral neuropathy are usually of the IgM class. These antibodies are frequently directed against myelin associated glycoprotein (MAG), and the neuropathy in such cases is frequently demyelinating and predominantly sensory.

INFECTIOUS AND POSTINFECTIOUS NEUROPATHIES

Herpes Zoster (Shingles)

Herpes zoster is the most frequent infectious neuritis in adults and is due to reactivation of the varicella-zoster virus in the ganglia and associated sensory axons. It is associated with dermal pain, frequently in the thoracic area, with or without a vesicular rash along the course of the affected nerve. Less frequently one branch of the fifth cranial nerve can be involved. Acyclovir (Zovirax), 800 mg five times a day for 7 days, shortens the time of scabbing, healing, and pain and possibly reduces the incidence of postherpetic neuralgia.

Human Immunodeficiency Virus Infection (Acquired Immune Deficiency Syndrome)

Peripheral neuropathy is the most frequent neurologic disorder in infection with human immunodeficiency virus (HIV). The type of neuropathy correlates with the stage of infection. In the early asymptomatic stages an inflammatory demyelinating neuropathy and a Guillain-Barré–like syndrome can occur. CSF pleocytosis and laboratory evidence of HIV infection differentiate these neuropathies from the idiopathic ones. In the early symptomatic phase of infection a vasculitic syndrome that is probably due to immune complex deposits in the blood vessel can produce some mononeuropathies or multiple mononeuropathy.

During the late immunocompromised stage the most frequent form is the distal symmetric polyneuropathy. This is typically a painful sensory polyneuropathy involving the feet and distal leg. At this stage also a cytomegalovirus infection (CMV) is frequently found and produces a radiculopolyneuropathy or myelopathy.

Leprous Neuropathy

Leprous neuropathy is a disease endemic in tropical areas and is due to direct invasion of the nerve by *Mycobacterium leprae*. The neuropathy is frequently associated with skin lesions and is a mixed sensori-motor neuropathy with features of multiple mononeuropathy predominantly affecting cool areas of the skin. Painless injury as a result of sensory loss is the main manifestation of the disease. Nerve enlargement is a prominent finding. The organisms can be demonstrated in skin or nerve biopsies. Antibiotic treatment (dapsone, clofaximine, and rifampin) arrests the progression of the disease.

Acute Inflammatory Demyelinating Polyneuropathy (Guillain-Barré Syndrome)

Acute idiopathic polyneuritis is an immunologically mediated demyelinating polyneuropathy of world-wide distribution that affects all ages and both sexes equally. The disease is usually preceded by an acute infectious illness, including Campylobacter jejuni, viral or *Mycoplasma* infection, surgery, or immunization (rabies, swine influenza) or can occurring patients with malignant disease (lymphomas) or lupus erythematosus. The disease is characterized by rapidly progressive motor weakness, frequently symmetrical, with or without mild ataxia at the onset and frequently of ascending nature beginning distally in the legs, progressing to the upper extremities, and ending with severe respiratory paralysis. There can be involvement of portions of the cranial nerves causing facial paralysis, which is found in one half of the patients, and external ophthalmoplegia with sixth nerve palsy, which is the most frequent extraocular finding. Progression of the weakness varies from 3 days to 4 weeks. Areflexia is usually generalized and occurs early; this is an almost constant feature. Although paresthesias are frequently an early complaint, sensory signs are mild. Autonomic dysfunction can cause cardiac arrhythmias and postural hypotension, but bladder or bowel dysfunction at the onset or persisting during the disease is rare. Functional recovery usually begins 2 to 4 weeks after stabilization of the symptoms and is complete in most patients. Areflexia can be a permanent residual finding. A variant of the disease includes acute onset of ophthalmoplegia, ataxia, and areflexia with or without weakness of the extremities (Fisher syndrome). Rapid onset of symmetrical cranial nerve dysfunction (polyneuritis cranialis) can also be a variant. Pure pandysautonomia of rapid onset with full recovery is considered another variant, and in some cases predominant autonomic symptoms can precede the typical course of Guillain-Barré syndrome. The autonomic symptoms can cause sudden death. The increase in CSF protein with less than 10 cells/ml (albuminocytologic dissociation) strongly supports the diagnosis when found after the first week of symptoms or when a progressive rise of protein content is demonstrated from several lumbar punctures. Nerve conduction studies confirm a demyelinating process by showing a reduction in conduction velocity, a conduction block or abnormal temporal dispersion in a motor nerves, prolonged distal latencies, and absent F-waves. Treatment consists of maintaining adequate respiratory function and instituting respiratory assistance when vital capacity falls below 12 to 15 ml/kg or when there is decreased oxygen saturation in the blood. Cardiovascular status should be monitored to control autonomic dysfunction when present. Passive bedside physiotherapy should be started immediately and followed throughout the recovery of the patient. There is convincing evidence that plasmapheresis early in the course of the disease reduces the duration of acute hospital care, shortens the duration of ventilator dependency, and hastens motor recovery. One session every other day with an exchange of 40 to 50 ml/kg should be done to achieve a cumulative exchange of 200 to 250 ml/kg. Intravenous immune globulin in a dosage 0.4 gm per kilogram per day for 5 days is as effective as or superior to plasma exchange. The Dutch Guillain-Barré Study Group has recently reported that treatment with high-dose immune globulin as described, combined with 0.5 gm of methyprednisolone/day, is more effective than treatment with immune globulin alone.

Chronic Inflammatory Demyelinating Polyneuropathy

Chronic recurrent inflammatory demyelinating polyneuropathy is a rare form of both motor and sensory polyneuropathy or polyradiculoneuropathy that affects distal and proximal limbs. The onset of symptoms is usually insidious, and the course is slowly progressive, either stepwise or relapsing. Motor weakness predominates, but sensory loss is found in most patients. The muscle atrophy is of a lesser degree than would be expected from the amount of weakness. The CSF protein is elevated as much as four times the normal value without an increased cell count. Respiratory involvement is less frequent than in Guillain-Barré syndrome, and there is greater fluctuation of functional impairment. The treatment is similar to the treatment for GBS. Intermittent intravenous immune globulin treatment with or without methylprednisolone, intermittent plasmapheresis, chronic steroid therapy, or immunosuppression with cyclophosphamide (Cytoxan) or azathioprine (Imuran) may be necessary.

Sensory Neuronopathy

Sensory neuronopathies are pure sensory syndromes without motor deficit produced by damage to the nerve cell bodies in the spinal dorsal root or trigeminal ganglia. Sensory manifestations include both positive (dysesthesia) and negative phenomena (hypesthesia). Severe sensory ataxia, caused by deafferentation, is the main clinical manifestation. Dependence on visual input for the maintenance of postural stability is strong and helps to differentiate this type of ataxia from the cerebellar type. Pseudo-athetosis of the upper limbs is frequent, and areflexia is a constant feature. The clinical presentation can be acute, subacute, or chronic. The acute form is rare, and the few cases described may have been produced by the use of synthetic antibiotics. The subacute form has been associated with carcinoma, pyridoxine abuse, or cisplatin therapy. This form often begins asymmetrically and can first appear in the upper limbs or the trigeminal distribution. Pain and dysesthesias are followed by proprioceptive loss. The chronic forms are sporadic and of unknown cause, and there is a group of hereditary disorders. The prognosis of this group of disorders is poor except for the toxic ones, which can improve if the diagnosis is made early and the toxic agent is discontinued.

Neuropathies Associated with Connective Tissue Disorders

Neuropathies associated with connective tissue disorders are usually of ischemic vascular origin caused by arteritis. Clinical evidence of neuropathy in *rheumatoid arthritis,* other than carpal tunnel syndrome, is not frequent but when present is due to arteritis and occurs in patients with longstanding disease (approximately 10 years), destructive joint disease, rheumatoid nodules, and high titers of rheumatoid factor. The disease can appear as a progressive, distal (legs first), sensorimotor polyneuropathy or can have the features of multiple mononeuropathy. Neuropathy in *polyarteritis nodosa* occurs in 50% of patients with this disease and can be the initial manifestation. The neuropathy appears as a multiple mononeuropathy with involvement of two or more nerves in an acute fashion, with pain and paresthesias in the distribution of the affected nerve, followed by weakness. The distribution can also be that of a diffuse, distal, and symmetrical sensorimotor polyneuropathy. Treatment consists of corticosteroids and immunosuppression. Neuropathy in *systemic lupus erythematosus* occurs in only 11% of patients; it can be the initial symptom of the disease and indicates diffuse vasculitis and a poor prognosis. The disease appears as a progressive symmetrical, distal, sensorimotor neuropathy with elevated CSF protein suggestive of Guillain-Barré's syndrome. More rarely the disease can also appear as a multiple mononeuropathy.

Cranial Neuropathies

Cranial nerves can be affected by several disease processes without involvement of spinal nerves. They can be individually affected (cranial mononeuropathies), or else several nerves can be involved (cranial polyneuropathies). When cranial mononeuropathies or polyneuropathies are associated with impaired function in the corticospinal, spinothalamic, or cerebellar tracts, the lesion is within the brain stem. Pure mononeuropathies or polyneuropathies localize the lesion outside the brain stem. The most common cranial neuropathy is discussed here.

Bell's Palsy (Idiopathic Facial Paralysis)

Bell's palsy is an acute disease of the facial (seventh cranial) nerve of unknown causes that produces edema and compressive ischemia of the nerve within its bony canal. Onset is sudden or can develop in a few hours or days. It occurs in either sex and at any age. Ten percent of patients are diabetic. Facial palsy can develop in patients with basilar meningitis (sarcoid; neoplastic, including leukemia). The most significant finding is infranuclear (peripheral) facial palsy, which can be partial or complete and can be associated with or preceded by retroauricular (mastoid) pain in 50% of patients and decreased taste in 30% of patients. Some patients can have hyperacusis and excess or decreased lacrimation. Recovery tends to be rapid (weeks) and complete in 80% of patients. Prognostic indicators for delayed or partial recovery include age over 44, complete paralysis with decreased tearing, decreased taste, retroauricular pain, and electromyographic evidence of denervation 10 days after onset of symptoms. Treatment consists of protecting the cornea with an eye patch during sleep or when going outdoors and facial exercises. Corticosteroids can have a beneficial effect when used within 72 hours of onset (60 mg/day for 4 days, then taper to

5 mg/day in 10 days.) No evidence exists that surgical decompression improves the outcome.

Brachial Neuritis (Neuralgic Amyotrophy)

Brachial neuritis is a disease of undetermined causes that can be associated with the use of foreign sera (tetanus antitoxin) or vaccines. However, most commonly it is idiopathic. Males are predominantly affected. The disease is characterized by sudden, severe, and often nocturnal pain in the shoulder, arm, forearm, and hand. This pain is usually severe and is followed within a few days or 2 weeks by weakness. In 50% of the patients the weakness is confined to the shoulder girdle, mainly the axillary and suprascapular nerves (upper brachial plexus). Partial brachial plexus involvement in one or both sides may be noted usually in an asymmetrical fashion. Nerves derived from the lower plexus are rarely involved alone. An EMG shows denervation in the distribution of affected nerves but nerve conduction velocity (NCV) is usually normal. All other tests including CSF studies are normal. The diffuse nonsegmental signs, the lack of radicular pain, and normal CSF findings argue against cervical radicular involvement. The prognosis is excellent in most cases with complete recovery in 80% of patients at the end of 2 years. Treatment consists of symptomatic relief of pain and physical therapy. Corticosteroids have been used in the acute phase for relief of pain.

▨ TOXIC NEUROPATHIES

A great variety of toxic agents produce damage to the peripheral nerves usually to the distal portion of the axon (dying-back neuropathies). Only a few that have rather specific features are discussed here.

Heavy Metals

Lead produces a pure motor neuropathy of the radial nerve (wristdrop), which can be unilateral or bilateral. Arsenic poisoning is characterized by mixed polyneuropathy with predominant sensory symptoms usually affecting the lower extremities. Thallium produces a mixed polyneuropathy with marked synesthesia and is associated with severe hair loss.

Drugs

Streptomycin affects the cochlear part of the eighth nerve. Isoniazid produces polyneuropathy by creating a pyridoxine deficiency. Ethambutol and amphotericin can also produce polyneuropathy. With longstanding use anticonvulsants such as phenytoin frequently produce subclinical symptoms. Antineoplastic agents including vincristine and nitrogen mustard can produce neuropathies. Cisplatin commonly causes sensory neuronopathy. Industrial agents, mainly solvents including n-hexane and related compounds, acrylamide, or organophosphates can produce an axonal neuropathy.

▨ INHERITED PRIMARY PERIPHERAL NEUROPATHIES

Heriditary Motor and Sensory Neuropathies or the Charcot-Marie-Tooth Polyneuropathy Syndrome

These are a genetically and clinically heterogeneous group of disorders of the peripheral nerves characterized by an insidious onset and slowly progressive weakness of the distal muscles and mild sensory impairment. The symptoms can appear in the first decade or early in the second decade. Children with the disease often walk on their toes, and adults complain of abnormalities of gait, foot deformities, or loss of balance. Pes cavus develops as the disease progresses. Atrophy of the distal legs can be a prominent feature ("stork leg" or inverted champagne bottle appearance). Tripping over objects on the floor and ankle sprains are frequent as a result of weakness of dorsiflexion of the foot produced by weakness of the peroneal and anterior tibialis muscles. Weakness of the intrinsic hand muscles usually occurs late but may not be related to the degree of leg weakness or atrophy. The most frequent complaints concerning hand involvement are difficulty using zippers, difficulty buttoning and unbuttoning, and difficulty manipulating small objects when using fine finger movements. In severe cases the wasting of the hand muscles gives the appearance of claw hands. Muscle stretch reflexes disappear early at the ankle and later on at the patella. The plantar reflex is flexor or absent. Sensory involvement to any significant degree is rare, but decreased pain to pricking in a stocking distribution is seen in most patients. *Electrophysiological* studies distinguish two major forms of Charcot-Marie-Tooth (CMT) that have the same clinical phenotype and some variable clinical features. *CMT type 1* (CMT1) is a demyelinating neuropathy with moderate to severely decreased motor NCV, absent reflexes, and, in some slender patients, enlarged (hypertrophic), visible, or palpable nerves. Patients with *CMT type 2* (CMT2), the neuronal form, have normal NCVs, normal muscle stretch reflexes, and normal size nerves.

Genetics of CMT

CMT1 can be inherited as an autosomal-dominant (AD), autosomal-recessive (AR), or X-linked disorder.

AD CMT1 is the most frequently observed pattern, whereas AR CMT1 is rare. In 70% of AD CMT1 patients the disease locus shows DNA duplication in a segment of chromosome 17 (17p11.2p12) that encodes a membrane-associated myelin protein with an apparent molecular weight of 22 kd (PMP22). CMT 1 B is linked to markers on chromosome 1 (1q21.2q23) that encode for the protein zero (Po) myelin. The dominant X-linked form, CMTX (sq1213), has a missense mutation in the segment of the X chromosome that encodes the conexin-32 protein (Tables 16-1 and 16-2). All these proteins are found in peripheral nerve myelin and seem to play a role in keeping the compaction of the myelin layers.

TABLE 16-1 Genetic Classification of CMT

Disease	Locus	Mutation	Gene/Protein
AD CMT1A	17p11.2p12	1.5-Mb duplication	PMP22
AD CMT1A	17p11.2p12	Missense mutation (including Dejerine-Sottas)	PMP22
AD CMT1B	1q21.q23	Missense mutation (including Dejerine-Sottas)	Po
AD CMT1C	—	—	—
AR CMT1A	8q13q21.1	—	—
CMTX	Xq1213	Missense mutations	Conexin-32
HNPP	17p11.2p12	Deletion	Deletion of PMP22
AD CMT2	1p35p36	—	—
AR CMT2	—	—	—

Hereditary Neuropathy with Liability to Pressure Palsies

This disorder, which is also called familial recurrent polyneuropathy or tomaculous neuropathy, was originally described in a family in which three generations had recurrent peroneal neuropathy after digging potatoes in a kneeling position. Hereditary neuropathy with liability to pressure palsies (HNPP) can cause periodic episodes of numbness, muscular weakness, atrophy, and in some cases palsies that follow relatively minor compression or trauma of the peripheral nerves. Carpal tunnel syndrome and other entrapment neuropathies are frequent manifestations of HNPP. Electrophysiologic studies sometimes show mildly slow nerve conduction velocity in clinically affected individuals as well as in asymptomatic carriers. Conduction blocks can also be seen. Peripheral nerves show segmental demyelination and remyelination with tomaculous or sausagelike focal thickening of the myelin sheath. HNPP is associated with a 1.5-Mb deletion in 17p11.2p12. All of the DNA markers known to be duplicated in patients with the CMT1A duplication are deleted in patients with HNPP. Commercially available blood tests to detect either the duplication of CMT1A or the deletion of HNPP are available and show high diagnostic specificity.

Refsum's Disease (Heredopathia Atactica Polyneuritiformis)

Refsum's disease is a hereditary metabolic disorder transmitted as an autosomal recessive trait as a result of deficiency of phytanic acid a-hydroxylase and accumulation of phytanic acid in tissues and blood. The disease starts in childhood and is manifested by chronic polyneuropathy associated with cerebellar

TABLE 16-2 Clinical and Genetic Correlations

	Onset	Weakness Hands	Legs
CMT1	1st or 2nd decade	Late	Early
AD CMT2	2nd decade	Mild	Severe
AR CMT2	At birth or infancy	Severe	Severe

MSR: muscle stretch reflexes
NCVs: nerve conduction velocities
*: may be decreased and are absent in late stages of the disease

ataxia, retinitis pigmentosa, deafness, and pupillary abnormalities. The disease responds to a diet low in phytanic acid.

Hereditary Sensory Neuropathies

Hereditary sensory neuropathies are rare hereditary disorders characterized by sensory loss of a dissociated type resembling syringomyelia. These neuropathies can appear early or late in life and are frequently associated with painless traumatic deformities, ulcers of the extremities, and autonomic dysfunction.

DISEASES OF MOTOR NERVES

Amyotrophic Lateral Sclerosis, Motor Neuron Disease, Lou Gehrig's Disease

Amyotrophic lateral sclerosis, also known as motor neuron disease and often referred to as Lou Gehrig's disease, is a devastating paralytic and fatal disorder of adult patients caused by degeneration of large motor neurons of the brain and their corticospinal tract, motor

Nerves	MSR	NCVs	Wheelchair
Can be enlarged	·Absent	Prolonged	Rare
Normal	Normal*	Normal	Rare
Normal	Normal*	Normal	2nd decade

neurons of the brain stem, and anterior horn cells of spinal cord. The cause of the disorder is undetermined, and there is no treatment currently available to prevent, slow, or stop the progression of the disease. The disease is characterized by progressive weakness and early wasting (amyotrophy) of muscles with fasciculations and upper motor neuron signs. There is striking sparing of bladder and bowel control, sparing of sensation, and preservation of sexual function, intellect, and eye movements. In spite of severe paralysis late in the disease, decubiti are rare. The clinical presentation varies according to the group of neurons or tracts affected. It usually consists of progressive, usually symmetrical, distal weakness of legs or hands. Leg muscle cramps are a frequent early complaint. Weight loss and progressive wasting of muscles associated with fasciculations in the upper and lower limbs indicate anterior horn cell involvement. Spasticity of the legs with hyperreflexia and bilateral Babinski signs indicate corticospinal tract involvement. Weakness progresses proximally and affects neck muscles and bulbar musculature to cause difficulty swallowing and speech impairment. Respiratory muscle paralysis is the terminal effect of the disease. Emotional lability with uncontrollable bouts of laughing or crying, dysarthria, difficulty swallowing, spastic tongue without fasciculations, and hyperactive jaw jerk can occur and is known as pseudobulbar palsy. The course is relentless, progressing to death within 3 to 7 years or more. There are no specific biologic markers for amyotrophic lateral sclerosis, and electrophysiologic and radiologic studies are necessary to exclude other disease processes. Electromyographic evidence of widespread denervation with reinnervation should be found. Muscle biopsy shows severe denervation (fascicular) atrophy. The differential diagnosis includes mainly cervical spondylitic myelopathy and other cervical cord lesions including tumors, disk herniations, syringomyelia, or foramen magnum lesions that can be diagnosed by myelography or CT/MRI scanning. Lead and mercury intoxications, thyrotoxicosis, and familial or tropical spastic paraparesis should also be excluded.

Progressive bulbar palsy can be the first manifestation of motor neuron disease. Speech impairment and difficulty swallowing are early signs associated with tongue atrophy and fasciculations. The symptoms progress to respiratory impairment or aspiration pneumonia. The clinical course usually lasts less than 3 years. Progressive bulbar palsy is the final stage of most patients with amyotrophic lateral sclerosis. In *progressive spinal muscular atrophy,* predominant findings are progressive muscle atrophy and fasciculations with lack of corticospinal tract involvement. The progression of this type of motor neuron disease is slower. However, most patients eventually develop upper motor neuron signs and follow the regular course of amyotrophic lateral sclerosis. Some patients with *primary lateral sclerosis* (PLS) have a progressive spastic paraparesis (PLS) that later affects the upper limbs and that eventually shows signs of lower motor neuron involvement. Rarely the clinical presentation remains as pure upper motor neurons signs. Care of the patient with amyotrophic lateral sclerosis requires a multidisciplinary approach. Physical therapy to increase the usefulness of preserved muscles is important. Feeding gastrostomy improves the general nutrition of the patients with dysphagia and prevents aspiration pneumonia. Ventilatory assistance when necessary should be discussed with the patient and the family early in the disease. There is no effective therapeutic agent at the present time, but randomized trials are being done with nerve growth factors, mainly ciliary neurotrophic factor, glutamate antagonists (Riluzole), and antioxidant vitamins including vitamins E and C and betacarotene. Five to 10% of the cases are familial cases transmitted in an autosomal dominant pattern. There is evidence that the genetic defect in some families is linked to chromosome 21 (D21S58) segment that encodes for Superoxide Dismutase 1, an important neuronal antioxidant.

A clinically heterogeneous group of hereditary lower motor neuron diseases that predominantly affect infants and young patients is known as *progressive spinal muscular atrophy* (SMA). Regardless of the age of onset, they all are linked to chromosome 5. The disease is inherited through an autosomal recessive gene. This heterogeneous disease has several clinical presentations with different ages of onset. When present at birth (Werdnig-Hoffman) it is manifested by floppiness, abdominal breathing, fasciculations of the tongue, and evidence of denervation on electromyography and muscle biopsy. An intermediate form of spinal muscular atrophy appears in infancy. Patients with this form have a longer survival span. Another intermediate type of spinal muscular atrophy with the same type of inheritance but with onset in adolescence is characterized by predominantly proximal muscle involvement and a normal life span (*Kugelberg-Welander type*). In this form of SMA weakness and atrophy are frequently proximal and simulate myopathy; however, in contrast with a myopathy muscle stretch reflexes are usually absent in Kugelberg-Welander syndrome. Electrophysiologic studies and muscle biopsy are necessary for the diagnosis. Bracing and physical and occupational therapy to stretch or prevent contractures and to prevent scoliosis improves the quality of the patient's life.

▦ SUMMARY

Disorders of the peripheral nerves (neuropathy) can cause motor, sensory, and autonomic symptoms. Motor features include weakness and wasting in a distal distribution (feet, hands). Sensory disturbances include numbness or painful paresthesias in a stocking-glove distal distribution. Autonomic features include bladder, sexual, and gastrointestinal dysfunction and skin, hair, and nail changes. Stretch reflexes are decreased early in most neuropathies. The diagnosis of neuropathy is confirmed by nerve conduction velocity slowing. The neuropathy can be generalized (polyneuropathy) or focal as occurs with compressive (entrapment) neuropathies. Patients with motor neuron disease develop distal weakness with signs of corticospinal tract and anterior horn cell involvement. The presence of fasciculations in weak and wasted muscles indicates anterior horn cell disease.

Suggested Readings

Neuropathy—General

Asbury AK, Johnson PC: *Pathology of peripheral nerve* Philadelphia, 1985, WB Saunders.

Dyck PJ, et al: *Peripheral neuropathy,* ed 3, Philadelphia, 1993, WB Saunders.

England JD, Sumner AJ: Neuralgic amyotrophy: an increasingly diverse entity *Muscle Nerve* 10:60, 1987.

McLeod JG: Investigation of peripheral neuropathy, *J Neurol Neurosurg Psychiatry* 58:274, 1995.

Malamut RI, et al: Postsurgical idiopathic brachial neuritis, *Muscle Nerve* 17:320, 1994.

Guillain-Barré Syndrome

Gibbels E, Giebisch U: Natural history of acute and chronic monophasic inflammatory demyelinating polyneuropathies, *Acta Neurologica Scand* 85:282, 1992.

McKhann GM: Plasmapheresis and the Guillain-Barré Syndrome, *Ann Neurol* 22:762, 1987.

Ropper AH: Guillain-Barré syndrome, *N Engl J Med* 326:1130, 1992.

The Dutch Guillain-Barré Study Group: Treatment of Guillain-Barré syndrome with high dose immune globulins combined with methylprednisolone: a pilot study, *Ann Neurol* 35:749, 1994.

Van der Meche FGA, Schmitz PIM, the Dutch Guillain-Barré Study Group: A randomized trial comparing intravenous immune globulin and plasma exchange in Guillain-Barré syndrome, *N Engl J Med* 326:1123, 1992.

Motor Neuron Disease

Bradley WG: Recent views on amyotrophic lateral sclerosis with emphasis on electrophysiological studies, *Muscle Nerve* 10:490, 1987.

Leigh PN, Chaudhuri KRT: Motor neuron disease, *J Neurol Neurosurg Psychiatry* 58:886, 1994.

Rowland LP: Amyotrophic lateral sclerosis: theories and therapies, *Ann Neurol* 35:129, 1994.

Siddique T, Figlewicz DA, Pericak-Vance MA: Linkage of a gene causing familial amyotrophic lateral sclerosis to chromosome 21 and evidence of genetic-locus heterogeneity, *N Engl J Med* 324:1381, 1991.

Tandan R, Bradley WG: Amyotrophic lateral sclerosis: 1. Clinical features, pathology and ethical issues in management, *Ann Neurol* 18:271, 1985.

Tandan R, Bradley WG: Amyotrophic lateral sclerosis: II. Ethiopathogenesis, *Ann Neurol* 18:419, 1985.

Williams DB: Motor neuron disease (amyotrophic lateral sclerosis), *Mayo Clin Proc* 66:54, 1991.

Inherited Neuropathy

Bergoggen J, et al: Connexin mutations in X-linked Charcot-Marie-Tooth disease, *Science* 262:2039, 1993.

Kaku DA, et al: Uniform slowing of conduction velocities in Charcot-Marie-Tooth polyneuropathy type 1, *Neurology* 43:2664, 1993.

Lupski JR, et al: DNA duplication associated with Charcot-Marie-Tooth disease type 1A, *Cell* 66:219, 1991.

Lupski JR, Chance PF, Garcia CA: Inherited primary peripheral neuropathies, *JAMA* 270:2326, 1993.

Diseases of Muscle and Neuromuscular Junction

17

▦ MYOPATHIES

Clinical Features

Myopathies are diseases that primarily affect the muscles and are usually characterized by weakness, fatigue, or stiffness (myotonia) or a combination of the three. They are not due to peripheral nerve damage or central nervous system (CNS) lesions. They are usually characterized by symmetrical proximal muscle weakness, normal sensation, and normal stretch reflexes. More than 50% of muscle bulk must be lost before functional weakness can be demonstrated. Limb pain of the aching type or muscle cramps sometimes precipitated by exercise can be present. The patient's complaints usually localize the weakness to a certain group of muscles. The questions listed in Box 17-1 should be answered.

The neuromuscular examination (see Chapter 5) should give the examiner a good idea of the muscle groups affected, the acuteness (no atrophy) or chronicity (atrophy) of disease, the progression of the disease, and the inheritance pattern in familial myopathies.

BOX 17-1

1 Is it an acute (days), subacute (weeks), or chronic (months to years) process?

2 Is the weakness symmetrical, proximal, distal, or generalized?

3 What muscles were affected first, and what has been the progression of the weakness? Relentlessly worse or fluctuating?

4 Does exercise make the symptoms worse (fatigability in myasthenia), or do the symptoms improve with muscle activity (as in myotonias)?

5 Are the ocular or bulbar muscles predominantly affected, as in myasthenic or mitochondrial disorders?

6 Are the neck muscles involved?

7 Is there difficulty chewing, swallowing, or breathing?

8 Does exercise produce cramps or weakness? Is there an associated change in the color of the urine suggestive of myoglobinuria?

9 Is there a family history? If so, what is the inheritance pattern? A pedigree of the family should be drawn.

Laboratory Tests

The laboratory tests should be done in a selected and methodical way, beginning with measurement of serum electrolytes and enzymes. Serum tests include electrolyte determination of mainly potassium, magnesium, and calcium. Electrolyte alterations can produce weakness or irritability of the muscle. The ischemic forearm exercise test to measure lactic acid combined with an electromyography (EMG) is necessary in certain metabolic myopathies. The most reliable and helpful serum muscle enzyme is the creatine kinase (CK). Patients should avoid heavy exercise, injections, and muscle trauma before blood sampling for muscle enzymes. Serum CK isoenzymes (MM band) are highly specific and sensitive and usually indicate skeletal muscle destruction. DNA studies are at this time commercially available for Duchenne-Becker, myotonic muscular dystrophy, and mitochondrial disorders. Electrophysiologic studies such as EMG, nerve conduction velocities, and repetitive nerve stimulation, when indicated, should precede the muscle biopsy. Needle insertion into the muscle or sampling of the muscle tends to elevate the muscle enzymes artificially. Electrophysiologic studies can also help to select the appropriate muscle for biopsy. In symmetrical myopathies, the electrophysiologic studies can be done on one side and the biopsy on the other side to avoid needle tracks that can produce artifactual alterations. An EMG demonstrates functional activity in the muscle, more specifically in the motor unit and neuromuscular junction. Gallium nuclide scanning, computed tomography, and magnetic resonance imaging can be used to detect muscle abnormalities that can help select the site of the biopsy. The muscle biopsy, when done in the properly selected patient and properly selected muscle, can confirm the clinical impression, differentiate denervation from primary myopathies, demonstrate metabolic diseases, and support diagnoses of inflammatory myopathies and some mitochondrial disorders. A portion of muscle can be used for biochemical analysis, immunohistochemistry, deoyribonucleic acid (DNA) studies, and diagnosis in metabolic myopathies.

Inflammatory Myopathies

Inflammatory myopathies are a large and heterogeneous group of disorders characterized by different morphologic alterations of the muscle tissue with variable amounts of inflammatory reactions as a response to injury. The injurious agent can be easily found or traceable, as is the case with bacterial (pyomyositis) or parasitic myositis, or it can be elusive and indeterminate, as in the idiopathic forms. The inflammatory myopathies can be acute in onset and rapidly progressive (bacterial and some viral forms) or can be insidious in onset and slowly progressive (idiopathic forms). They can be localized to a muscle or a group of muscles (pyomyositis, some viral forms) or can be more diffuse and symmetrical (idiopathic forms). They can be benign and transient (some viral forms) and can respond to therapy (pyomyositis and some parasitic and autoimmune forms), whereas others can be disabling, resistant to therapy, and even fatal. Recent advances in the development of new medications and treatments have been beneficial for treating some of the bacterial, parasitic, and idiopathic forms. However, immunodysfunction, either produced during cancer therapy or seen as part of other disorders, including human immunodeficiency virus, seems to have increased the frequency of opportunistic muscle infections. Immunodysfunction also seems to play an important role in the production of idiopathic myositis. We will only deal here with the idiopathic forms: dermatomyositis, polymyositis, and inclusion body myositis.

Dermatomyositis and Polymyositis Syndromes

Dermatomyositis (DM) and polymyositis (PM) are the most common acquired myopathies. Both share the same diffuse and symmetrical involvement of muscles, elevation of muscles enzymes, response to immunosuppressive therapy in some patients, and unknown causes. However, there are striking differences in the immunologic mechanism and in the pathologic changes besides the obvious skin involvement in dermatomyositis. Both diseases can occur at any age, and both occur predominantly in females. Most cases of DM occur between 5 and 14 years of age, and most cases of PM occur in the 50s and 60s. Polymyositis is rare in childhood. Both can be associated with connective tissue disorders, and predominantly the adult form of DM can be associated with malignancies (Table 17-1).

Childhood and juvenile dermatomyositis. Childhood and juvenile dermatomyositis, as the name implies, affects children and young adults. It frequently has an insidious onset and a rapid progression and lacks a precipitating factor. Facial erythema, fatigue, general malaise, and muscle weakness are the most frequent complaints.

Muscle weakness is a constant feature. It is usually proximal in distribution, involving the shoulders and pelvic muscles, but can be severe and generalized. Neck muscles, predominantly the flexors, are frequently affected. In approximately half of the patients the weakness is associated with muscle pain and tenderness.

Dysphagia and dysphonia are frequent and indicate involvement of the muscles of deglutition and phonation.

Skin involvement is variable according to the stage of the disease but consistently affects the face and extensor surfaces on the joints. The facial lesion affects predominantly sun-exposed areas and consists of an erythematous rash in butterfly distribution over the malar regions and a lilac discoloration (heliotrope) and edema of periorbital surfaces. The rash can extend

TABLE 17-1 Inflammatory Myopathies Clinical Features

	Age	Site of Weakness
DM	5–14	Prox. limbs & neck muscles
	40–50	Prox. limbs & neck muscles
PM	40–60	Prox. limb & neck muscles
IBM	After 50	Prox. & distal limbs

DM, Dermatomyositis; *PM*, polymyositis; *IBM*, inclusion body myositis.

to the neck and upper thoracic areas. Erythematous discoloration also affects the extensor surfaces of the elbows, keens, and knuckles (Gottron's sign). Scalp involvement includes a diffuse scaly dermatosis with erythema, atrophy, and often a nonscarring alopecia.

Periungual hyperemia and telangiectasis are frequent, seem to correlate with the disease activity, and are early signs of recurrence or exacerbation of the disease. Subcutaneous nodules and ulcerations occur in prolonged and severe disease or in partially treated patients. Subcutaneous calcification (calcinosis) is a late event and is frequently associated with joint contractures. Ulceration and perforation of the gastrointestinal tract as a result of vasculitis can be the cause of death and are usually seen in severe and chronic cases. Cardiac involvement and restrictive pulmonary disease have also been described.

Laboratory findings include nonspecific elevation of the sedimentation rate in half of the cases and elevation of CK in most cases. The elevation of CK, predominantly the MM isoenzyme, and the elevation of serum myoglobin occur in active disease and can be used along with the clinical improvement of weakness as a guide for the progression of the disease and

Calcinosis	Malignancy	CK
Frequent	No association	Elevated
Rare	Found in 10–20%	Elevated
Absent	Rare	Elevated
Absent	No association	Normal

response to therapy. The EMG shows increased insertional activity, fibrillation potentials, and a train of positive sharp waves indicating abnormal spontaneous activity. There can also be myopathic features such as a decrease in the duration of the motor unit potentials and short duration polyphasic motor units. Complex repetitive discharges and myotonic discharges are occasionally seen.

Pathology of the muscle biopsy shows endothelial hyperplasia of intramuscular blood vessels and segmental perivascular and intravascular mononuclear cell infiltration with and without thrombosis. In most children's biopsies and in a few adult biopsies some intramuscular arteries and veins show deposition of IgG, C3, and C9 immune complexes. There is also necrosis and a decreased number of capillaries surrounding individual muscle fibers. This microvasculopathy is due to deposition of neoantigens of the C5b-9 complement membrane attack complex early in the disease. Small areas of infarction in the center of some fascicles and necrosis or atrophy of muscle fibers in the periphery of the fascicles (perifascicular atrophy) with little or no inflammatory reaction are prominent features. The vasculitis, the perifascicular atrophy, and the reduced capillary density are the most important and specific histologic diagnostic features of the disease (Table 17-2).

Treatment consists of general supportive care including rest, passive physical therapy oriented toward preventing contractures, and immunosuppressive therapy. Prednisone, 2 mg/kg in divided daily doses, should be given for at least 1 month after the disease is clinically and enzymatically inactive. Intravenous gamma globulin has been tried with great success. Cytoxan pulse therapy along with steroids speeds the recovery of the weakness and decreases the side effects of the steroids.

Polymyositis and dermatomyositis of the adult. The skin lesions of *adult dermatomyositis* are similar to those seen in the childhood type except for calcinosis. Also contractures and skin ulcers are rare in the adult type. The skin lesions in the adult can be seen without muscle weakness and with normal CK for 2 or more years ("amyopathic dermatomyositis"). However, EMGs and muscle biopsies reveal muscle involvement in most of these cases. DM of the adult is more frequently associated with a manifested or occult tumor than with polymyositis. The DM and malignancy develop within a year of each other. The muscle biopsy, the immune mechanism, and the treat-

TABLE 17-2 Inflammatory Myopathies Histopathology

	Arteries and Arterioles	Capillaries
DM	Vasculitis, immune complex	Decreased
PM	Perivascular inflammation	Normal
I.B.M.	Normal	Increased

ment are similar for both childhood and adult DM. When associated with malignancy, eradication of the tumor should be the priority.

Adult polymyositis has an insidious onset and progresses over weeks or months. Weakness usually starts in the hip muscles, exhibited by difficulty arising from a sitting or squatting position and difficulty climbing stairs. At this time or later the patient notices difficulty combing the hair or doing anything that requires raising the arms above the head. Neck flexor muscle weakness is also a prominent feature. Dysphagia and respiratory muscle weakness occur in 30% of patients. There is preservation of strength in distal muscles and in ocular and facial muscles. Muscle pain or tenderness is not a prominent finding. Visceral involvement includes cardiac arrhythmias and interstitial pneumonitis. The muscle biopsy and the immune mechanisms in PM differ from those seen in DM. In PM the muscle biopsy shows scattered necrotic and regenerating fibers. The prominent perimysial and endomysial inflammatory mononuclear infiltrate is predominantly composed of T cells, particularly activated CD8, and macrophages. There is no perifascicular atrophy and the capillary density is normal (see Table 17-2).

Therapy. The treatment is variable, and the response is not always good. Prednisone, 60 to 80 mg

---

Muscle Fascicles

Perifascicular atrophy, necrosis, & microinfarcts

Single fiber necrosis, T cells around normal fibers

Atrophic fibers, rimmed vacuoles, inclusions

daily, in divided doses until the disease is stablized or improved according to clinical findings and the CK level is stabilized, followed by alternate-day doses of 60 to 80 mg for at least 6 months, seems to be effective. Azathioprine (Imuran), 2 mg/kg/day, can be added to the treatment of patients who are nonresponsive to steroids. Cyclophosphamide (Cytoxan) pulse therapy, once a month for 6 months, has been used with good results in some corticosteroid-resistant patients and can be the first line of therapy to avoid the side effects of the steroids. Other therapeutic modalities include plasmapheresis and total body, low dose irradiation.

Polymyositis associated with connective tissue disorders. One third of adult polymyositis patients have a connective tissue disorder associated with the polymyositis. The associated connective tissue disorder can be rheumatoid arthritis, scleroderma, mixed connective tissue disorders, lupus erythematosus, polyarteritis nodosa, or Sjögren's syndrome. Clinical features such as arthritis, sclerosis of the skin, renal disease, multiple mononeuropathies, or salivary gland enlargement should suggest an associated connective tissue disorder.

Viral polymyositis. Viruses including influenza types A and B and Coxsackie virus have been associated with acute local or diffuse myositis that is similar clinically and morphologically to the idiopathic form. The exact relationship between the viral infection and the myositis is still unknown, but the possibility exists that viruses elicit and perpetuate the autoimmune response responsible for most cases of PM and DM.

Inclusion body myositis. Inclusion body myositis is a disease predominantly seen in males. The age of onset varies from 16 to 68 years, but the disease rarely starts before the age of 50. The disorder is relatively benign, has an insidious onset, and runs a slow course of several years duration characterized by progressive weakness, which is usually proximal but can also involve the distal musculature. There is frequent but not consistent muscle atrophy. Muscle pain and association with other connective tissue disorders is rare. Dysphagia is unusual, and cardiac abnormalities have not been described. The CK is mostly normal but when elevated is usually less than 1000 IU. The EMG shows both myopathic and neurogenic patterns. The muscle biopsy shows variable amounts of endomysial inflammatory mononuclear exudate that frequently invades nonnecrotic muscle fibers. The main histologic differentiating feature is the presence of single or multiple vacuoles within the muscle fibers that contain small basophilic granules in their lumen or against their wall ("lined" or "rimmed vacuoles"). Eosinophilic masses can be seen in the sarcoplasm often near the rimmed vacuoles. There is an increased number of capillaries around individual muscle fibers. The inclusions are masses of filaments found in the nucleus or cytoplasm or both. The inclusions or some material associated with them are congophilic and immunoreact for beta amyloid protein and ubiquitin. There are often atrophied angular fibers, which suggest denervation. Familial cases inherited as autosomal dominant have been reported. These familial cases have the same clinical and histologic features as the sporadic cases. Currently there is no effective therapy for the disease. The response to steroids, high-dose intravenous immunoglobulin, azathioprine, and methotrexate have been variable and not very encouraging.

Dystrophic Myopathies

Muscular dystrophies are diseases of undetermined causes, are usually hereditary, and are characterized by weakness caused by progressive degeneration of muscles. The dystrophies are best classified according to the inheritance pattern, age at onset, progression of the disease, and muscles affected (Table 17-3).

Dystrophinopathies

Dystrophinopathies are a group of disorders produced by either absence or abnormalities of the dystrophin protein encoded in the X chromosome (Xp21). Dystrophin is a subsarcolemmal cytoskeletal protein of skeletal muscle. It has also been found in other cells such as neurons, glia, Schwann cells, and cardiac cells. Dystrophin is concentrated in transverse riblike rings, or costameres, on the cytoplasmic side of the sarcolemma and attaches the myofibrils to the sarcolemma. Dystrophin has a tight membrane association via the dystrophin-associated protein complex (DAP), and both provide mechanical support for the muscle membrane. Absence or deficiency of dys-

TABLE 17-3 Muscular Dystrophies

Type	Inherit	Onset
Congenital	A-R	Birth
Limb girdle	A-R	Teens
FSH	A-D	Variable
Emery-Dreifuss	X Linked AD	First decade
Oculopharyngeal	A-D	>Fourth decade

FSH, Facioscapulohumeral muscular dystrophy.

trophin produces weakness of the muscle membrane that ruptures under mechanical stress. Dystrophin is encoded by a large gene on the X chromosome (Xp21). Mutations in this gene produce different allelic disorders as described in Table 17-4.

Duchenne (pseudohypertrophic) muscular dystrophy. This lethal disorder is the most common dystrophy in children. It is inherited through an X-linked recessive gene that because of its large size has a high spontaneous (30%) mutation rate. This gene is located in band I of region 2 of the short arm of the X chromosome (Xp21). This gene encodes for dystrophin. Deletions or mutations in this gene are the cause of the absence of dystrophin in Duchenne patients. Most of the patients are boys, but the disease can be seen in girls who have Turner's (XO) or Turner mosaic syndromes. Also some female carriers can manifest some of the symptoms of the disease (manifesting carriers). In most patients with Duchenne's dystrophy there is a delay in reaching motor developmental milestones, and most of these patients never learn to walk normally. The onset of

Progression	Intellect and Others
Early improvement Later slow progression	Normal intellect
Normal life span	Normal intellect
Slow	Normal intellect
Slow	Cardiac involvement
Slow	Normal intellect

TABLE 17-4 Dystrophinopathies Xp21

Duchenne	Becker	Manifesting Carrier
2–5	5–12 yrs	Second decade
Fatal in 20s	Slow progression	Slow progression
Cardiac involvement	Cardiac involvement	No cardiac involvement
Intellectual deficit	Color blind	Normal intellect
Absent dystrophin	Decreased or abnormal dystrophin	Patchy dystrophin

symptoms is variable but usually begins around age 4, when it is noted that the child walks on his toes, becomes clumsy, falls frequently, and has difficulty rising from the floor. Characteristic findings include a waddling gait, toe walking with external foot rotation, and difficulty going up stairs, running, and rising from a sitting position. There is early neck muscle involvement. When the child is examined early in the disease there is abnormal posture when standing, with marked lumbar lordosis, a protuberant abdomen, and overextended knees. These children can have a husky appearance with herculean features and enlarged rubbery calves mainly as a result of infiltration and replacement of muscle fibers by fat and connective tissue (pseudohypertrophy). The thighs and tongue can be enlarged. Pain in the calf muscles can be triggered by exercise. When asked to get up from the floor or a chair, the patient uses his arms to push himself up (Gower's maneuver). The progression of the disease is variable but relentless. Most patients stop ambulating independently by 8 to 12 years of age. Shortening and contracture of the Achilles tendons occur early, but most of the contractures of other joints are accelerated by immobilization and are related to a sitting posture, especially after the child has been in a wheelchair. At this stage the muscles become severely atrophic, and the stretch reflexes are lost. Progressive kyphoscoliosis with severe deformity late in the disease causes a restrictive pulmonary deficit that along with cardiac fibrosis is often the cause of death at the end of the second or early in the third decade. Intellectual impairment of a nonprogressive type is also part of the disease. Levels of serum muscle enzymes including aldolase and CK are elevated. Early in the disease the CK value can be as high as 50 times normal. Enzyme elevations can precede clinical symptoms and decline as the disease progresses. EMG shows myopathic features. Muscle changes vary with the stage of the disease but consist of type I fiber predominance, variation in fiber size with degeneration and regeneration, rounding and splitting of the fibers, and central migration of nuclei. Fibrosis and fatty infiltration of muscle are frequent findings. Absence of dystrophin by immunostains are diagnostic of the disease. The correct diagnosis is made by the combined analysis of DNA, immunoblot, and immunostain methods. In new cases without family history of the disease, polymerase chain reaction (PCR) analysis identifies most deletional cases (65% of the dystrophinopathies) but cannot determine frameshift mutations and cannot differentiate between Duchenne and Becker dystrophies. Southern blotting analysis is more accurate than PCR for detection of partial gene duplications and for frame shift deletions or duplications. If these two tests fail, immunostain analysis on the muscle biopsy identifies most cases of

Duchenne and Becker dystrophy, detects manifesting carriers, and diagnoses other myopathies.

Treatment: Management of the patient includes intensive physical and occupational therapy and bracing to prolong ambulation and to delay the development of contractures and deformities.

Carrier detection: Carrier detection begins with pedigree analysis and manual muscle testing of a suspected carrier. An elevated CK can help detect a few cases in childhood, but the CK gradually decreases with age and pregnancy. Once the dystrophin mutation is discovered in an affected child (the proband), the carrier status is easier to determine in the patient's sisters, mother, and aunts by DNA testing done on their blood cells. If the proband shows no deletions, the use of genetic markers can be offered. Finally carrier status can be determined by obtaining a muscle biopsy from the suspected carrier for immunoblotting and immunostaining.

Prenatal diagnosis: Cells from amniocentesis or chorionic villus sampling can be obtained to look for DNA dystrophin mutations. Fetal muscle biopsy can be used when DNA dystrophin mutations have not been identified in the family.

Becker dystrophy. This is a less severe form of dystrophinopathy with clinical features similar to Duchenne dystrophy and the same inheritance pattern. The abnormal gene (Xp21) is the same as for Duchenne dystrophy (allelic disorders), but the dystrophin in partially present or defective rather than absent. However, the symptoms usually start later, the weakness is less severe, and the patient ambulates beyond the twelfth year of life. Marked hypertrophy of the calves is a prominent feature. Skeletal deformities are not as prominent. Cardiac symptoms can occur, but mental retardation does not occur.

Other dystrophinopathies can manifest as exercise intolerance, myoglobinuria, muscle cramps and myalgias, quadriceps myopathy, asymptomatic elevation of CK, and minimal limb girdle weakness. Also a cardiomyopathy with mild weakness and a fatal X-linked cardiomyopathy without weakness have been described.

Muscular Dystrophies

Congenital muscular dystrophy. Congenital muscular dystrophy (CMD) is an autosomal recessive disorder (affects both boys and girls) seen at birth or infancy. The affected patients are floppy at birth and frequently have contractures. Intellectual functions are normal. Improvement in muscle strength is seen in the first few years, and some patients become able to walk. The CK is elevated, and the muscle biopsy shows severe dystrophic changes similar to those seen in the Duchenne type. In CMD the biopsy shows more fibrosis, less necrosis, and normal dystrophin immunofluorescence. The distinction between this disorder and severe childhood autosomal-recessive muscular dystrophy (SCARMD) is controversial, but SCARMD is linked to chromosome 13q. Some congenital forms are associated with brain abnormalities (Fukuyama), and other forms are associated with other somatic abnormalities.

Limb-girdle dystrophy. Limb-girdle dystrophy is inherited through an autosomal recessive gene. Both males and females are affected. In some patients the disorder starts in childhood or adolescence, the progression is slow, and the patients are still able to ambulate into their 40s or 50s. In other patients the disease begins in the 40s but progresses faster. The weakness begins in the hip, quadriceps, and hamstring muscles. Waddling gait, back-kneeing, and Gowers' sign are striking features. Shoulder girdle weakness can start early but is usually less striking than hip involvement. Early biceps involvement is followed by involvement of other muscles. Deltoid muscle weakness is also prominent. Neck muscles are affected, but facial and ocular muscles are spared. Usually there is no cardiac involvement or mental changes. Joint contractures are rare and late. Except for lordosis, skeletal deformities are rare. The serum CK level is elevated, and the EMG shows myopathic low-amplitude polyphasic potentials. Muscle biopsy shows variation of muscle fiber size, evidence of degeneration and regeneration, splitting of fibers, and migration of nuclei and should allow exclusion of denervation and inflammatory changes. Dystrophin immunofluorescence is normal. Management should include physical therapy and bracing, encouraging ambulation.

Facioscapulohumeral muscular dystrophy (FSH). Facioscapulohumeral muscular dystrophy is inherited as an autosomal dominant disorder with variable penetrance. Linkage to chromosome 4 (D4S139 and D4S163) has been found. Subclinical cases in one parent of severely affected patients can be found. Onset of the disease is variable but rarely is in infancy. In most cases the weakness begins at the end of the first decade or in adolescence. Progression of the disease is very slow, beginning usually in facial or scapular muscles. Muscle involvement can be asymmetrical. Inability to whistle, drink through a straw, or blow are early symptoms of facial weakness. In severe cases (usually the infantile form) the face is smooth and without expression, the mouth is open, and the lips are usually prominent. Patients are unable to wrinkle their foreheads or close their eyes. They demonstrate Bell's phenomenon (upward movement of the eyeball seen through partially open lids), mimicking an infranuclear bilateral seventh nerve palsy. Mild facial weakness can be demonstrated by an inability to bury the eyelashes. Scapular weakness is usually early and severe with an inability to raise the arms above the head. There is drooping of the shoulders and poor scapular fixation. The scapulae wing easily and are displaced upward above the shoulders. The deltoid muscles are strikingly preserved, a characteristic differentiating this disorder from limb-girdle dystrophy. Preservation of the forearm muscles, which frequently become hypertrophic, causes a "Popeye" appearance. Hip weakness can also be an early sign of the disease and is usually associated with lumbar lordosis and prominent abdominal protrusion. Skeletal abnormalities, cardiac involvement, and mental changes are not features of the disease. The serum CK level is usually mildly elevated. Muscle biopsy can show early and minimal myopathic features in spite of severe disability. Marked inflammatory changes as in polymyositis or denervation can also be seen. Management includes genetic counseling, physical and occupational therapy, and bracing when needed.

Emery-Dreifuss muscular dystrophy. This is an X-linked (Xq28) or autosomal dominant inherited disorder. Early onset of elbow and ankle contractures, even before there is a significant weakness, is the most prominent clinical feature. The intellectual functions are not impaired, and there can be cardiac involvement. The weakness affects first the triceps and biceps in the upper limbs and the anterior tibial and peroneal muscles in the legs (humeroperoneal distribution) and then becomes more generalized. The CK is elevated, and the muscle biopsy shows nonspecific dystrophic changes with normal dystrophin immunofluorescence.

Oculopharyngeal muscular dystrophy. Oculopharyngeal dystrophy is a rare disease described in people of French-Canadian or Spanish-American origin but has been found in all races and geographic locations. It is transmitted through an autosomal dominant gene and is late in onset, usually in the fifth decade. The disease begins with ptosis followed by pharyngeal weakness in the 40s or 50s. Inability to swallow can be a prominent features. The facial, neck, and hip girdle muscles can be involved. The serum CK level is mildly elevated. The EMG shows myopathic features. Muscle biopsy reveals small angulated fibers and "rimmed vacuoles" within the muscle fibers. Management includes genetic counseling, physical therapy, surgical correction of the ptosis in severe cases, and gastrostomy in some cases. A rare form of pure ocular muscular dystrophy has been described. This form of the disease is slowly progressive and self-limited to extraocular muscles.

Myotonic Disorders

Myotonia. This is an involuntary painless delay in relaxation of skeletal muscle after contraction, associated with spontaneous bursts of high-frequency and high-amplitude electrical discharges on EMG. The patients usually describe the symptoms as stiffness that is worse at the onset of activity, improves with repeated muscle contraction, and worsens in cold weather. Myotonia can be elicited by voluntary contraction (contraction or active myotonia) or by muscle percussion (percussion myotonia). Percussion myotonia can be elicited by tapping the thenar eminence causing adduction and flexion of the thumb; tapping the tongue, producing a temporary dimple in the contracted muscle; or tapping the radial side of the forearm with the hand flexed in pronation, producing extension of the hand with a very slow relaxation time. Myotonia should be differentiated from the electrically silent myoedema of hypothyroidism. Paramyotonia congenita (Eulenberg's disease) is a rare familial type of myotonia in which patients exposed to cold suffer flaccid paralysis. Although myotonia is the predominant symptom in myotonic dystrophy, myotonia congenita, and paramyotonia, it can also be seen in metabolic myopathies and in patients who have had therapy with some cholesterol lowering agents.

Myotonic dystrophy. Myotonic dystrophy is the most frequent dystrophy in adults. It is an autosomal dominant inherited disorder. Genetic linkage analysis has shown the locus to be situated in the central region of chromosome 19. The disorder is characterized by myotonia, muscle weakness that is usually late and distal in distribution, endocrine abnormalities, and cardiac and central nervous system involvement. The age at onset is usually in the late teens or early adulthood. The disease progression, the severity of the symptoms, and the age of onset correlate with the size of a repeat CTG sequence in the DNA. Anticipation of the disease, in which affected members of the youngest generation have an earlier onset and more severe disability than those in the older generation, has been confirmed in the disease and is explained by the progressive expansion of the unstable DNA sequence. Myotonia is a predominant early symptom. This can be manifested by muscle stiffness, difficulty starting movements, or aching low back pain. The facial features are characterized by premature balding, marked temporal and masseter muscle atrophy and weakness ("hatchet face"), and inability to close thick and protuberant lips. There is usually mild ptosis and weakness of the orbicularis oculi muscles manifested by inability to bury the eyelashes on maximal effort. The neck muscles are atrophic and weak, mainly the flexor group (sternocleidomastoid), and there is accentuation of the normal cervical lordosis causing the appearance of a swan neck. Weakness in the extremities when present is predominantly late and distal with atrophy and weakness of hand muscles and foot drop. Later on there is quadriceps muscle weakness with recurvation of the knee and weakness at the hips. The voice becomes nasal, and the speech is dysarthric and rapid. Smooth muscle involvement is frequent in the gastrointestinal tract and can also involve the urinary tract, uterus, and iris. Dysphagia, abdominal pain, and constipation are frequent complaints. Dilatation of the esophagus and colon can occur. Gallbladder disease with cholelithiasis seems to be more frequent in myotonic patients than in the general population. Mental changes are frequent and consist of low intelligence with a hostile and demanding personality. Hypersomnia is a frequent feature. Cardiac abnormalities caused by lesions in the conduction system are frequently detected in electrocardiograms and consist of left bundle branch block and atrial flutter, which explains "sudden cardiac death" in some of the patients. Testicular or ovarian atrophy and abnormalities of carbohydrate metabolism (diabetes mellitus) are not unusual. Low serum testosterone levels have been found in myotonic males. Eye abnormalities consist of cataract, retinal degeneration, and low intraocular pressure. There is no elevation of muscle enzymes.

An EMG detects the myotonic discharge. Muscle biopsy is usually not necessary for the diagnosis but shows characteristic dystrophic changes, type I fiber hypotrophy with a striking increase in the number of central nuclei, and frequent ring fibers. Management consists of genetic counseling and symptomatic treatment. No treatment modifies disease progression. Phenytoin and acetazolamide reduce myotonic symptoms in some patients. Although quinine and procainamide improve myotonia, they can affect ventricular conduction and myocardial function in patients who may already have conduction defects. Tonocard (tocainide) does improve myotonia. Most patients are not as concerned about the myotonia as they are about the weakness. Cardiac pacemakers are useful in some patients. Cataract extraction should be done under local anesthesia because of the risk of complications of general anesthesia. Testosterone replacement has been used in male patients.

Congenital myotonic dystrophy. Congenital myotonic dystrophy is present at birth and is seen in children of either sex born of a mother who has overt or subclinical evidence of myotonic dystrophy. Quantification of the unstable CTG triplet repeat shows around 2000 copies. (Normal is as many as 30 repeats.) Characteristically the child is severely hypotonic at birth and has facial diplegia associated with an open, triangular, tent-shaped mouth with a high-arched palate. The children have difficulty sucking and swallowing. They also have talipes and other joint contractures. No evidence of myotonia is seen at birth, but the floppiness improves with age only to be transformed into myotonia. Developmental motor milestones are delayed, and mental retardation of varying degree is frequent.

Nondystrophic myotonias

Myotonia congenita. Myotonia congenita is a rare non-progressive disease manifested by myotonia and inherited as an autosomal dominant disorder (Thomsen's disease) or autosomal recessive (Becker myotonia). Both types share common clinical features, and both are linked to the same gene that encodes a chloride channel on chromosome 7. The disease can be seen at birth or in the first two decades. The patients have muscle hypertrophy. There is no mental, cardiac, or endocrinologic abnormality. There is no baldness. The myotonia is more pronounced at rest and improves with exercise. The EMG shows myotonic discharge but no myopathic features, and the muscle tissue is normal. Most patients respond to Tonocard (tocainamide).

Paramyotonia congenita and the periodic paralyses. This rare group of disorders is usually hereditary and due to sodium channel deficiencies (channelopathies). They all have in common the periodicity of the attacks of weakness that can last from minutes to several days. The weakness can be generalized or focal and is associated with hyporeflexia or areflexia. Paramyotonia congenita is characterized by paradoxical myotonia. The myotonia, which affects predominantly the face and upper limbs, appears with exercise, increases with continuous exercise, and is aggravated by cold exposure. Attacks of weakness can occur spontaneously or be precipitated by cold. The periodic paralyses are usually autosomal dominant inherited disorders, but sporadic cases can occur. The paralysis is due to inexcitability of the sarcolemma produced by sodium channel deficiencies. During the weakness there is a shift of potassium, chloride, sodium, and water into the muscle cells.

Periodic paralyses are classified according to the serum potassium levels during the attacks and can be hypokalemic, hyperkalemic, or normokalemic. Prevention of the attacks can be achieved by avoiding precipitating factors and the use of diuretics.

Congenital Myopathies

Congenital myopathies are heterogeneous hereditary disorders transmitted in different inheritance patterns. Although they are called congenital and frequently appear early in life as floppiness or delayed motor development, muscle weakness can appear later or even in adulthood. Improvement of the weakness can occur in the cases seen in infancy. The earlier the age of onset, the worse the motor deficit will be. The muscle mass is constantly small, and there can be associated dysmorphic features such as elongated face, scoliosis, pigeon chest, and hip and foot deformities. When the disease manifests in adulthood the muscle weakness is slowly progressive, usually self-limited, and very rarely leads to a wheelchair-bound or bedridden state. The serum muscle enzymes and the EMG are usually normal.

Central Core Disease and Malignant Hyperthermia

Central core disease (CCD) and malignant hyperthermia are autosomal dominant allelic disorders caused by missence mutations in the ryanodine receptor gene (sarcoplasmic reticulum calcium release channel) mapped to chromosome 19 (19q13.1). Patients with CCD have a high risk of malignant hyperthermia (MH) during general anesthesia. However, not all patients who have MH have CCD. Malignant hyperthermia is produced by potent volatile anesthetic agents or succinylcholine used during surgery. These agents produce increased oxygen and lactate production resulting in exaggerated heat production, muscle rigidity, and cellular permeability. The syndrome is most likely produced by the inability of the muscle cells to control calcium concentration as a result of a mutation in the ryanodine receptor gene. CCD is manifested by early childhood hypotonia and proximal muscle weakness. The CK is usually normal, and the EMG is not specific. The muscle biopsy shows characteristic cores in the muscle fibers devoid of mitochondrial enzymatic activity. There is no treatment for CCD. Malignant hyperthermia can be prevented by avoiding the use of precipitating agents. The treatment of the acute episodes consist of (1) immediate discontinuation of the precipitating agent; (2) use of dantrolene 2 mg/kg intravenously each 5 minutes to reach a total of 10 mg/kg; (3) a rapid intravenous infusion of 2 to 4 mEq/kg of sodium bicarbonate; and (4) aggressive cooling if the temperature is above 40.6° C. Subsequent treatment is based on arterial blood gases and acid-base values.

Nemaline Myopathy

Nemaline myopathy is a genetically heterogeneous disorder that is transmitted by autosomal dominant or recessive inheritance. The symptoms can appear in the neonatal period with severe hypotonia, facial diplegia, and joint contractures. This type of myopathy carries a poor prognosis. When the symptoms appear in childhood, the weakness is slow or nonprogressive and is associated with skeletal deformities and dysmorphic facial features. The adult onset type has variable weakness, and the patients have Marfan-like phenotypic features. The CK is normal, and the EMG is nonspecific. Only one report of the adult onset autosomal dominant type has shown linkage to chromosome 1 (1q21–q23), the same site as that of Charcot-Marie-Tooth 1B. The diagnostic histologic features in the muscle biopsy consist of subsarcolemmal nemaline rods in small muscle fibers. No treatment currently is available.

Centronuclear (Myotubular) Myopathy

Centronuclear (myotubular) myopathy can appear in either of two forms, a neonatal or a late onset form. The neonatal X-linked form is characterized by severe weakness, dysmorphic facial features, and skeletal abnormalities. Ptosis and limitation of ocular movements are frequent. The late onset form appears before the third decade. The ptosis and the limb weakness are less marked than in the neonatal form. No linkage has been described yet. The characteristic histologic features consist of the presence of round muscle fibers, type I fiber predominance, and central nuclei in 30% to 95% of the fibers. In the neonatal X-linked form, numerous small fibers with central nuclei resemble myotubes.

Metabolic Myopathies

Metabolic myopathies are rare familial muscle diseases in which an enzymatic defect, an endocrine dysfunction, or a metabolic abnormality is associated with transitory or permanent muscle weakness as part of a multisystem disease or a primary muscle disorder.

Diseases of Carbohydrate Metabolism

At least seven different enzymatic defects of glycogen metabolism have been described. Only a few affect muscles, and of those only two are discussed here.

Acid maltase deficiency. Pompe's disease (glyco-genosis type II) is a rare disease that is due to acid maltase (1,4-glucosidase) deficiency and is inherited as an autosomal recessive disorder. Acid maltase is a lysosomal alfa-glucosidase that releases glucose from maltose, glycogen, and oligosaccharides. The gene that codes for acid maltase has been mapped to region 2 of the long arm of chromosome 17 (17q 21–23 or 17q 23–25). In the infantile or classic form, the disease appears as severe hypotonia with car-diorespiratory problems. There is associated vis-ceromegaly including enlarged heart, liver, and spleen. The muscle weakness is due to accumulation of intracytoplasmic glycogen. It is usually fatal in infancy. The childhood type starts somewhat later, does not usually involve the heart, causes proximal muscle weakness that is difficult to differentiate from limb-girdle or Duchenne's dystrophy, and is fre-quently associated with mental changes. The adult form appears after the age of 20 with very slowly progressive proximal muscle weakness. In 30% of adult cases respiratory failure is the first manifesta-tion of the disease. The enzymatic defect in all types is the same. The muscle is characterized by vacuolar degeneration, in which accumulated glycogen can be detected. Biochemical analysis of the muscle shows the enzyme defect. Enzyme replacement has not modified the course of the disease.

McArdle's disease. McArdle's disease (glycogenosis type V), a nonlysosomal glycogenosis, is a rare dis-ease produced by deficiency of myophosphorylase. This enzyme initiates glycogen breakdown. Myo-phosphorylase along with the debrancher enzyme degrades glycogen completely into glucose-1-phos-phate and glucose. Deficiency of myophosphorylase produces accumulation of subsarcolemmal glycogen. The disease has an autosomal recessive inheritance. Six mutations that cause the disease have been identified in the gene that encodes the enzyme localized on chromosome 11. The disease is more frequently seen in males, varies in intensity, and is manifested early by fatigability followed by muscle cramps precipitated by exercise. The amount of exercise needed to produce cramps seems to shorten with the progression of the disease. Exercise can trigger myoglobinuria. The diagnosis should be confirmed by a muscle biopsy demonstrating the subsarcolemmal vacuoles, glycogen accumulation, and lack of myophosphorylase. Treatment consists of decreasing activity, warming the muscles before activity, or the second wind effect. Oral loading with glucose or fructose has inconsistent effects.

Diseases of Lipid Metabolism

Diseases of lipid metabolism are rare disorders that cause accumulation of excessive lipid that can often be seen on muscle biopsy sections. They can be caused by defective transport of fatty acids substrates into mitochondria, defects in the beta oxidation of fatty acids, defects in the respiratory chain, and defects in the use of endogenous triglycerides. The histologic diagnosis is not always certain because some defects of lipid metabolism do not result in lipid storage myopathy. Ischemia and obesity increase the muscle fiber lipid content, and diseases of lipid metabolism affect the heart, liver, and other organs.

Carnitine deficiency. Lipids are an important source of skeletal muscle energy during fasting or prolonged exercise. Diet provides 75% of body carnitine requirements; the rest is endogenously synthesized.

Carnitine deficiency is believed to be produced by defective transport in tissues. It has two forms, one with progressive cardiomyopathy and the other with episodes of hypoketotic hypoglycemia. In both cases there is consistent muscle weakness and an excess of lipid in skeletal muscle. Myoglobinuria can occur. There are normal or slightly decreased serum concentrations of carnitine. A muscle biopsy shows vacuolar myopathy with accumulation of lipids. Biochemical analysis of muscle demonstrates low skeletal muscle carnitine. The patients have a dramatic response to 2 to 6 g of oral L-carnitine daily supplementation, with improvement of cardiac and skeletal muscle function.

Carnitine palmitoyltransferase deficiency. Carnitine palmitoyltransferase deficiency is a rare disease with an autosomal recessive X-linked inheritance. Myoglobinuria not preceded by muscle cramps is the hallmark of the late onset form of the disease, which becomes symptomatic in the second or third decade. The myoglobinuria is precipitated by fasting or exercise. Biochemical studies of muscle demonstrate decreased carnitine palmitoyltransferase. Therapy consists of a high-carbohydrate, low-fat diet and regulation of exercise to reduce the number of attacks. In the infantile form hepatic failure and nonketotic hypoglycemic coma occur. The response to treatment of this form is not as good as in the adult form.

Mitochondrial Myopathies

Mitochondrial myopathies are a clinically, biochemically, and genetically heterogeneous group of disorders that affect multiple systems, including the skeletal muscles, and are characterized by nonspecific structural abnormalities of affected tissue mitochondria. The diagnosis needs to be confirmed by biopsy, biochemical analysis of skeletal muscle, and determination of mitochondrial DNA (mtDNA) delections or mutations. In most mitochondrial myopathies the muscle histologic abnormalities consist of the presence of ragged-red fibers, which are seen with the modified Gomori's trichrome stain. Transmission electron microscopy of muscle can show mitochondria abnormalities, including the presence of crystalline or paracrystalline mitochondrial inclusions ("parking lot" appearance), or excessive accumulation of glycogen or lipid droplets. A variety of defects of mitochondrial metabolism have been identified, but none is associated with a specific or consistent clinical syndrome. More than 15 different syndromes with more than 35 biochemical abnormalities have been described as being associated with mitochondrial abnormalities. Three distinctive clinical encephalomyopathies will be described here. The first, *Kearns-Sayre syndrome,* is characterized by onset before age 15, progressive external ophthalmoplegia, pigmentary degeneration of the retina, heart block, cerebellar dysfunction, and variable limb weakness. Elevated cerebrospinal protein and peripheral neuropathies have also been described. Spongy degeneration of the brain has been found in autopsied cases. However, chronic progressive external ophthalmoplegia and proximal muscle weakness can be the early or only manifestations of late-onset mitochondrial myopathies. The muscle biopsy confirms the diagnosis by showing the ragged red fibers. *Myoclonus epilepsy with ragged-red fibers* is a familial disorder characterized by myoclonus, ataxia, weakness, generalized seizures, and in most cases onset before age 20. A syndrome that includes *mitochondrial myopathy, encephalopathy, lactic acidosis, and strokelike episodes* appears early in life with episodic vomiting, seizures, and recurrent strokes.

Other mitochondrial disorders include Leber's hereditary optic neuropathy, Alpert's syndrome, and Leigh's syndrome. For further information, the reader is referred to the neuropediatric or neuromuscular literature.

Corticosteroid Myopathy

Corticosteroid myopathy is one complication of prolonged high-dose corticosteroid therapy, usually appearing after months or years of therapy. Although fluorinated corticosteroids are more frequently implicated, any corticosteroid can produce the same effect. Corticosteroids produce muscle protein catabolism. This catabolism is enhanced by disuse or during sepsis producing the muscle disorder. The myopathy appears as proximal shoulder and hip girdle muscle weakness. The CK level is usually normal or slightly elevated. Muscle biopsy reveals nonspecific type II fiber atrophy. Cushing syndrome can cause the same symptoms as corticosteroid myopathy. Acute quadriplegic myopathy has recently been described in patients who had received large doses of intramuscular or intravenous doses of glucocorticoid. Most of these patients had also received neruomuscular blockade agents and mechanical ventilation. The treatment consists of discontinuing the steroids. Recovery following discontinuation is slow.

◼ DISEASES OF THE NEUROMUSCULAR JUNCTION

Myasthenic Disorders

Acquired autoimmune myasthenia gravis is a disorder of neuromuscular transmission that is due to acetylcholine receptor (AChR) deficiency at the myoneural junction. The disease is manifested by abnormal and objective (pathologic) fatigability and weakness after repeated or sustained muscle activity with recovery of strength after rest or anticholinesterase medication. The disease is more frequent in young females but can occur at any age and in either sex. Male patients predominate when the disease appears later in life. The onset is usually insidious but can appear acutely after allergic episodes or febrile illnesses. The disease invariably involves the most frequently used muscles such as the eyelids and extraocular and bulbar muscles. Ptosis or diplopia as a result of involvement of one or more extraocular muscles is seen in 90% of myasthenics. Eye muscle involvement is frequently asymmetrical and can resemble internuclear ophthalmoplegia. Although the disease is initially purely ocular, it remains confined to ocular muscles in less than 15% of the patients after 1 year of the onset of the symptoms. The bulbar muscles affected include those of mastication, deglutition, and phonation. Speech becomes nasal, and the jaw can hang on so loosely that the patient must hold it up by using the hands. Facial expression and facial mobility are lost, and the smile can become a snarl. In advanced cases weakness can become generalized and involve the intercostal and diaphragmatic muscles, impairing respiratory function. In spite of severe weakness, atrophy of muscle is unusual and is seen only late in the course of the disease, and stretch reflexes are preserved. Muscle pain is not frequent. When present it usually involves the extraocular or neck muscles and is probably secondary to muscle fatigue. The progression of the disease is variable. There are rare spontaneous remissions. There is some association of myasthenia gravis with other autoimmune diseases including hyperthyroidism, lupus erythematosus, rheumatoid arthritis, and polymyositis. Rare familial cases have been reported. The diagnosis is made by history and clinical findings and by demonstrating fatigability if clinical signs are not obvious. When the patient looks upward forcibly and for a prolonged period of time, there is a progressive eyelid droop. Counting rapidly and loudly brings a progressively nasal quality to the speech. Walking or running can demonstrate extremity weakness. This weakness should improve after rest. When objective signs are present or are precipitated by the examiner, edrophonium chloride (Tensilon) improves weakness. The Tensilon test is an important diagnostic test, but there are false-positive (see Clinical Myasthenic Syndromes, p. 533) and false-negative responses. The test is performed by intravenous injection of edrophonium chloride, 2 to 10 mg (0.2–1.0ml). After 2 mg (0.2 ml) infusion the patient is observed for a response or cholinergic sign (tearing or fasciculations of eyelids); then the rest of the injection can be given very slowly. The response, in affected patients, appears in 10 to 30 seconds, and a positive effect (improved muscle strength) lasts no more than 5 minutes. Atropine should be available to counteract unfavorable cholinergic side effects. Edrophonium chloride is a fast acting anticholinesterase that reduces the hydrolysis of acetylcholine, making acetylcholine available in larger quantities and for a longer period of time at the neuromuscular junction.

The next step in the diagnosis consists of the repetitive nerve stimulation test. Repeated supramaximal nerve stimulation at a rate of 3 Hz while recording the M waves from muscles innervated by the nerve produces a more than 10% decremental response in myasthenic patients. Single fiber EMG shows an abnormal response (jitter) in myasthenic patients. Both studies are nonspecific but indicate abnormal neuromuscular transmission. Antibodies to the acetylcholine receptor have been found in the serum of 87% to 93% of myasthenic patients and are highly specific. The titer of antibodies does not correlate with the disease severity. Moreover, antibodies can be absent in 25% of patients with ocular myasthenia. Antibodies to striated muscle have also been found in myasthenia gravis but are less specific and less sensitive. They are found in 84% of myasthenics with thymoma. The thymus is frequently abnormal and shows germinal hyperplasia (thymitis) in 75% of the patients. A thymoma is present in 10% to 15% of myasthenic patients. Tissue typing has shown that young female myasthenics (under age 40) have a high prevalence of HLA A1, B8 or DRw3, or both, and these patients have higher acetylcholine receptor antibody titers, have a higher incidence of associated autoimmune disorders, have no thymoma, and respond faster and better to thymectomy. Older (over age 40) myasthenic patients without thymoma are frequently males; have a higher prevalence of HLA A3, B7 or DRw2, or both; and have low titers of acetylcholine receptor antibodies. In patients with MG and thymoma there is no sex or HLA association, AChR antibody titers are high, and 84% have striated muscle antibodies.

Pathogenesis. There is good evidence that the antibodies to the AChR are important in causing myasthenia gravis. These polyclonal antibodies recognize one immunogenic region of AChR. There is also electron microscopic evidence of damage of postsynaptic folds with deposition of IgG, C3, and C9. Antiidiotypic antibodies have been found in 20% to 50% of myasthenics, and these antibodies seem to regulate the immune response to acetylcholine receptor antibodies and affect the clinical expression of myasthenia gravis. There is a high prevalence of thymic abnormalities in myasthenic patients, and there is often a favorable response after thymectomy. The normal thymus gland contains myoid cells. Some incompletely characterized thymus cells express AChR molecules. The hyperplastic thymus of myasthenic patients contains an increased number of B cells, and thymocytes of MG patients secrete anti-AChR antibodies. What triggers and regulates the production of the antibodies, how many different antibodies to acetylcholine receptors there are, why some myasthenic patients have no antibodies to acetylcholine receptors, and why there is no correlation between clinical symptoms and titers of antibodies are questions that remain to be answered.

Treatment is directed toward improving the symptoms and immunosuppressing the patient. The symptomatic treatment consists of the use of anticholinesterase drugs, mainly pyridostigmine (Mestinon). The dosage varies according to individual patient response and severity of weakness. The use of pyridostigmine should be as required by the patient's symptoms. In bulbar involvement, 60 mg should be given 30 to 45 minutes before each meal to avoid aspiration. It should also be used to improve diplopia and limb weakness. Most patients learn when they need the Mestinon and when to take it. When the dosage reaches more than eight tablets a day (an arbitrary number) the patient should be put on immunosuppressive medication. Unreliable absorption makes use of timespan tablets undesirable. Plasmapheresis reduces antibodies and produces a dramatic but temporary improvement of symptoms. It is indicated in myasthenic crisis and should be used along with other therapeutic measures. It can also be used intermittently as an adjuvant in patients who are not responding well to immunosuppression. Intravenous gamma globulin has also been used with mixed results and should be used along with immunosuppressive treatment. Immunosuppressive measures include transsternal thymectomy with complete removal of the thymus. This is particularly important when there is a thymoma. Complete remission is more likely if thymectomy is done early in the disease. Improvement can continue for a number of years (at least 5) after thymectomy. The best response is achieved in young females without a thymoma. High doses of prednisone (60 to 80 mg on alternate days) can be used, but treatment should be initiated with smaller (20 mg) doses that are gradually increased by 10 mg every third dose to avoid exacerbation of weakness. After optimal results have been obtained, the dosage should be continued for at least 6 months and then gradually reduced over a period of 12 to 16 months. Response to corticosteroids is quite dramatic in most patients. Whether prednisone should be started before or after thymectomy depends on the severity of the disease. Undesirable secondary effects of high-dose corticosteroids can appear in some patients and should be carefully monitored and managed. Azathioprine (Imuran) in a dosage of 2.5 mg/kg/day can help bring about a remission and reduce antibodies. Results are better in males who do not have HLA-B8 and who have high titers of antibodies. Careful observation is necessary. Imuran is usually added to the therapy of patients who are not responding well to prednisone. When thymectomy should be done, if and when corticosteroids should be used (before or after thymectomy), and when azathioprine or plasmapheresis are indicated are debatable issues. Therapy should be individualized. It is important to remember that myasthenic patients can suffer worsening of symptoms during pregnancy, menstruation, and hyperthyroid states. Drugs that are contraindicated in myasthenics include antibiotics of the amino glycoside group that inhibit release of acetylcholine such as gentamicin, kanamycin, neomycin, polymyxin, and streptomycin and antiarrhythmic drugs such as quinine (including tonic water), quinidine, procainamide, lidocaine, beta-adrenergic blockers, and phenytoin (Dilantin) (Box 17-2).

Transient neonatal myasthenia is a transient (1 to 6 weeks) form of myasthenia seen in approximately

---

BOX 17-2   **Drugs Reportedly Inducing or Exacerbating Myasthenic Weakness**

Antibiotics Contraindicated in MG

Inhibition of presynaptic release of Ach

Gentamicin	Streptomycin
Neomycin	Kanamycin
Tobramycin	Erythromycin

Depression of postjunctional sensitivity

Bacitracin	Netilmicin
Clindamycin	Polymyxin B
Colistin	Tetracycline (rare)
Lincomycin	Ampicillin* (rare)
Neomycin	*Ca++ reverses weakness

Other Medications

D-penicillamine	Phenytoin
Verapamil	Beta-blockers
Quinine	Chloroquinequinidine
Procainamide	Chlorpromazine
Lithium	K-wasting diuretics
Curare	Gallamine
Pancuronium	Ether

15% of newborns born to mothers with myasthenia gravis and is due to transplacental passage of antibodies to acetylcholine receptors. Symptoms improve with spontaneous or therapeutic reduction of antibodies (plasmapheresis).

Clinical Myasthenic Syndromes

Congenital Myasthenic Syndromes

Congenital myasthenia is a familial heterogeneous disorder of nonimmune causes that is possibly inherited as an autosomal recessive gene. It is seen predominantly in male children. The disease appears in the newborn period in infants of nonmyasthenic mothers. Although the symptoms are similar to those of myasthenia gravis, they do not respond well to anticholinesterase therapy or thymectomy, and there is no increase of antibodies to acetylcholine receptors. The symptoms do not seem to progress. Although the pathogenesis in this disorder is not clear, both presynaptic and postsynaptic defects have been described, including a defect in acetylcholine synthesis or packaging, congenital end-plate acetylcholinesterase deficiency, slow channel syndrome, and congenital end-plate acetylcholine receptor deficiency.

Drug-Induced Myasthenia

Drug-induced myasthenia appears in patients with rheumatoid arthritis who have been treated with penicillamine for several months. It does not usually occur in patients receiving penicillamine for Wilson's disease. The symptoms and antibodies to acetylcholine receptors are the same as in myasthenia gravis, and symptoms improve when AChR antibody titers decrease after discontinuation of the drug.

Eaton-Lambert Syndrome

This is an acquired autoimmune myasthenic syndrome produced by autoantibodies that deplete the voltage sensitive calcium channels (VSCCs) of the motor nerve terminal (presynaptic). It is frequently but not always associated with the presence of a malignant tumor, usually a small (oat) cell carcinoma, and rarely with other tumors. The syndrome is more frequent in males and is characterized by fatigability and weakness, predominantly of the limb-girdle musculature and less prominently of the ocular and bulbar muscles, and is associated with areflexia. Strength improves and reflexes reappear after maximal voluntary contraction. There is no increase of acetylcholine receptor antibodies. The diagnosis is confirmed by electromyography. Stimulation of a nerve at or above 10 cps evokes incremental responses of the muscle. The response to the anticholinesterase edrophonium (Tensilon) is positive but not as dramatic as in myasthenia gravis. The discovery of the malignancy can be delayed by several years after the diagnosis of the syndrome. Therapy consists of eradication of the tumor when present and administration of guanidine (15 mg/kg/day) to increase the release of acetylcholine from nerve terminals. Symptoms also respond to plasmapheresis and immunosuppressive therapy.

Botulism

Botulism is a disease of neuromuscular transmission produced by the exotoxin of *Clostridium botulinum,* an anaerobic microorganism that can contaminate improperly prepared canned or bottled foods. The toxin interferes with the release of acetylcholine and produces acute and progressive weakness within 72 hours. There is ocular, bulbar, and generalized muscle weakness with loss of stretch reflexes and no sensory abnormalities. Botulism, unlike myasthenia gravis or Guillain-Barré syndrome, causes dilated unreactive pupils. Treatment consists of cardiorespiratory support and administration of antiserum, 10,000 U intravenously, followed by intramuscular doses of 50,000 U daily, until strength improves. Guanidine has been beneficial in some cases.

Tick Paralysis

Tick paralysis is an ascending paralysis probably produced by a neurotoxin liberated by the female tick (*Dermacentor andersoni* or *D. variabilis*). Although the mode and site of action of the toxin are not known, there are reductions in motor nerve conduction velocities and myoneural junction abnormalities. The disease causes ascending paralysis with bulbar involvement, areflexia, and facial weakness but no pupillary abnormalities. The symptoms improve soon after the engorged tick is removed.

◼ SUMMARY

Disorders of muscle (myopathies) are characterized by proximal muscle weakness and wasting. The neck and bulbar muscles can also be weak. Muscle enzymes including CK and aldolase are elevated as a result of muscle destruction. Electromyography confirms abnormal function of the muscle fiber, and the specific pathologic feature of the myopathy can be determined by muscle biopsy. Disorders of the neuromuscular junction are manifested by abnormal fatigue and weakness after sustained muscle activity with recovery of strength after a period of rest. Myasthenia gravis is the most characteristic disorder of neuromuscular junction transmission. The eye muscle can be initially involved. This can result in ptosis and diplopia. The diagnosis of myasthenia gravis can be established by improvement in strength following intravenous injection of edrophonium (Tensilon) and demonstration of serum antibodies to the acetylcholine receptor.

Suggested Readings

Muscle Disease—General

Brooke MH: A clinician's view of neuromuscular diseases, ed 2, Baltimore, 1986, Williams & Wilkins.

Di Mauro S, et al: Mitochondrial myopathies, *Ann* Neurol 17:521, 1985.

Dubowitz V: Muscle disorders of childhood, Philadelphia, 1978, WB Saunders.

Engel AG, Francini-Armstrong C: Myology: basic and clinical, ed 2, New York, 1994, McGraw-Hill.

Harper PS: Myotonic dystrophy, ed 2, Philadelphia, 1989, WB Saunders.

Muscle Disease

Bunch TW: Polymyositis, *Mayo Clin Proc* 65:1480, 1990.

Dalakas MC: Polymyositis, dermatomyositis, inclusion body myositis. *N Engl J Med* 325:1487, 1991.

Mastaglia FL, Ojeda VJ: Inflammatory myopathies, *Ann Neurol* 17:215, 317, 1985.

Neville HE, et al: Familial inclusion body myositis: evidence for autosomal dominant inheritance, *Neurology* 42:897, 1992.

Myasthenia Gravis

Drachman DB: Myasthenia Gravis, *N Engl J Med* 330:1797, 1994.

Engel AG: Myasthenia gravis and myasthenic syndromes, *Ann Neurol* 16:519, 1984.

CHAPTER

Infectious Diseases
of the Nervous System

18

ACUTE BACTERIAL MENINGITIS

Purulent meningitis represents an inflammatory reaction of the pia and arachnoid (leptomeninges), which surround the spinal cord and brain. The pathologic response includes congestion of superficial cerebral and pial vessels, thickening of the meninges, reduced cerebral blood flow, cerebral edema of vasogenic and cytotoxic types, elevated intracranial pressure, exudate in basal cisterns and cortical subarachnoid spaces, exudate in ventricles (ependymitis, ventriculitis), vascular thrombosis (of arteries, veins, and dural sinuses), and hydrocephalus. Following treatment of meningitis the neurologic outcome correlates with the physician's ability to control intracranial pressure and prevent herniation and to prevent reduced cerebral blood flow that can lead to cerebral ischemia.

The most frequent etiologic agents are listed by age in Table 18-1. In neonates, Group B streptococcus, *Escherichia coli, Klebsiella pneumoniae,* and *Listeria monocytogenes* cause the most cases of bacterial meningitis. In young children, *Haemophilus influenzae*

> **TABLE 18-1 Etiology of Acute Bacterial Meningitis by Age**
>
> | Neonatal Organisms | Percentage | Infants and Children Organisms | Percentage |
> |---|---|---|---|
> | *H. influenza* | 5 | *H. influenzae* | 70 |
> | | | *S. pneumoniae* | 15 |
> | Group B streptococci | 48 | *N. meningitides* | 10 |
> | *S. pneumoniae* | 2 | | |
> | *N. meningitides* | 1 | Group B streptococci | 2 |
> | Others | 44 | Others | 3 |
> | *L. monocytogenes, E. coli,* other Enterobacteriaceae | | | |

is the most common microorganism with *Streptococcus pneumoniae* and *Neisseria meningitides* next in frequency. As *Haemophilus* vaccines become more readily available this microorganism will become a less common meningitis cause. In immunocompromised patients (diabetics, alcoholics, pregnant women, sepsis, acquired immune deficiency syndrome [AIDS], medication use including corticosteroid and chemotherapeutic agents), *L. monocytogenes* must be considered a potential etiologic agent. Parameningeal infections (ear, sinus, face, eye, head trauma with cerebrospinal fluid [CSF] leak) can cause bacterial infection as a result of *Pseudomonas aeruginosa, Staphylococcus aureus,* or multiple diverse pathogens.

Adults		Elderly Adults	
Organisms	Percentage	Organisms	Percentage
S. pneumoniae	20–40	H. influenzae	3
		S. pneumoniae	50
S. aureus	5–15	N. meningitides	2
N. meningitides	10–40	Group B streptococci	3
Group B streptococci	3	Others including L. monocytogenes E. coli	42
Streptococci	5–10		
Gram-negative bacilli	1–10		
H. influenzae	5–10		
Others	3		

In children over 5 years old and adults (including elderly patients) *S. pneumoniae* and *N. meningitides* are the most common; however, *H. influenzae, L. monocytogenes, S. aureus,* and *P. aeruginosa* must be considered.

Clinical features of bacterial meningitis usually develop rapidly (within 6 to 24 hours); however, in certain cases they develop more insidiously over several days. Signs and symptoms include headache, fever, nausea, vomiting, photophobia, and stiff neck caused by meningeal irritation. In children younger than 1 year with meningitis, central nervous system (CNS) signs can be absent, and the only findings may be fever, failure to thrive, irritability, or lethargy. In elderly patients diagnostic clues can be limited—febrile response and headache can be minimal or absent, and meningeal signs may not be convincingly demonstrated. An altered mental state can be the only diagnostic clue to meningitis, and this is nonspecific as it can occur in other conditions in elderly patients. In both neonates and elderly patients the index of suspicion for meningitis must be high, and lumbar puncture (LP) should be performed early. In other meningitis patients, clinical findings include nuchal rigidity (demonstrated by placing the examiner's hand beneath the occiput (back of the head) and passively flexing the head to elicit neck extensor muscle spasm), Brudzinski sign (passive flexion of the patient's head causes flexion of thighs and legs), and Kernig sign (with hip and knee flexed, legs cannot be straightened without hamstring spasm and pain). Cranial nerve palsies can result from basal meningeal exudate infiltrating the cranial nerves. Disturbances of consciousness result from the effects of bacterial toxins, cerebral edema, hydrocephalus, vasculitis, and cerebral ischemia. Seizures, focal neurologic deficit, or papilledema do not usually occur in bacterial meningitis unless there are complicating neuropathologic conditions. These include cerebral infarction resulting from inflammatory arteritis or cortical vein thrombosis, focal suppurative cerebritis or brain abscess, subdural or epidural empyema, and hydrocephalus.

LP with CSF examination (Table 18-2) is necessary to establish the diagnosis of meningitis and to identify the etiologic agent(s). Untreated bacterial meningitis is usually a fatal disorder; delay in initiating therapy can result in irreversible neurologic sequelae. If focal neurologic signs are present, LP should be avoided until computed tomography (CT)

TABLE 18-2 Differential Diagnosis of Abnormal CSF Using Cell Count, Cell Type, and Sugar Concentration

Group	Predominant Cell Type
1 Thousands of cells, decreased sugar*	
Bacterial meningitis	PMN
Ruptured brain abscess	PMN
Partially treated bacterial meningitis	PMN or mononuclear
Naeglerial (amebic) meningitis	PMN
2 Thousands of cells, normal sugar†	
Early or partially treated bacterial meningitis	PMN
"Chemical" meningitis	PMN
3 Hundreds of cells, decreased sugar	
Bacterial meningitis	PMN
Granulomatous meningitis‡	Mononuclear
Meningovascular syphilis	Mononuclear
Sarcoidosis	Mononuclear
Neoplastic meningitis	Mononuclear and/or tumor cells
Spontaneous subarachnoid hemorrhage	Mononuclear or PMN
Rare association with viral meningitis (mumps, and lymphocytic choriomeningitis)	Mononuclear
Rare association with *Herpes hominis* type 1 encephalitis	Mononuclear
4 Hundreds of cells, normal sugar	
Early bacterial meningitis	PMN
Partially treated bacterial meningitis	PMN
Early granulomatous meningitis	Mononuclear
Parameningeal infections	Mononuclear or PMN
Meningovascular syphilis	Mononuclear
Aseptic "viral" meningitis-encephalitis	Mononuclear
Lead poisoning (children)	Mononuclear
Bacterial endocarditis	Mononuclear or PMN

PMN, Polymorphonuclear.

*A CSF cell count > 10/mm^3 or more than 1 PMN/mm^3 is considered abnormal. A decreased sugar concentration is less than 40% of a simultaneous blood sugar concentration.

†Least common category.

‡Tuberculous, fungal, brucellar, listerial, and parasitic.

is done and shows no lesion that might precipitate cerebral herniation. Risk of transtentorial or tonsillar herniation as a result of cerebral edema and intracranial hypertension following LP is low in uncomplicated meningitis. If bacterial meningitis is suspected but delay in diagnostic LP is warranted, initiation of antibiotic therapy (after several blood cultures are obtained) should be done. This empirical treatment is warranted if the patient's clinical condition is critical and delay in initiating antibiotics could be disastrous. Because bacterial meningitis can progress rapidly, immediate initiation of antibiotics should be considered even when immediate LP is carried out because the time required for performance of LP and subsequent CSF analysis can use up precious hours during which time neurologic deterioration can occur.

In bacterial meningitis CSF pressure is usually elevated; this finding is of unknown prognostic significance. CSF can appear clear, turbid, or cloudy. Cloudy CSF indicates pleocytosis of at least 200 white blood cells. The CSF white cell count can contain as few as 10 or as many as 10,000 cells/mm^3, of which 60% to 90% are polymorphonuclear (PMN) leukocytes; however, there are usually more than 1000 white blood cells. There can be minimal CSF pleocytosis in meningitis; this is particularly true for early meningococcal meningitis. If meningitis is strongly suspected clinically but there are equivocal CSF findings, a repeat CSF study should be performed 4 to 6 hours later to follow the possible evolution of abnormal CSF findings.

CSF protein content is usually elevated. When increased (excess of 1 g/dl), the fluid appears yellow tinged (xanthochromic). A peripheral blood glucose specimen should always be drawn just before LP because the stress of LP can elevate blood glucose concentration. If there is peripheral hypoglycemia or hyperglycemia, the CSF glucose concentration can be normal, but the CSF/blood glucose ratio (normal 0.5 to 0.6) can be altered. CSF glucose content is decreased in bacterial meningitis as well as in other conditions (subarachnoid hemorrhage, meningitis caused by *Mycobacterium tuberculosis,* fungi, sarcoid, syphilis, carcinoma, rarely viral meningitis as a result of mumps or herpes simplex virus) (Table 18-3). Decreased glucose content can be spurious and result from deterioration of CSF (5 mg decrement per hour) if the determination is not performed immediately after obtaining CSF.

Gram stain of CSF suggests the causative organism in two thirds of cases of bacterial meningitis; however, this is often misinterpreted because of observer inexperience or faulty preparation of smear. The culture should confirm presence of the causative microorganism(s); delay in plating the culture can result in false negative results. Because bacterial meningitis is sometimes caused by multiple agents, cultures for both aerobic and anaerobic organisms should be considered if the Gram stain shows more than one morphotype. If the cause of meningitis is not defined by the Gram stain and culture, other CSF studies should include acid-fast stain and culture for *Mycobacterium tuberculosis;* India ink preparation for *Cryptococcus neoformans;* latex particle agglutination to identify capsular antigens (*Cryptococcus neoformans, H. influenzae, N. meningitides*); counterimmunoelectrophoresis for *S. pneumoniae, H. influenzae,* and *N. meningitides;* serologic tests for syphilis; cytologic examination for malignant cells; viral cultures (including acute and convalescent serum samples 7 to 14 days apart); and fungal cultures.

TABLE 18-3 Antibiotic Therapy in Bacterial Meningitis

Drug	Route	Child's Daily Dose	Adult's Daily Dose
Ampicillin	IV	75–100 mg/kg	12 g
Penicillin G	IV	50,000 U/kg	20–24 million U
Nafcillin	IV	50–75 mg/kg	12 g
Chloramphenicol	IV	25–50 mg/kg	6 g
Carbenicillin*	IV	400–500 mg/kg	30–40 g
Ticarcillin*	IV	200–300 mg/kg	18–24 g
Metronidazole	PO or IV	Not FDA approved for children	15 mg/kg loading dose, then 7.5 mg/kg
Gentamicin†	IV	5 mg/kg	5 mg/kg
Tobramycin†	IV	5 mg/kg	5 mg/kg
Amikacin†	IV	15 mg/kg	15 mg/kg
Cefotaxime	IV	50 mg/kg	2–3 g
Ceftriaxone	IV	50 mg/kg	2–3 g
Ceftizoxime	IV	50 mg/kg	12 g
Vancomycin	IV	10 mg/kg	2 g
Oxacillin	IV	300 mg/kg	12 g

*Combined with aminoglycoside antibiotic in the therapy of gram-negative meningitis.
†These aminoglycoside antibiotics must be given intrathecally or intraventricularly as well to obtain adequate levels in the CSF. Gentamicin and tobramycin, 5 mg/day intrathecally. Amikacin, 20 mg/day intrathecally (CSF levels should be monitored).

Frequency	Indication
Every 6 hours	*N. meningitides* *S. pneumoniae* *H. influenzae* *S. agalactiae* *L. monocytogenes*
Every 4 hours	*S. pneumoniae* *N. meningitides* *S. agalactiae*
Every 4 to 6 hours	*S. aureus*
Every 6 hours	*H. influenzae* *E. coli* Anaerobes
Every 4 hours	*P. aeruginosa*
Every 4 hours	Proteus—mirabilis *E. coli*
Every 6 hours	Anaerobes
	Pseudomonas and other aerobic gram- negative bacilli
Every 6 hours	*H. influenzae* *S. pneumoniae* Enterobacteriaceae *P. aeruginosa*
Every 12 hours in children; once daily in adults	*H. influenzae* *S. pneumoniae* Enterobacteriaceae *P. aeruginosa*
Every 6 hours in children; every 8 hours in adults	*H. influenzae* *S. pneumoniae* Enterobacteriaceae *P. aeruginosa*
Every 6 hours	*S. aureus*
Every 4 hours	*S. aureus*

Patients with subarachnoid hemorrhage, toxic metabolic encephalopathy, and meningismus (clinical features of meningeal irritation, but normal CSF findings) can have clinical findings to simulate meningitis; differentiation is established by the CSF findings. In patients whose CSF shows pleocytosis without evidence of infectious causes, other conditions must be considered (see Table 18-3). If patients with bacterial meningitis are treated with inadequate doses of antibiotics or inappropriate antibiotics, there can be a sufficient reduction in the number of microorganisms such that the Gram stain and culture are negative but a complete cure has not been achieved (partially treated bacterial meningitis). At this stage the CSF formula including cell count and differential (ratio of lymphocytes to polymorphonuclears [PMNs]), sugar, and protein content is variable. In cases of partially treated bacterial meningitis, tests for capsular antigens are most useful. Certain patients with neoplasm have CSF pleocytosis with PMN cell preponderance, elevated protein, and decreased glucose; all studies for infectious causes and malignant cells are negative. This is consistent with parasympathetic reaction caused by parameningeal focus; however, despite these negative studies, infectious and carcinomatous meningitis cannot be completely excluded, and periodic reevaluation must be considered.

In bacterial meningitis treatment with intravenous antibiotics is usually determined by the Gram stain and culture results. If the CSF shows PMN predominance but the initial Gram stain is negative and no identifiable systemic source is defined, the initial empiric treatment depends on the patient's age and other epidemiologic data: for newborns, ampicillin plus an aminoglycoside or cefotaxime; for children 1 to 5 years old, ampicillin or third generation cephalosporin; for children older than 5, adolescents, and adults, penicillin, ampicillin or third generation cephalosporin; and for immunocompromised patients, ampicillin plus third generation cephalosporin. If CSF shows mixed pleocytosis with a negative Gram stain and normal sugar content, latex particle agglutination or counterimmunoelectrophoresis can be helpful in detecting capsular bacterial antigens; positive results are consistent with partially treated bacterial meningitis. Latex particle agglutination, if available, can define the cause of meningitis more reliably than the Gram stain and much more rapidly (within minutes) than a culture, which requires 48 hours to complete.

Antibiotics used to treat bacterial meningitis are listed in Table 18-3. Following initiation of therapy, the CSF analysis can be repeated 48 hours later; the Gram stain and culture should revert to negative if the organism causing meningitis is susceptible to antibiotics. Cellular reaction begins to decrease, and the shift to lymphocytic predominance occurs. There should be a normalization of sugar content, and this is an important prognostic parameter. Reduction of elevated protein content can occur slowly, and unless protein is markedly elevated protein content has little prognostic significance. Following 2 weeks of antibiotics, the cell count usually normalizes; however, slight pleocytosis can persist for several months. In patients whose initial CSF shows mixed pleocytosis with normal sugar content and a negative Gram stain and there is no history of prior antibiotic therapy, antibiotic therapy is usually initiated but is stopped if the culture is negative 48 hours later. Recurrent bacterial meningitis (usually caused by *S. pneumoniae*) suggests abnormal communication into subarachnoid spaces (skull fracture) or, less frequently, parameningeal infection focus. Blood cultures can be helpful in determining the cause. Bacterial meningitis should be treated with intravenous antibiotics. For *H. influenzae* and *N. meningitides,* 7 to 10 days is probably adequate, but as many as 21 days can be needed for neonatal meningitis. The length of treatment should be determined by the patient's clinical response.

In acute bacterial meningitis, overhydration should be avoided because cerebral edema and inappropriate secretion of the antidiuretic hormone can complicate this condition. Corticosteroid medication was not routinely used unless there was symptomatic intracranial hypertension or herniation syndromes; however, recent studies have reported that dexamethasone (0.15 mg/kg administered intravenously every 6 hours for 4 days) can improve the neurologic outcome, especially for children with *H. influenza meningitis*. Dexamethasone should be administered immediately before the initial antibiotic dose. The effectiveness of dexamethasone in adults with bacterial meningitis is not yet established. Other treatment for symptomatic cerebral edema includes hyperosmolar agents (mannitol, glycerol).

Potential neurologic sequelae of poorly or late treated bacterial meningitis includes blindness, deafness, seizures, cerebellar dysfunction, mental changes, cranial nerve palsies (most commonly third, sixth, seventh), and motor disturbances (hemiparesis, quadriparesis). Symptoms as a result of hydrocephalus can develop in early or delayed stages of bacterial meningitis. These occur more commonly in meningitis cases when the diagnosis was delayed or the organism was drug resistant; however, it can occur unpredictably in other cases of bacterial meningitis. CSF findings that often correlate with poor outcomes include the number of bacteria seen on the Gram stain, the amount of capsular antigen detected (greater the amount, worse the prognosis), and very low CSF sugar content.

■ TUBERCULOUS MENINGITIS

This can develop from dissemination of miliary tuberculosis to disseminate throughout the meninges. Nodules are encapsulated by the surrounding tissue; these break down, and bacilli are discharged into subarachnoid spaces. Thick white exudate forms in basal cisterns. Pathologic findings include proliferative arachnoiditis with thick proteinaceous exudate in basal cisterns infiltrating cranial nerves, vasculitis with arterial wall inflammation and thrombosis resulting in cerebral ischemia, hydrocephalus caused by inflammatory exudate obstructing cisterns, and tuberculomas (caseating granulomas). Using CT or MRI multiple small parenchymal and basal meningeal focal lesions can be visualized; however, these usually resolve with adequate medical treatment.

Symptomatology of tuberculous meningitis usually develops insidiously. Ask the patient for a history of any possible tuberculosis contact. Evaluate patients for systemic tuberculosis (positive chest radiogram, urinary tract involvement, abnormal liver function tests). Clinical findings of tuberculous meningitis include fever, headache, stiff neck, focal neurologic deficit, and behavioral or mental changes. There may be no evidence of active systemic tuberculosis: skin test (intermediate strength purified protein derivative) is usually positive (50% to 75% of patients), or the chest roentgenogram can show pulmonary involvement but frequently does not, especially among older adults. CSF cultures for *M. tuberculosis* are positive in 90%, whereas acid-fast stains of CSF finding *M. tuberculosis* are positive in 30%. If the initial CSF culture and acid-fast stain are negative, repeat the LP three additional times using specimens that contain at least 20 ml of CSF.

If tuberculous meningitis is suspected, initiate treatment on an empiric basis. Treatment regimens vary but include isoniazid (300 mg/day), usually in combination with ethambutol (15 mg/kg/day), rifampin (600 mg/day), or pyrazinamide (25 mg/kg/day). When drug resistance is suspected, for example, on the basis of prior drug treatment, streptomycin (750 to 1000 mg intramuscularly per day) is used. After the initial diagnosis is established, a repeat CSF study is performed 1 week after initiating treatment. If the patient is clinically improving and the CSF formula is normalizing, LP should be performed before hospital discharge and several weeks after the completion of therapy to confirm that relapse has not developed. Streptomycin (750 mg/day) can be used instead of ethambutol for the initial 8 weeks of therapy. Some experts recommend the addition of pyrazinamide (25 mg/kg/day) because of its bacterial activity against dormant *M. tuberculosis*. Dexamethasone should be used to reduce cerebral edema, intracranial hypertension, and inflammatory response (prevent hydrocephalus or vasculitis). There is no evidence that dexamethasone delays the elimination of tuberculosis if adequate antituberculous treatment is initiated. The duration of treatment for tuberculous meningitis is not established; 12 to 24 months of treatment is probably necessary to avoid relapse. Primary antituberculous drugs are potentially toxic:

- Streptomycin causes eighth nerve damage with hearing loss and vestibular disturbances that can be irreversible.
- Ethambutol causes optic nerve damage with early impairment of color vision, but this usually is not seen if a dosage of 15 mg/kg/day is not exceeded.

- Isoniazid can cause peripheral neuropathy and rarely encephalopathy; these side effects are dose dependent and preventable if supplemental pyridoxine is administered. Hepatotoxicity occurs in 3% of older patients.
- Rifampin has no known neurotoxicity but is potentially hepatotoxic.
- Pyrazinamide can cause hyperuricemia and gout.

CRYPTOCOCCAL MENINGITIS

Cryptococcal meningitis is the most common CNS fungal infection. One half of patients are immunologically suppressed (diabetes mellitus, transplant patients, lymphoma, leukemia, AIDS); in the others no predisposing factor is identified. The usual finding is basilar granulomatous meningitis; granulomas or cysts rarely develop intracerebrally. Clinical onset of symptoms is insidious; patients complain of headaches for several weeks to months. CSF findings include lymphocytic pleocytosis (100%), decreased sugar content (50%), elevated protein content (90%), positive India ink preparation (50%), presence of the cryptococcal antigen (90%), and positive fungal culture (95%). The initial CSF analysis may show only pleocytosis; it may be necessary to perform several studies or obtain fluid by cisternal or ventricular tap to diagnose cryptococcal meningitis. Removal and culturing of large CSF volumes (15 to 25 ml) increases success. If the serum cryptococcal antigen is negative, it is highly unlikely that the patient has cryptococcal meningitis. In AIDS patients CSF can show minimal lymphocytic pleocytosis as a result of systemic lymphopenia. In these patients, if CSF is acellular with normal protein and sugar content, perform cryptococcal antigen and fungal cultures because of a high index of suspicion of this disorder.

Initial treatment consists of systemic amphotericin B and flucytosine. Amphotericin B is administered intravenously in dosages of 0.3 to 6 mg/kg/day mixed in a 5% dextrose and water solution during a 2- to 3-hour interval. Untoward effects include fever, hypotension, nausea, and vomiting; renal toxicity with impaired tubular function; anemia due to bone marrow depression; phlebitis; and hypokalemia. Treatment is continued for 6 to 10 weeks or until the total dose is 2.5 g. Intrathecal amphotericin B is used for patients showing poor response to systemic drugs or with impaired renal function. Flucytosine is an antifungal agent administered orally in a dosage of 150 mg/kg/day divided into six hourly doses and continued for 6 weeks. It is synergistic with amphotericin B. Flucytosine is toxic to bone marrow; thrombocytopenia or leukopenia can also result. In AIDS patients, fluconazole (diflucan) is used in a dosage of 200 mg per day for lifelong suppressive treatment. It is not used alone because organisms rapidly become resistant. A repeat course of treatment is necessary if the CSF shows increased cell count, decrease in glucose content, or elevation of cryptococcal antigen titer.

NEUROSYPHILIS

CNS infection by *Treponema pallidum* can cause several clinical patterns: latent (asymptomatic), basilar meningitis, granuloma (gumma), meningovascular, parenchymal (general paresis), and tabes dorsalis. CSF should be analyzed in all patients having positive serum treponemal tests who have not received adequate antibiotic therapy for syphilis or if nontreponemal serum titers are elevated above posttreatment levels.

In latent neurosyphilis the patient is neurologically normal; the CSF shows positive syphilis serology. Serodiagnosis of syphilis is established by demonstrating two types of antibodies: nonspecific reagin (VDRL, RPR) and specific treponemal, including *T. pallidum* immobilization test (TPI), fluorescent treponemal antibody-absorption test (FTA-ABS), and microhemagglutination assay for *T. pallidum* (MHA-TP). Reagin antibody tests can have false-negative results; furthermore, these tests lack specificity, and false-positive results can occur in certain conditions including systemic lupus erythematosus, bacterial endocarditis, rheumatoid arthritis, and pregnancy. In active neurosyphilis, serologic titers are elevated; they become low or negative following treatment. Specific reagin antibody tests are the "scarlet letter" of syphilis and remain positive even with adequate treatment. Serologic tests for syphilis can become negative spontaneously with late CNS involvement for unknown reasons.

Patients with syphilitic meningitis can have meningeal signs. The CSF findings include mononuclear pleocytosis, elevated protein content, decreased glucose content, and positive serology (VDRL test of CSF should be performed) in blood and CSF. In AIDS patients with neurosyphilis, CSF may not show abnormalities, and there must be high index of suspicion. The presence of confusion, seizures, hemiparesis, and cranial nerve palsies suggests parenchymal involvement; stroke can be an indication of syphilitic vasculitis. CSF findings in parenchymal and vasculitic neurosyphilis include mononuclear pleocytosis, elevated protein content, reduced sugar content, and positive serology. General paresis usually develops as the most advanced form. Clinical findings include dementia, neurobehavioral abnormalities, postural tremor, and seizures. CSF findings include pleocytosis, elevated protein (with increased gamma-globulin component) content, and positive serology. CT/MRI show brain atrophy. Pathologically the cerebral gyral pattern is atrophic, the meninges are thickened, and the sulci are widened.

Tabes dorsalis is syphilitic involvement of nerve roots and spinal cord. Clinical findings include recurrent lancinating and paroxysmal lightninglike pains of burning, electrical, or cramping quality involving the legs or abdomen; visceral crises consisting of abdominal pain, nausea, and vomiting; sensory defects and paresthesias with loss of vibration and position sense in lumbosacral region; neurogenic bladder; sensory ataxia; and trophic joint changes. The finding of small, irregularly shaped miotic pupils nonreactive to light with normal response to accommodation (Argyll Robertson pupil) is pathognomonic of neurosyphilis.

For neurosyphilis many physicians prefer to hospitalize for treatment with aqueous crystalline penicillin G (2 million units every 4 hours, 12 million units/day for 14 days). Benzathine penicillin (24 million units administered intramuscularly by weekly injection for 3 consecutive weeks) does not provide adequate CSF levels to treat neurosyphilis. If recurrence is suspected, indications for a repeat antibiotic course include clinical progression of neurologic findings, CSF pleocytosis persisting 1 year after the initial treatment, fourfold increase in VDRL titer, and initially high titer that fails to decrease fourfold within 1 year. Unfortunately, no good data exist regarding the efficacy of alternative forms of therapy for the penicillin-allergic patient. Recommendations include tetracycline, 2 g per day for 30 days; doxycycline, 100 mg twice per day for 30 days; or intramuscular ceftriaxone, 1g per day for 14 days.

▰ LYME DISEASE

Lyme disease is caused by a spirochete referred to as *Borrelia burgdorferi* and is carried by specific genus of wood tick (Ixodes). It is endemic in the northeastern United States, the upper Midwest states including Minnesota and Wisconsin, and wooded Pacific coast areas. Pathologic involvement includes skin, joints, eyes, the cardiac system, and the peripheral nervous systems. Lyme disease has several stages: flulike illness (headache, stiff neck, fever, myalgias) with skin lesion erythema chronicum migrans (circular-shaped at the tick bite with lesions later disseminating), meningitic syndrome with prominent cranial and peripheral radiculoneuropathy, polyarthritis, and symptoms simulating multiple sclerosis or diffuse encephalopathy. Antibodies to this spirochete can be determined by immunofluorescent or enzyme-linked immunosorbent assay. The diagnosis of Lyme infection is established by positive *B. burgdorferi* culture or the presence of anti–*B. burgdorferi* antibodies in serum or CSF. CSF abnormalities include monnuclear pleocytosis and the presence of anti–*B. burgdorferi* antibodies, but CSF findings can be negative. In some clinically suspected cases the CSF may show no abnormalities. The diagnosis of CNS involvement in Lyme disease can be quite difficult as there can be false-positive and false-negative laboratory findings.

Treatment includes doxycycline 100 mg three times daily for 30 days, amoxicillin 500 mg three times daily for 30 days, or azithromycin 500 mg daily for 7 days. For neurologic symptoms use parenteral antibiotics. These include a 2-week course of ceftriaxone 2 g intravenously daily, penicillin G 20 million units intravenously daily, and cefotaxime 2 g three times daily intravenously. Following successful treatment, post–Lyme disease syndrome including disabling fatigue, headache, dizziness, impaired memory and concentration, myalgia, sleep disturbances, and arthralgias can occur. These symptoms should be treated symptomatically and do not require further antibiotic treatment unless there are definite laboratory findings of incomplete treatment or recurrence. Recently many patients with vague and nonspecific symptoms have been diagnosed as having Lyme disease without definitive clinical or laboratory findings, and they have received long-term and high-dose antibiotics indiscriminately. This practice should be discouraged!

SUBDURAL EMPYEMA

Subdural empyema (SDE) can develop from an infected contiguous source (paranasal sinusitis, orbital cellulitis, mastoiditis, skull osteomyelitis, meningitis). SDE is defined as pus collection between the dura and arachnoid. The most common location is over frontal convexities or in the interhemispheric fissure. Cortical vein and dural sinus thrombosis or brain abscess can complicate SDE. Clinical features of SDE include headache, fever, and stiff neck; however, altered mentation, focal neurologic deficit, and papilledema occur later. Rapid neurologic deterioration can occur; lumbar puncture is potentially hazardous procedure with SDE, sometimes precipitating transtentorial herniation. CSF findings are nondiagnostic and include elevated intracranial pressure, sterile pleocytosis, elevated protein, normal sugar, and negative culture. The diagnosis is established by CT/MRI showing lenticular-shaped extracerebral lesions or by angiography showing medial inward displacement of superficial cortical vessels. The choice of initial antibiotics depends on the SDE source. Following head trauma, *S. aureus* is common; with ear infections, *Proteus mirabilis, Pseudomonas aeruginosa,* or anaerobic streptococci; with sinus infection, Bacteroides fragilis, gram negative aerobes and sometimes mixed infections. SDE patients are frequently very ill, and the CT/MRI should be immediately performed. Early initiation of empiric antibiotics and surgical drainage should be carried out. Subsequent antibiotic therapy is continued by 4 to 6 weeks; the choice of subsequent antibiotics is determined by the results of a bacterial Gram stain and culture obtained from surgery.

■ CRANIAL EPIDURAL EMPYEMA

Cranal epidural empyema (CEE) is localized pus collection in the preformed space between skull and dura. CEE occurs in settings similar to that of SDE. Expansion of CEE occurs as the dura is torn away from the inner skull table, forming a well-circumscribed pus collection; this contrasts with the diffuse extracerebral pattern of SDE. Clinically there can be tenderness over skull, ear, or sinus with specific tenderness over the CEE site. These patients develop cranial nerve paresis as the CEE extends into the foramen of cranial nerves through which they exit the dura and bone. For example, with temporal bone involvement trigeminal and abducens paresis can develop with tenderness over the temporal bone, and there can be facial pain and paresthesias. The diagnosis is established by a CT or MRI showing *localized* extracerebral collection, frequently with evidence of bone or sinus involvement. Treatment includes bone and dural surgical debridement and antibiotic therapy.

FOCAL SUPPURATIVE CEREBRITIS AND BRAIN ABSCESS

Suppurative brain reaction can result from local contiguous extension or hematogenous dissemination of systemic infection (endocarditis, bronchiectasis) or sepsis. Hematogenous dissemination frequently results in multiple noncontiguous lesions, usually in areas supplied by the middle cerebral artery, whereas direct local extension always causes solitary or directly contiguous multiple lesion(s). In focal suppurative cerebritis the initial pathologic reaction includes edema, tissue necrosis, PMN cellular infiltration, and multiple petechial brain hemorrhages. Brain abscess is defined as a sharply demarcated focus of suppuration within brain tissue with surrounding capsule. In the region surrounding the necrotic core there is fibroblastic response with granulation tissue developing within the capsule. Because the vascular supply is better formed in the superficial cortex, this portion of the capsule is thicker than the capsule on the ventricular surface. If an abscess rupture occurs, it is usually through the thinner ventricular portion rather than into subarachnoid spaces due to the protective effect of the thicker capsule on the cortical (superficial) surface.

In the early stage of focal suppurative cerebritis, patients show meningeal signs and altered mentation; focal neurologic deficit and papilledema are uncommon. The value of conventional neurodiagnostic studies is limited: an EEG shows slow wave focus, an isotope scan shows localized abnormal uptake, the CSF shows sterile pleocytosis with normal sugar content, and an angiogram is normal or shows only minimal mass effect. CT findings are usually positive but nonspecific. There is a hypo-dense lesion with significant mass effect, and a post-contrast study shows incomplete ring enhancement (Figure 18-1). The MRI can show the central necrotic core, surrounding edema, and mass effect; the postgadolinium MRI can show ring enhancement similar to CT. Both CT and MRI have a high degree of sensitivity but low specificity for cerebritis-abscess diagnosis as other inflammatory and neoplastic conditions can have similar CT/MRI appearances. It is important to differentiate cerebritis (in which there is an absent or poorly formed capsule) from abscess (containing a well-formed capsule). This is *usually* possible with CT/MRI if the clinical history indicates an infectious condition. From the treatment perspective antibiotics can penetrate a cerebritis or thin-wall abscess, and surgical treatment can be avoided; however, in the case of a thick-wall abscess, surgery is inevitable as antibiotics do not penetrate the capsule.

Treatment of focal suppurative cerebritis includes intravenous antibiotics; this can be supplemented by corticosteroids to reduce cerebral edema. Surgery is not of value because the infection is not encapsulated. Many cases of brain abscess are caused by multiple microorganisms. Initial antibiotics include penicillin and/or chloramphenicol plus metronidazole. Metronidazole penetrates the blood-CSF and blood-brain barrier and exhibits bactericidal activity against anaerobic bacteria. Adequate coverage against anaerobic bacteria is necessary because these are present in 90% of nontraumatic abscesses and can be the sole causal organism in 50% to 66% of abscesses. If a cerebritis-abscess has resulted from open head trauma or develops following a neurosurgical procedure, coverage for

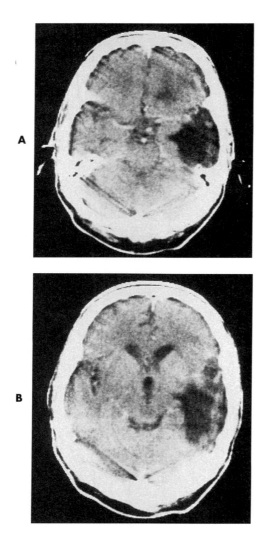

FIGURE 18-1. A and B, Irregular marginated nonenhancing hypodense left temporal lesion; suppurative cerebritis was evident at autopsy.

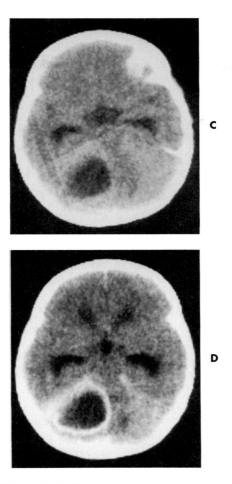

FIGURE 18-1, cont'd. **C,** Sharply marginated hypodense left cerebellar lesion that effaces the fourth ventricle and is causing obstructive hydrocephalus. **D,** Following contrast infusion there is a thin peripheral enhancing rim. An encapsulated brain abscess was identified at surgery.

Staphylococcus aureus and aerobic gram-negative bacilli is necessary. Following antibiotic treatment clinical recovery is expected with normalization of CT/MRI findings. In certain cases the area of suppuration becomes encapsulated. In these cases clinical and CT resolution do not occur, and the CT/MRI shows dense ring enhancement consistent with firm nonpenetrable capsule; surgical drainage is necessary at this stage.

If an encapsulated abscess forms, clinical findings include altered mentation, focal neurologic deficit, and papilledema. Symptoms and signs associated with brain abscesses are nonspecific, and an infectious condition may not be initially considered because fever is absent (30% to 50%), and peripheral white cell count is normal (40%). Headache (64%) is the most common complaint. The most characteristic clinical picture consists of a headache, recent seizure, altered consciousness, low-grade fever, papilledema, and focal neurologic deficit.

CT and MRI are the safest, most sensitive, and most specific procedures to detect brain abscess (see Figure 18-1), being positive in 95%. This shows a ring-enhancing lesion representing encapsulation; angiography shows an avascular mass. MRI is equally effective for detecting brain abscesses. The abscess capsule is sometimes thick enough that it is relatively impermeable to antibiotics; however, in other cases the capsule is completely formed but remains thin and can be permeable to antibiotics.

The outcome for suppurative cerebritis and brain abscess was associated with 25% to 30% mortality before CT/MRI despite antibiotic treatment. With CT/MRI it is possible to determine three crucial features: (1) presence of single or multiple lesions;

(2) the stage of capsule development, for example, cerebritis, early abscess with thin wall, or late abscess with thick wall; and (3) the degree of mass effect. With CT/MRI mortality has decreased to less than 5%, probably because of earlier diagnosis, better localization, and earlier and more precise determination of need for medical or surgical management. If multiple abscesses are present, medical therapy is indicated. The primary therapy for a certain single (solitary) brain abscess consists of antibiotics and surgical drainage, especially if the CT/MRI shows a thick-walled abscess. In certain single or multiple abscess(es), antibiotics and corticosteroids cause resolution of the abscess without surgery, especially if abscess wall appears thin. This represents a major advance because before CT/MRI all patients would have required surgery. Corticosteroids are used to decrease cerebral edema, but their effect on the pathologic process (immunologic suppression and fibroblastic proliferation) is not known. The initial antibiotic therapy for abscess(es) includes intravenous penicillin (20 million units daily) and chloramphenicol (1 g every 6 hours). The choice of empiric therapy is based on the most likely bacterial source. If there is septicemia or endocarditis, antibiotics are selected on the basis of results of the blood culture. Brain abscesses developing as a result of head trauma can require coverage for *S. aureus* using penicillinase-resistant, semisynthetic penicillin. Treatment is usually continued for 4 to 6 weeks after the surgical drainage of a brain abscess. A serial CT/MRI is helpful in monitoring response to therapy. The pathologic process as visualized by the CT/MRI can take several additional months to resolve after antibiotics have been discontinued.

VIRAL MENINGOENCEPHALITIS

Acute viral meningoencephalitis represents a major manifestation of systemic viral infection. There is hematogenous infection; the virus enters the CNS across the endothelial cell. Certain viruses infect meninges and ependyma (meningitis), others infect neurons and glial cells (encephalitis), and some viruses infect both meninges *and* brain to cause meningoencephalitis. Initial symptoms of meningoencephalitis are headache, nausea, vomiting, and changes in behavior. Findings include altered mentation, seizures, and focal neurologic deficit. CSF findings are pleocytosis (lymphocytic predominance), normal sugar content, and elevated protein content. The causal virus is isolated in only 25% of cases of viral meningoencephalitis. The viruses most likely to cause encephalitis are arbovirus and herpes simplex virus type 1. The course is monophasic; improvement begins within 2 to 3 weeks; however, in some cases significant residual neurologic deficit can persist. Most viral encephalitis appears as a diffuse encephalitic condition; however, herpes simplex type 1 appears as focal temporal-frontal cerebritis.

Arthropod-Borne (Arbovirus)

Most cases of arbovirus encephalitis occur during summer and fall and are transmitted to humans by mosquitoes. Mosquitoes are responsible for St. Louis encephalitis (SLE), Western equine encephalitis (WEE), and Eastern equine encephalitis (EEE). WEE is usually a mild viral encephalitis with minimal neurologic sequelae; the mortality rate is 10%. EEE is a more severe disease characterized by high fever, altered mentation, convulsions, and permanent neurologic impairment (dementia, retardation, psychoses, motor deficit, seizures). It has a mortality rate of 70%. Patients with SLE have confusional states, head tremor, and prominent primitive reflexes; neurologic residua persists in 10%. The overall case-fatality of arbovirus encephalitis is 10%; however, in elderly patients this can reach 30%. The diagnosis is established by a fourfold rise in acute and convalescent blood antibody titer or by viral isolation from CNS tissue (almost never from CSF culture). There is no specific therapy for arbovirus encephalitis, but supportive therapy is important.

Herpes Simplex Virus

Herpes simplex virus type 1 attacks the skin, mucous membranes, and the CNS. It is thought to enter the CNS through the olfactory or trigeminal nerve(s). Patients have fever, headaches, meningeal signs, altered mentation, papilledema, and focal neurologic deficit with prominent temporal lobe dysfunction (aphasia, visual field defect, amnesia). CSF findings include pleocytosis with lymphocyte predominance, red blood cells (500 to 1000 mm^3), elevated protein, and normal sugar (rarely CSF glucose is decreased). Because serum antibodies to herpes simplex are present in 40% to 60% of normal subjects, an elevated titer is not helpful in establishing the diagnosis of CNS infection. This is established only by a brain biopsy with analysis for immunofluorescent antibody staining for herpes simplex, intranuclear inclusion bodies, and isolation of herpes virus. In patients with clinical signs of temporal lobe dysfunction and systemic signs of infectious illness who have CT/MRI and EEG evidence of temporal abnormalities, the presumptive diagnosis includes herpes simplex encephalitis (Figure 18-2). Pathologic findings include hemorrhagic necrosis

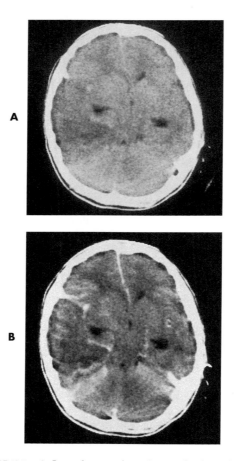

FIGURE 18-2.   **A,** Irregular marginated extensive hypodense in left frontal temporal lesion causing marked mass effect. **B,** Following contrast infusion, there is irregular or diffuse enhancement. Herpes simplex encephalitis was diagnosed at surgery.

localized to the inferior medial temporal lobe. When idoxuridine, a highly toxic antiviral agent, was used, treatment was never undertaken without an initial brain biopsy. Since the introduction of vidarabine, which is much less toxic, treatment can be initiated if there is strong clinical suspicion of herpes simplex encephalitis. The disadvantage of vidarabine treatment is that the drug must be mixed in a large fluid volume; this can worsen cerebral edema. Acyclovir (Zovirax) has been proved effective in treating herpes simplex encephalitis and has minimal toxicity. In patients with suspected herpes simplex encephalitis, initiate empiric antiherpes simplex treatment with acyclovir in a dosage of 10 mg per kgm intravenously for 10 days. Treatment should be initiated immediately to minimize brain inflammatory reaction. If clinical deterioration occurs with acyclovir or the CT/MRI shows evidence of worsening despite treatment, a brain biopsy should be carried out to exclude alternative causes of temporal lobe lesions, for example, neoplasm or other infectious-inflammatory disorders. If the diagnosis is initially uncertain because of atypical features, initiate acyclovir therapy, then perform brain biopsy.

Myxovirus

CNS disorders can be part of mumps infections. Mumps meningoencephalitis can rarely occur in patients without clinical parotitis. The diagnosis is established by mumps virus CSF isolation and a fourfold increase of the antihemagglutin antibody titer in the acute and convalescent stages. The CSF can display lymphocytic pleocytosis, elevated protein, and sometimes low sugar content (hypoglycorrhachia).

Rabies

Rabies is a neurotropic myxovirus that can be present in the saliva of an infected animal (dog, wolf, bat) and is usually but not always transmitted through the bite. The incubation period is 1 to 4 weeks. Initial symptoms are paresthesias and pain at the bite site. Within 7 to 14 days features of rabies include irritability, agitation, inability to swallow, hydrophobia, painful spasms, and coma. The diagnosis is established by finding fluorescent antibodies in the brain at the necropsy of an infected animal or human; the presence of Negri bodies is a relatively specific finding. Prophylactic treatment must include both rabies immune globulin (passive immunity) and human diploid cell rabies vaccine (active immunity). Use of human diploid cell rabies rather than duck vaccine has decreased the neurotoxicity of treatment. Rabies immunoglobulin should be given with the initial vaccine dose. After being bitten by potentially rabid animal, meticulous wound cleansing with soap and water followed by 70% ethanol is necessary.

Enterovirus

Enterovirus group includes coxsackie and echo viruses. These are spread by the fecal-oral route. The clinical pattern is usually mild meningitis symptoms; the CSF shows sterile lymphocytic pleocytosis. The diagnosis is established in the following manner: the virus is isolated from the CSF, throat, or stool to determine the subtype involved, then, if this test is positive, acute and convalescent blood titers for neutralization and complement fixation antibodies are performed. Treatment is symptomatic.

Poliomyelitis is caused by enterovirus. The virus enters through the pharynx, and viremia then develops. Initially, these patients have a febrile illness with myalgias; they subsequently fully recover. The CSF shows lymphocytic pleocytosis. The virus attacks large spinal and cranial bulbar motor neurons nerves; this causes rapid onset of weakness in limbs and bulbar muscles. There is sudden onset of asymmetrical (frequently unilateral) lower motor neuron type weakness with no sensory disturbances or incontinence. Certain patients progress to quadriparesis with respiratory failure and do not recover; others have mild motor weakness and fully recover. It is presumed that in these patients who recover fully, the anterior horn cells were only partially injured and were capable of recovery. Recently, postpoliomyelitis syndrome has been described. This can develop 20 to 30 years after the initial acute poliomyelitis. It is characterized by limb pain and increased weakness (in limbs that were initially affected). It is not known if this represents the normal aging process or is due to an immunologic condition characterized by further attack on motor neurons. Since the development of the Salk and Sabin immunizations, this paralytic disease is almost never seen.

Varicella Zoster

Rarely encephalitis can follow chicken pox. This usually develops 1 week after the rash appears. Encephalitis can involve the cerebellum to cause acute ataxia, dysarthria, and incoordination. This cerebellar ataxia usually resolves completely. In other cases encephalitis causes impaired consciousness, seizures, and motor weakness. In this postvaricella encephalitis, recovery is less complete.

Measles

Following measles there can be a postinfectious disorder characterized by fever recurrence, altered consciousness, seizures, motor deficit, and myoclonus. There is white matter demyelination; this occurs as the rash fades. This is an uncommon measles complication, but the neurologic morbidity is high. The CT/MRI can show multiple focal white matter lesions that can be confused with white matter demyelinating disorders such as multiple sclerosis.

Herpes Zoster

The varicella (chickenpox) zoster virus causes inflammatory lesions in dorsal (sensory) root ganglia and cranial nerve (ophthalmic branch of trigeminal and geniculate) ganglia. Initial symptoms of zoster infection are vesicular skin lesions occurring in distribution of involved ganglia. The patient can later develop dysesthetic pain. These lesions and the resultant pain syndrome most commonly involve the thoracic region. In certain cases there can be ophthalmic involvement; this can result in corneal scarring. In otic zoster infection there is involvement of the geniculate ganglion. Vesicles can be seen on the eardrum, and unilateral facial paralysis can then develop. In rare cases bandlike thoracic pain caused by herpes zoster can occur in the absence of vesicles. Acyclovir is used in both immunologically competent and incompetent patients. It is most effective in immunocompromised patients with disseminated herpes zoster. Use acyclovir, 5 mg/kg intravenously three times per day for 5 to 7 days, for these patients. In immunologically intact patients use acyclovir 800 mg five times per day orally for 7 days. Postherpetic pain is characterized by sponteneous burning pain, developing at the site of previously visualized vesicles. Postherpetic pain may respond to amitriptyline, phenytoin, or carbamazepine. There is some evidence that corticosteroids can reduce postherpetic neuralgia; however, there is a risk that corticosteroids could adversely alter viral dissemination and cause generalized viremia.

■ SLOW VIRAL INFECTIONS

Creutzfeldt-Jakob Disease

Creutzfeldt-Jakob disease (CJD) is characterized by rapidly progressing dementia and myoclonus. As the disease progresses there can be motor signs, for example, ataxia and in-creased limb tone. The CSF shows no abnormal cellular response, but protein can be elevated. EEG shows periodic (0.5 to 2.0 seconds) high-voltage spikes or slow wave patterns. The CT/MRI shows enlarged ventricles and subarachnoid spaces. Pathologic findings are vacuolated spongiform neurons and astrocytes in the cerebral cortex and basal ganglia; however, despite evidence that this is due to a transmissible agent, there is no brain inflammatory change. The agent causing CJD is different from usual viruses and is believed to be a proteinaceous infectious particle not containing nucleic acids; this has been referred to as "prion." Disorders caused by prions are not contagious. The exact mechanism of transmission of the disease is not known, but tissue transmission (corneal transplants, human pituitary growth hormone, inadequately sterilized brain surgery equipment, for example, electrodes, sterotactic equipment) has occurred. The transmissible agent is resistant to physical and chemical treatment (heat, ionizing and ultraviolet radiation); therefore, autoclaving or bleach is necessary. There is no effective treatment. Patients rapidly progress to coma and die.

Kuru

Kuru occurs in natives of New Guinea highlands. Cannibalism is major transmission mode. Clinical symptoms include ataxia followed by mental deterioration. There is progression to coma and death in less than 2 years. Pathologic changes include neuronal and astrocytic spongiform degeneration.

Progressive Multifocal Leukoencephalopathy

Progressive multifocal leukoencephalopathy (PML) is demyelinating disease caused by papovavirus. It is most common in patients with impaired cellular immunity. Clinical symptoms include rapidly progressive dementia, visual impairment and hallucinations, ataxia, weakness, and cranial nerve dysfunction. This disorder rapidly worsens, and these patients die. The CSF and EEG show no abnormalities. The CT/MRI can show symmetrical bilateral subcortical hemispheric white matter lesions. These demyelinated lesions can initially occur in the occipital-parietal region; they subsequently enlarge and spread anteriorly. Pathologic findings are multifocal demyelinated areas, loss of oligodendrocytes, and eosinophilic intranuclear inclusion bodies. Viral particles consistent with papovavirus have been recovered from these patients. Treatment with antiviral agents (cytosine, arabinoside, interferon, acyclovir) has not been successful.

Subacute Sclerosing Panencephalitis

Subacute sclerosing panencephalitis (SSPE) is caused by rubeola (measles) virus; it occurs in children. The initial clinical symptoms include slowly progressive dementia, ataxia, and myoclonus. The disease usually progresses to coma with quadriplegia, dystonia, and seizures; however, rarely a patient's condition stabilizes. The CSF shows no pleocytosis or elevated protein content, but there is elevated gamma-globulin content. The EEG shows periodic high-voltage slow waves followed by an isoelectric (burst suppression) pattern. Measles antibodies are elevated in the serum and CSF. Pathologic findings include perivascular cortical and white matter infiltration with mononuclear cells. There is demyelination in white matter. Intranuclear and intracytoplasmic inclusion bodies are found in neurons and astrocytes; the measles virus can be isolated from brain tissue.

▨ PARASITIC INFECTIONS

Toxoplasmosis

Toxoplasmosis is discussed in Chapter 22.

Cerebral Malaria

Cerebral malaria occurs rarely in patients affected by *Plasmodium falciparum*. The diagnosis is established by demonstration of the organism on thick and thin blood smears. Neurologic symptoms include acute encephalopathy (altered consciousness, seizures) and are due to capillary occlusion by parasites and infected red blood cells. The CSF is usually normal. Treatment includes chloroquine and quinine.

Primary Amebic Meningoencephalitis

Primary amebic meningoencephalitis is caused by free-living amoeba (including *Naegleria* and *Acanthamoeba* species). These parasites are usually found in freshwater lakes and pools. They enter nasal mucosa and travel along the cribriform plate and olfactory nerves to the undersurface of frontal lobes.

Clinical features include fever, meningeal signs, and frontal headache. CSF findings include polymorphonuclear pleocytosis. Motile amoeba can be identified by wet-mount CSF preparations; stained amoeba can be demonstrated by Wright's or Giesma stain. Amoeba will not be demonstrated by routine bacterial stains because heat fixation degenerates these organisms. Treatment includes amphotericin B, ketoconazole, or metronidazole.

Trichinosis

Trichinosis is caused by the roundworm *Trichinella spiralis*. Infection occurs in humans if raw or poorly cooked pork is ingested. The parasite is contained in striated muscles of pigs. Trichinosis can cause acute febrile illness, rash, conjunctivitis, eyelid edema, gastrointestinal symptoms, and myalgias. Subcutaneous and muscular nodules can be palpated. There can be muscle tenderness and weakness; muscle biopsy can show encysted *Trichinella* organisms. This organism can spread to the brain to cause encephalitis. The diagnosis is established by a history of pork ingestion, the presence of eosinophilia in the blood count, and muscle biopsy findings showing the parasite. Treatment includes thiabendazole.

Cysticercosis

Cysticercosis is caused by encystment of larvae of *Taenia solium* (pork tapeworm) in human tissues. Humans ingest the ova of *Taenia solium* from contaminated food or water, as well as being infected by fecal-oral transmission of ova derived from intestinal parasite. Ova are digested in the stomach and release oncospheres that extend through gastrointestinal wall to reach the CNS and muscle by hematogenous dissemination. When cysticercosis dies there can be an active inflammation in the brain, meninges, or ventricles. After the active inflammatory response has terminated, intracranial gliosis, calcification, and cyst formation occur. Larval forms develop in skeletal muscle and the brain. Cysticercosis can enlarge in the meninges, ventricles, or brain parenchyma to form multiloculated cysts. Symptoms depend on the cyst location: meningitic with obstruction of basal cisterns cause intracranial hypertension and meningitic reaction, intraventricular form mass lesions within lateral ventricles and obstructive hydrocephalus, and parenchymal cause mass lesions or seizures as a result of cortical cysts. Intracranial calcification is commonly due to cysticercosis occurring in the inactive stage. The diagnosis can be made by biopsy of a subcutaneous nodule if any are present. In certain cases the CSF shows PMN or eosinophilic pleocytosis. Serologic CSF tests can demonstrate antigens or antibodies for cysticercosis, but these are not diagnostic. The CT/MRI can show hydrocephalus, parenchymal lesions, or calcifications (these probably represent dead organisms). Therapy includes shunting for hydrocephalus and corticosteroids to reduce edema associated with inflammatory reaction. Praziquantal, an anthelmintic, is effective to kill live larva. It is used at a dosage of 50 mg kg daily for 14 days. This can exacerbate the inflammatory response and worsen clinical symptoms transiently.

▨ TETANUS

Tetanus is caused by the toxin of anaerobic bacterium *Clostridium tetani*. This organism is frequently found in soil, and it can contaminate wounds. The toxin spreads along the neural sheath or by hematogenous dissemination to invade the spinal cord and brain stem. Tetanus toxin blocks interneurons. The earliest symptoms of tetanus include muscle spasms in the thoracic and lumbar paraspinal muscles, which can gradually spread to involve the jaw (lockjaw), face (risus sardonicus), pharynx (dysphagia), or larynx (respiratory stridor). Initial mild intermittent muscle spasms can progress to persistent muscle rigidity and tetanic spasms. Treatment includes identification and adequate debridement of wound; passive immunization with 12,000 units of tetanus-immune globulin; active immunization with tetanus toxoid; tracheostomy to provide adequate ventilation support for the prolonged 6- to 12-week course of intense generalized muscle spasms; central venous line for hyperalimentation; cardiac monitoring to prevent arrhythmias caused by sympathetic overdischarge; curare to suppress severe tetanic contractions, which if not controlled lead to muscle breakdown with myoglobinuria; and skin care to prevent decubitus ulcers. Mortality from generalized tetanus can be 60% despite adequate supportive care. If complications are prevented, toxin is released from the interneurons after several weeks, and the patient gradually recovers.

▨ SUMMARY

CNS infection can be caused by bacteria, virus, fungi, tuberculosis, spirochetal organisms, or parasites. The pathologic process can be diffuse (meningitis, encephalitis) or focal (cerebritis, abscess, subdural or epidural empyema). The diagnosis of meningitis and encephalitis is established by performing lumbar puncture with CSF analysis; the diagnosis of focal CNS infection is best established by CT or MRI, and

LP can be dangerous if a focal CNS infectious-inflammatory lesion is present. CNS infection results in damage to the blood-brain barrier, and this loss of integrity of the barrier permits antibiotics to penetrate into the CNS. Treatment with appropriate antibiotics must be by parenteral route and in high dose to treat the CNS infection completely. Early diagnosis of CNS infection is mandatory to prevent irreversible brain injury. In patients with HIV infection CNS infectious-inflammatory and neoplastic disorders occur as a result of immunosuppression of the patients' natural defense mechanisms.

Suggested Readings

Acute Bacterial Meningitis

Anderson M: Management of cerebral infection, *J Neurol Neurosurg Psychiatry* 57:1243, 1994.

Dodge PR, Swartz MN: Bacterial meningitis—a review of selected aspects, *N Engl J Med* 272:725, 779, 842, 898, 954, 1003, 1965.

Smith A: Neurologic sequela of meningitis, *N Engl J Med* 319:1012, 1988.

Tauber MG, Sande MA: General principles of therapy of pyogenic meningitis, *Infectious Dis Clin North Am* 4:661, 1990.

Tunkel AR, Wispelwey B, Scheld WM: Bacterial meningitis: recent advances in pathophysiology and treatment, *Ann Intern Med* 112:610, 1990.

Welsby PD: Meningococcal meningitis, *Br Med J* 300:1150, 1990.

Tuberculous Meningitis

Falk A: Tuberculous meningitis in adults with special reference to survival, neurological residuals and work status, *Am Rev Respir Dis* 91:823, 1965.

Sheller JR, DesPrez RM: CNS tuberculosis, *Neurol Clin North Am* 4:143, 1986.

Wilhelm C, Wilner JJ: Chronic meningitis, *Neurol Clin North Am* 4:115, 1982.

Molavi A, LeFrock J: Tuberculous meningitis, *Med Clin North Am* 69:315, 1985.

Cryptococcal Meningitis

Lyons RW, Andriole WT: Fungal infections of the CNS, *Neurol Clin North Am* 4:159, 1986.

Sabetta JR, Andriole VT: Cryptococcal infections of the nervous system, *Med Clin North Am* 69:333, 1985.

Neurosyphilis

Hooshmand H, Escobar MR, Kopf SW: Neurosyphilis: a review of 241 patients, *JAMA* 219:726, 1972.

Pachner AR: Spirochetal disease of the CNS, *Neurol Clin North Am* 4:223, 1986.

Davis LE, Schmitt JW: Clinical significance of CSF tests for neurosyphilis, *Ann Neurol* 25:50, 1989.

Hook EW, Marra CM: Acquired syphilis in adults, *N Engl J Med* 326:1060, 1992.

Lyme Disease

Rahn DW, Malawista SE: Lyme disease: recommendations for diagnosis and treatment, *Ann Intern Med* 114:472, 1991.

Focal Suppurative Brain Infection

Kaufman DM, Miller MH, Steigbigel NH: Subdural empyema, *Medicine* 54:485, 1975.

Weisberg LA: Nonsurgical management of focal intracranial infection, *Neurology* 31:575, 1981.

Chun CH and others: Brain abscess: a study of 45 consecutive cases, *Medicine* 65:415, 1986.

Silverberg AL, DiNubile MJ: Subdural empyema and cranial epidural abscess, *Med Clin North Am* 69:361, 1985.

Viral Meningoencephalitis

Kennard C, Swash M: Acute viral encephalitis, *Brain* 104:129, 1980.

Whitley RJ: Viral encephalitis, *N Engl J Med* 323:242, 1990.

Whitley RJ: Herpes simplex virus infections of the central nervous system, *Am J Med* 85(suppl):61, 1988.

Huff JC, Bean B, Balfour HH: Therapy of herpes zoster with oral acyclovir, *Am J Med* 85(suppl.2A):84, 1988.

Slow Viral Infections

Prusiner SB: Prions and neurodegenerative diseases, *N Engl J Med* 317:1571, 1987.

Brooks BR, Walker DL: Progressive multifocal leukoencephalopathy, 2:299, 1984.

Brown P: Cruetzfeldt-Jakob disease of long-duration; clinico-pathological characteristics, transmissibility and differential diagnosis, *Ann Neurol* 16:295, 1984.

Parasitic Infections

Bia FJ, Barry M: Parasitic infections of the CNS, *Neurol Clin North Am* 4:171, 1986.

Sotelo J, Escobedo F, Penagos P: Albendazole vs praziquental for therapy of neurocysticercosis, *Arch Neurol* 45:532, 1988.

C H A P T E R

Lesions of the Spine and Spinal Cord

19

Diseases of the spine and spinal cord produce several distinct yet frequently overlapping clinical syndromes. A given patient can appear with one or a combination of the four major clinical pictures listed in Box 19-1.

Carefully performed spine and neurologic examinations are extremely important. The goals of the examination are to determine if the supporting tissues (i.e., disks, vertebrae, ligaments, muscles, and facet joints) are involved; to assess whether the spinal cord is damaged and, if so, at what level; and to establish whether the nerve roots are affected.

ANATOMY

The spinal cord, roots, intervertebral disks, vertebrae, and soft tissues supporting the spinal column are all subject to disease or injury. Because of the close interrelationship of these structures, disease in one can affect the function of another (e.g., the rupture of an intervertebral cervical disk can cause damage to the cervical spinal cord or cervical nerve roots). To understand the clinical syndromes fully the physician must know the anatomic relationship of the spine, cord, and roots. Figure 19-1 is a superior view of cervical vertebra with cord and roots. Figure 19-2 is a lateral view, and Figure 19-3 is a posterior view with spines and transverse processes removed.

BOX 19-1

1 Back pain
2 Nerve root symptoms
3 Spinal cord symptoms
4 Spinal injury

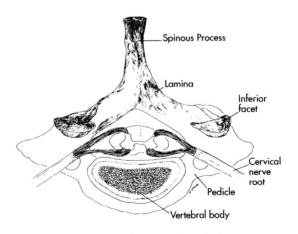

FIGURE 19-1. Cross-section of spine.

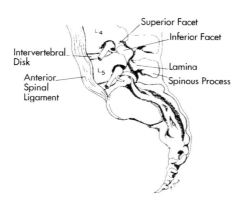

FIGURE 19-2. Lateral view of lumbosacral region. Note proximity of exiting nerve roots to both the facet joints and the disk. Disease in either the disk or facets can easily damage the roots.

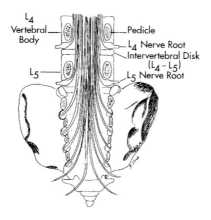

FIGURE 19-3. Posterior view of lumbosacral region with transverse processes and spines removed to expose the filum terminale. Note relationship between exiting nerve root and intervertebral disk; rupture of the disk (e.g., L4–L5) can damage the L4 root above, but often only affects the L5 root, which is passing the disk to exit below.

CLINICAL SYNDROMES

Back Pain

There are many causes of back pain, and the symptom must be viewed as a complex diagnostic problem. Boxes 19-2 through 19-4 outline the history, physical examination, and differential diagnosis of back pain.

Evaluation

The evaluation of back pain cases is individualized. Simple mechanical back pain rarely requires any imaging studies. Progressive unrelenting pain suggests a destructive lesion and does require extensive

---

BOX 19-2   History

1 Presence of trauma (see Spinal Trauma)
2 Character of onset and course
3 Location
4 Relief or exacerbation of pain with change in position
5 Radiation of pain around body or into limbs
6 Associated neurologic symptoms (e.g., weakness and paresthesias) or bladder dysfunction
7 Previous back surgery
8 History of cancer
9 Medical disease such as heart disease, ulcer, renal, or pelvic disease; all can produce referred pain to the back
10 Intermittent claudication (i.e., neurologic claudication: neurologic symptoms such as weakness and paresthesias that come on after walking a short distance)
11 Recent infection, particularly tuberculosis or pelvic inflammatory disease
12 Corticosteroid use or metabolic disease that can lead to osteoporosis with possible compression fracture

BOX 19-3   Physical Examination

1 Inspection of the back
   a Spasm in paraspinous muscles
   b Alignment (scoliosis, loss of normal lordosis—cervical or lumbar)
   c Dimples, sinus, or hair patch in lumbar area (might indicate underlying closure defect such as spina bifida with or without intraspinal tumor)

2 Palpation to identify spasm and tenderness

3 Percussion of spinous processes (start gently because percussion of an infected or damaged vertebra can be extremely painful)

4 Observation of the movement of the spine in all four directions and with rotation; note restrictions or production of pain or spasm

5 Neurologic examination with careful attention to spinal cord and nerve root signs

6 Maneuvers to evaluate low back pain:
   a *Patrick's maneuver.* With the patient supine and leg flexed, the leg is allowed to abduct fully until the knee lies on the bed laterally (frog-legged). Flexion of the leg relieves stretch on the root; therefore, pain elicited during this maneuver usually indicates hip joint disease.
   b *Straight leg raising.* With the patient supine, the examiner places a hand under one heel and slowly raises the leg to the 80- or 90-degree position. If there is root impingement, this maneuver will stretch and irritate the root and reproduce the radiating pain at the 30- to 60-degree position. If pain is present but equivocal, the examiner should dorsiflex the foot. This further stretches the nerve and should increase the pain if root pathology is present. This test is positive in a very high percentage of acute disk herniations, particularly in young persons (under age 30); in fact, a negative straight leg raising test almost completely eliminates the possibility of a disk lesion in that population.
   c *Pyriformis syndrome.* The pyriformis muscle can develop spasms and trap the sciatic nerve, causing back and leg pain. To test for these, have the patient lie supine with the

BOX 19-3—cont'd

    leg flexed, then adduct the leg and force the knee over the opposite leg. Sciatic pain is suggestive of a pyriformis syndrome.

  d Test for sciatic notch tenderness.

  e Observation for pelvic tilt. The pelvis can ride higher on the symptomatic side because this is an attempt to reduce pressure on this such that the weight is absorbed by the nonsymptomatic side.

7 Foraminal closure test for cervical root impingement
Have the patient extend the neck and tilt the head to the side. This will tend to close the neural foramen and produce root pain and paresthesias in a compromised root.

8 Abdominal examination

9 Rectal and pelvic examination (low back pain)

10 Peripheral pulses

study. Intermittent chronic back pain without nerve root or bladder symptoms rarely requires CT or MRI studies (Ellenberger, 1994). Given these general guidelines, the seven tests most commonly employed to evaluate back pain are listed in Box 19-5.

Root Lesions

Symptoms of nerve root compression or damage are often the initial and most prominent complaint of patients with spine disease or extramedullary spinal cord tumors. The principal symptoms are dermatomal pain, paresthesias, and sensory loss; selective motor loss; and bowel or bladder dysfunction if the cauda equina is involved.

Root (radicular) pain can also be seen from disease of the viscera, so a full medical history is advisable in patients with radiating pains. Disease of the

BOX 19-4   Differential Diagnosis (Excluding Trauma)

1 *Congenital abnormalities of the spine*
  a *Fusion of vertebrae.* This commonly occurs in the neck and can involve several levels of fusion. These en bloc vertebrae or Klippel-Feil deformities reduce neck mobility and can cause pain. There are often associated anomalies such as hemivertebrae and scoliosis. A short neck and reduced neck motion are common.
  b *Hemivertebrae.* Fusion of part of fifth lumbar vertebra to sacrum (sacralization of L5) can lead to a tilt of the spine with compensatory scoliosis and pain.
  c *Spondylolisthesis.* This is a congenital defect in the inter-articular process of the superior facet of L5 that can cause the L5 vertebral bodies to slip forward over S1. This slippage usually occurs in the mid teens and is characterized by back pain, muscle spasm, pain on straight leg raising, and often hamstring spasm with associated short stride gait. Sacral roots can be involved in severe cases. Surgery is necessary.
  d *Absent odontoid with instability of atlantoaxial joint.* This can give neck pain and neurologic symptoms if subluxation occurs.
  e *Basilar impression.* The base of the skull is flattened and the cervical spine is literally pushed upward. This can cause neck pain, cord compression, and lower cranial nerve abnormalities.
  f *Scoliosis (lateral spine curvature).* Scoliosis can be seen in association with spine abnormalities such as collapse or malformation of a vertebral body; spinal tumors, particularly those associated with neurofibromatosis; spinocerebellar degenerations; syringomyelia; and neuromuscular disease. The most common, however, is an idiopathic progressive variety, which can occur both in infancy or in juveniles. The problem is much more common in females and is usually thoracic in location. The deformity can be very marked, and surgery is often necessary.

2 *Diseases of the viscera that can produce back pain*
  a *Posterior wall cardiac ischemia or infarction.*
  b *Ulcer in posterior wall of stomach.* Pain in right posterior chest wall.
  c *Gallbladder, biliary tree, and pancreatic disease.*
  d *Retroperitoneal masses or hemorrhage.* Nerve root symptoms are often present at the level of the lesion.

BOX 19-4—cont'd

   e *Aortic or abdominal aneurysm* (can give acute back pain with dissection).

   f *Pelvic disease*. Tumor, mass, or inflammation can cause low back pain. The retroflexed uterus, however, probably does not.

3 *Osteoporosis* (bone softening)
This is a common problem in the elderly but is also seen in patients on chronic corticosteroid medication or with hormonal or neoplastic diseases that produce an imbalance between calcium absorption from bone and calcium deposition. Back pain is due to vertebral collapse or fracture; onset is often acute.

4 *Infectious disease*
Vertebral osteomyelitis is somewhat uncommon and predominantly affects adult diabetics. The major symptom is localized back pain. It is progressive, unremitting, and worse at night. Movement intensifies the pain, and paravertebral muscle spasm with spinal rigidity is common. The affected vertebrae can be extremely sensitive to percussion. Pain radiates around the chest if there has been some vertebral collapse and root impingement. Spinal cord findings can be present if vertebrae are collapsed and subluxed. The white blood cell count and erythrocyte sedimentation rate are elevated, but the temperature can be normal. Changes on the spine roentgenogram and bone scan are not demonstrated until 4 to 6 weeks after the disease onset.

   Tuberculosis of the spine (Pott's disease) is rare in developed counties. The disease has a more indolent course and less dramatic symptomatology than is seen with pyogenic infection. Long-term antimicrobial therapy is required in all types of osteomyelitis.

   Epidural spinal abscess can also appear with back pain. The origin of the infection is usually pelvic inflammatory disease. Signs of generalized infection and spinal cord findings are often early features.

5 *Neoplasm*
As with infection, the principal symptom is progressive, unremitting pain that is unrelieved by position change. Cramps of pain are common, and sudden exacerbations of the pain will occur with vertebral collapse. Scoliosis is often present. In young patients with back pain and scoliosis, tumor must always be ruled out. Fortunately, if discovered, most tumors are benign in young patients.

Continued.

BOX 19-4—cont'd

a *Multiple myeloma (plasmacytoma).* This is a common spine tumor. It is usually seen in males past the age of 50. There is often evidence of constitutional symptoms such as malaise and weight loss. The erythrocyte sedimentation rate is often increased, as are calcium, alkaline phosphatase, and uric acid. Bence Jones (light-chain) protein is seen in the urine on immunoelectrophoresis, serum electrophoresis often shows an increased globulin with an "M" spike, and immunoelectrophoresis shows an increase in light chain immunoglobulins.

b *Metastatic.* The spine is the most common site for skeletal metastasis. Roentgenographic findings are late because 30% of the vertebral mass must be destroyed before it is evident on plain roentgenography. Bone scan and MRI are more effective diagnostic tests. Metastatic disease can be osteolytic (hypernephroma, thyroid, and large bowel) or osteoblastic (prostate, lung, breast).

c *Intradural extramedullary tumors.* These tumors can also present with back pain (e.g., neurofibroma/schwannoma or meningioma).

6 *Collagen disease*
Ankylosing spondylitis and rheumatoid arthritis are both known to produce considerable back pain. Ankylosing spondylitis (predominantly males) commonly starts in the sacroiliac joints and is a cause of low back pain. Rheumatoid disease (predominantly females) has its most serious complications in the cervical spine where atlantoaxial dislocation can occur. Inflammatory pannus formation anterior to the cervical cord can also act like a mass lesion.

7 *Degenerative disk disease and arthritis of the facet joints*
Degenerative disease of the spine, both cervical and lumbar, is a major cause of back pain. This degeneration is often due to repeated trauma. Pain from disks and facets is not always midline or paraspinous; it can be referred to the hip (medial and lateral) and even to the anterior thigh.

8 *Hip or bursa pain*
If pain is much worse when the patient is lying on one side and radiates into thigh and calf, the clinician should carefully examine the hip; the patient may have a trochanteric bursitis. Also, if pain is much worse when walking, there is possibility of primary hip joint disease.

9 *Psychogenic back pain*
This diagnosis is suggested if there are no mechanical or neurologic (radiculopathy, myelopathy) signs. This is a complex problem and usually is associated with trauma.

BOX 19-5

1 Spine roentgenograms

2 Bone scan, especially in nontraumatic progressive pain

3 Erythrocyte sedimentation rate, collagen evaluation and rheumatoid factor, alkaline phosphatase, acid phosphatase (male), phosphate, calcium ions, fasting blood sugar, uric acid, serum electrophoresis, and immunoelectrophoresis

4 Urinalysis with immunoelectrophoresis if in an older patient

5 Selected cardiac, gastrointestinal, or pelvic studies as indicated

6 CT/MRI scan of spine

7 Myelogram with CT

ureter can give pain to the inner thigh and groin. Adnexal disease will often produce pelvic pain or anterior high pain from involvement of the femoral nerve in the pelvis. Coronary pain classically produces pain along the inner surface of the left arm.

Patients with symptoms of root disease can also have back pain and symptoms of spinal cord disease; thus a careful history and examination should be carried out to differentiate an isolated root lesion from a combined spine, cord, and root lesion. If no cord or spine findings are present, root disease must then be differentiated from peripheral nerve lesions. This task can be very difficult, but with the aid of the outlines in Chapters 1 and 16 plus nerve conduction and electromyographic (EMG) studies, this determination can usually be made. EMG studies, which include paraspinal muscle testing, are very sensitive in detecting nerve root involvement.

Disk Disease

Many conditions can cause root syndromes, but the most common is intervertebral disk disease, either acute herniation or chronic degeneration. In an acute herniation the annulus fibrosus of the disk tears and disk material (soft disk) extrudes either laterally to trap the exiting nerve root or centrally. Central herniation in the cervical region (Figure 19-4) will compromise the spinal cord, whereas in the lumbar area it can affect the lower sacral nerve roots (cauda equina) (Figure 19-5). In cases of chronic degeneration the disks age by becoming dry and less resilient. They flatten and eventually encroach both on the spinal canal and on the neural foramina. Calcium is deposited along their surfaces, and a protruding "hard disk" is formed. In addition to disk degeneration or spondylosis, the facet joints also can become hypertrophic and further compromise both the spinal canal and neural foramina (Figures 19-6 and 19-7). The clinical picture of root disease is similar whether the process is acute or chronic. Following are descriptions of the most common root syndromes. The lower cervical and lower lumbar disks are by far the most frequently involved. In the cervical area the root exits above its corresponding numbered vertebral body. In the lumbar area the root exits below the numbered vertebra. In the lumbar area the root exits quite high on the vertebra so an L4–L5 disk herniation will usually trap the L5 root (see Figure 19-3). Large disk protrusions can damage several roots. On occasion several disks can be involved; this is especially true with degenerative disease where multilevel involvement is common (Table 19-1, p. 596).

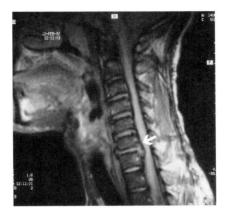

FIGURE 19-4. Lateral MRI of cervical spine demonstrating a herniated disk (*arrow*).

Lumbar Stenosis

In the lumbar area progressive hypertrophy of the facets and degeneration of disks can give rise to severe root encroachment at multiple levels (Figure 19-8). This condition, often referred to as lumbar stenosis, produces bilateral root symptoms in L4, L5, and S1 nerves. With extensive degeneration or multiple traumas the spine can also become unstable. With forward flexion one vertebra can ride forward over the one below then slip back with extension of the back. This retrolisthesis accentuates the spinal stenosis. In conjunction with their multiple root problems, these patients also experience a curious symptom often called lumbar claudication. When they walk or stand for a long time, they begin to develop pain and heaviness proximally in their legs. Paresthesias and

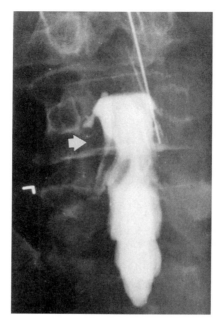

FIGURE 19-5. Lumbar myelogram demonstrating a herniated lumbar disk (*arrow*).

weakness follow if they cannot rest. These symptoms are due to the irritation of the roots because they are rubbed over the spinal spurs. Symptoms can also arise when the patient lies down. Antiinflammatory medications can help, but many of these patients require surgery to relieve their symptoms. Full evaluation including electromyography, flexion and extension lateral lumbar x-rays with the patient standing up (weight-bearing), and metabolic evaluation should

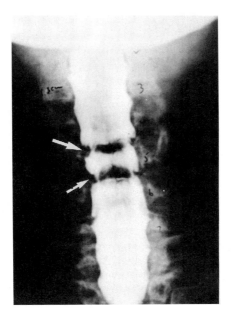

FIGURE 19-6. Anteroposterior view of cervical myelogram demonstrating cervical spondylosis. The impingement on the roots laterally (*arrows*) is demonstrated. The lack of contrast shadow in the center of the white contrast column indicates pressure from the disk anteriorly.

be carried out. Amyotrophic lateral sclerosis or peripheral neuropathy can mimic lumbar stenosis and must be included in the differential diagnosis in a patient with multiple radiculopathies.

Cauda Equina Syndrome

Cauda equina syndrome consists of damage to the roots of the sacral plexus. The cause can be an extruded central disk (as high as L1–L2 or, if very

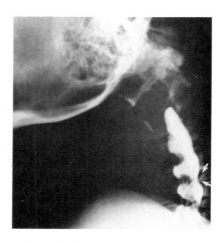

FIGURE 19-7. Lateral view of cervical myelogram demonstrating cervical spondylosis. The posterior protrusion of the calcified disk (*arrows*) is shown.

large, at L5–S1), tumor of the filum terminale (ependymoma), lipoma (common with spina bifida or other dorsal defects), or other masses in the lower lumbar canal. Clinical features are bowel and bladder incontinence, numbness in the perianal region, occasionally pelvic or buttock pain, and if the S1 root is involved, calf and leg weakness. On examination, the anus is atonic, sensation in the S2–S5 (perianal) region is decreased, and ankle jerks can be diminished.

Sciatica

Sciatica, or pain down the back of the leg, is another common yet multifaceted syndrome affecting the sci-

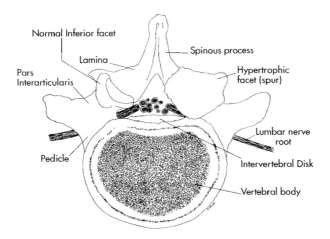

FIGURE 19-8. Superior view of a lower lumbar vertebral body at the level of the cauda equina. The facet at the left is normal, but the one on the right shows evidence of severe hypertrophic degenerative change. Note how this traps the nerve root exiting at that level. The disk below also shows evidence of degeneration and is encroaching on the spinal canal anteriorly.

atic nerve and its contributing roots. The differential diagnosis includes disk disease, tumor of roots, pelvic tumors or masses, spine disease in L5–S1, inflammatory disease in the pelvis, endometriosis, adnexal masses, sarcoma at the head of the femur, vascular malformation in the cord, or spasm of the pyriformis muscle.

Other Isolated Root Syndromes

Although disk disease is the most common cause of root symptoms, many other diseases must be considered in the differential diagnosis. Neurofibromas or schwannomas are not rare and are often multiple.

TABLE 19-1 Clinical Features of Major Radicular Symptoms

Root	Pain	Sensory Loss
C5	Neck, shoulder, and upper arm	Over deltoid
C6	Neck and arm to the thumb	Thumb pad and index finger
C7	Lateral arm to middle finger	Middle finger
C8	Lateral arm into little finger	Little finger
L4	Anterior thigh	Anteromedial thigh and knee
L5*	Lateral leg and lateral foot	Lateral leg and web of great toe
S1*	Back of leg to heel	Back to calf and lateral heel

*An L5 and S1 lesion can give a completely flail foot with the expected sensory changes.

Cysts of the root sleeves, although usually asymptomatic, can occasionally give rise to root symptoms, other tumors of the cord, vascular malformations, epidural abscess, vertebral disease with collapse (back pain usually prominent), and retroperitoneal or paravertebral tumors (primary or metastatic).

Evaluation

Box 19-6 shows the clinical and neurodiagnostic tests used to evaluate radiculopathy (nerve root disease).

Weakness	Reflex Diminished
Deltoid and external rotators of shoulders	None or partial biceps
Biceps and brachioradialis	Biceps
Triceps	Triceps
Intrinsic hand muscles	None
Quadriceps	Knee jerk
Dorsiflexion of great toe	None
Plantar flexion of foot and great toe (can be earliest sign)	Ankle jerk

Spinal Cord Lesions

The principal constituents of the spinal cord are the descending motor and autonomic fibers, ascending sensory fibers, the lower motor neurons (anterior horn cells), and the cell bodies of both the sympathetic chain and the spinothalamic sensory system. Disease of the cord or pressure on it from an external lesion can produce symptoms in one or more of the functions subserved by these elements. The neurologic deficit is frequently bilateral and produces symptoms only distal (caudal) to the lesion. *Myelopathy* is the general term for spinal cord dysfunction (Box 19-7).

BOX 19-6

1 Careful physical examination
2 Specific tests to determine which root is involved and the cause
3 Spine roentgenograms
4 Electromyogram
5 CT/MRI of spine
6 Myelography with postmyelogram CT scan

Because there is such a difference in the sense of urgency and also in the differential diagnosis between acute myelopathy and chronic, slowly progressive myelopathy, the two are discussed separately.

Acute Myelopathy

Acute myelopathy is usually vascular, infectious, or demyelinating, although occasionally it is neoplastic. The MRI is the study of choice and should be performed immediately.

Transverse myelitis. Transverse myelitis is an unusual condition that is probably of viral or postinfectious origin. It can also be seen after immunization and in vasculitis such as with systemic lupus. The cord symptoms evolve over 6 to 24 hours and involve motor, sensory, and autonomic functions. The lesion is usually in the upper to midthoracic level. Often an antecedent viral infection is reported. Pain is not prominent. Cerebrospinal fluid usually has some lymphocytes (50 to 200) and often increased protein. Myelin basic protein or oligoclonal bands can be present and suggest multiple sclerosis. An MRI is

BOX 19-7

1 Important symptoms to elicit during the history of patients suspected of having spinal cord disease:

   a *Speed of development of symptoms.* A rapidly progressing cord lesion (hours to days) is a true emergency. If cord function, particularly bowel and bladder control, is severely compromised for more than 24 hours from pressure, functional recovery is poor.

   b A level of dysfunction above which there are no symptoms but below which bilateral symptoms are present. Sensory symptoms are often vague and changing.

   c *Bowel, bladder, and sexual dysfunction.* The bladder is often "spastic" with low capacity and frequent spontaneous emptying. Clinically this can first appear as frequency and urgency, but soon incontinence is experienced.

   d *Back pain.*

   e *Root symptoms.*

   f *Absence of cranial nerve symptoms.*

   g *Family history of spinal cord disease.*

   h *General medical history:* Diabetes, stomach disease or surgery (possible vitamin B_{12} deficiency), atherosclerotic vascular disease, collagen disease, sarcoid, cancer, AIDS.

   i *Previous or recent trauma.*

2 Examination to establish both presence *and* level of spinal cord involvement:

   a *Cranial nerve examination.* This should be normal in isolated cord disease. In amyotrophic lateral sclerosis the patient can demonstrate spinal cord (anterior horn cell/motor neuron) signs plus cranial motor signs.

   b *Motor examination.* This should show decreased motor control, spastic gait, and hyperreflexia below the lesion (if a cervical cord lesion is suspected, check jaw jerk; if this is hyperactive the lesion can be above the pons) with clonus and pathologic reflexes.

   c *Sensory level.* Carefully examine for a sensory level (not always present, especially with intrinsic [intramedullary] tumors).

   d *Anal tone.*

   e *Inspection of back.* Examine back for tenderness, spasm, scoliosis, birthmarks, midline dimples, or hair patches.

almost always negative, although occasionally it shows a swollen cord with an increased signal on T2 at the level of the disease. The prognosis is variable. If recovery is to occur, improvement is usually seen in 3 to 4 weeks.

Epidural abscess. Patients with a spinal abscess usually have constitutional signs of infectious disease. Cutaneous and pelvic infections are frequent sites of origin. Neurologic signs evolve over one to several days. Focal, localizing back pain and spine tenderness are present and usually marked. There are usually rapidly evolving motor, sensory, and autonomic signs to indicate spinal cord compression. Cells are present in the cerebrospinal fluid, and the protein level is markedly elevated (particularly if a block exists).

Spinal cord tumors. Spinal cord tumors usually progress over weeks to months but can occasionally cause acute cord decompensation (malignant lesions such as metastases, lymphoma). Back and radiating root pain are often present in extramedullary tumors. There is no history of antecedent illness unless the tumor is metastatic or multifocal such as lymphoma.

Vascular Lesions

The following describes what happens with various vascular lesions:

- *Arteriovenous malformations.* When arteriovenous malformations rupture, the patient experiences sudden back pain, root pain at the level of the lesion, and cord symptoms. The neck is often stiff. Neurologic findings can be varied and often only involve partial cord ischemia (hemicord or anterior spinal/artery syndrome).

- *Spinal cord stroke.* Spinal cord strokes are rare but can be found in patients with severe aortic atherosclerosis or small vessel disease such as systemic lupus or diabetes. These disorders usually affect the anterior spinal artery and give the typical picture of arm flaccidity and leg spasticity (central cord syndrome).

- *Cord ischemia with a dissecting aortic aneurysm or after aortic aneurysm surgery.*

Acute cervical disk. An acute cervical disk is almost always seen with significant neck trauma and does not pose any diagnostic problem.

Collapse of diseased vertebrae. Vertebrae that have been weakened by osteoporosis, infection, or metastatic cancer can suddenly collapse and cause spinal cord compression. Back pain and root symptoms are also present. Myelopathy can be present as well.

Chronic Progressive Myelopathy

Cervical spondylosis (neurologic manifestations of radiculopathy or myelopathy as a result of arthritis of any cause) or degenerative disk disease. A degenerative disk can encroach on the spinal canal and press or rub on the cord; this process produces cord damage by direct pressure or ischemia secondary to pressure on the cord blood supply. The most common levels of the cord to be affected are C5–6 and C6–7. The clinical syndrome consists of progressive spasticity in the legs and frequently root symptoms in the hands with weakness, atrophy, and sensory loss. Complaints of arm and neck pain can also be present. Such patients are very vulnerable to forceful or prolonged neck extension, and neck trauma is poorly tolerated.

Treatment can be surgical with removal of the disk anteriorly or decompression posteriorly. Some return of function can be seen, although full restoration is not expected. Use conservative therapy with bed rest and intermittent cervical traction; antiinflammatory drugs can also be used.

Tumor. Fifteen percent of all tumors of the central nervous system occur in the spinal cord or spinal canal (see Chapter 15). Extramedullary (arising from tissue within the spinal canal but not in the spinal cord itself) tumors are the most frequent, with metastatic tumor being the most common, followed by schwannoma and meningioma. Intrinsic cord tumors (gliomas, sarcomas, lipomas) are less common. Most metastatic tumors spread to the bony spine, although some are epidural or intrinsic in the cord. Clinically there is usually a slowly progressive, often asymmetric spasticity with sensory loss below the level of the lesion. Bowel and bladder symptoms are often late to appear. Radicular pain and sensory

TABLE 19-2 **Signs and Symptoms of Intraspinal Tumors**

Signs and Symptoms	Extramedullary Tumors
Spontaneous pain	Radicular and early
Sensory changes	Brown-Séquard type or sharp sensory level distal to lesion
Anterior horn cell findings	Segmental pattern of atrophy and weakness
Paresis	Prominent and early
Hyperreflexia	Prominent and early
Babinski's sign	Unilateral or bilateral
Trophic changes	Mild
Spinal subarachnoid block and changes in cerebrospinal fluid (increased protein)	Early and marked

loss are common, particularly in the extramedullary tumors (Table 19-2). Mild to moderate back pain is often present and can precede neurologic symptoms. Pain is increased when lying down because of blockage of venous and CSF flow by the tumor.

Multiple sclerosis. Multiple sclerosis can present as an acute transverse myelopathy, but a considerable number of multiple sclerosis patients, particularly those with middle-age onset, experience a progressive myelopathy without a history of remissions and exacerbations. If the MRI is negative, the physician should obtain cerebrospinal fluid for special immunologic studies, oligoclonal bands, and increased immunoglobulin production in CSF because at least 50% of unexplained progressive myelopathy is due to demyelinating disease.

Intramedullary Tumors

Burning, poorly localized

Dissociation of sensation, "spotty" changes

Marked and widespread with atrophy and fasciculations

Moderate and late

Moderate and late

May not be present until late

Marked

Late and mild

Amyotrophic lateral sclerosis. Amyotrophic lateral sclerosis is a fairly common neurologic disease of middle-age that can often present primarily with spasticity and lower motor neuron findings but without sensory change. Early cases occasionally show a rather definite asymmetry.

Subacute combined degeneration. Subacute combined degeneration is the result of vitamin B_{12} deficiency. The condition can appear without evidence of pernicious anemia, although this is not common. Spasticity with loss of position and vibratory sense is the hallmark of the disease. Bowel and bladder findings are often present, with the loss of tone being the principal feature. At times diffuse paresthesias with signs of neuropathy can herald the onset.

Tabes dorsalis. Although uncommon, the late complications of parenchymatous syphilis must always be considered. Appropriate studies to rule out syphilis should be obtained on examination of the cerebrospinal fluid on any patient with spinal cord disease and a positive FTA-ABS in the serum.

Other medical disease. Systemic lupus erythematosus, sarcoid, cryptococcal meningitis, sickle cell disease, and other disorders can appear either as an acute or chronic myelopathy.

Syringomyelia. Syringomyelia is an interesting condition in which long cystic cavities are present within the spinal cord. The cavity, or syrinx, is usually in the cervical cord but can extend through the lumbar region. It is believed to be a nonobliterated and expanded central canal. In some cases the syrinx is part of a cystic astrocytoma of the cord or can be a late development after cord trauma. Symptoms can be asymmetrical, symmetrical, or strictly unilateral. Spasticity is present below the lesion. At the level of the syrinx there is segmental loss of pain and temperature with preservation of touch (sensory dissociation); this often produces insensitive hands that are subjected to repeated trauma and burns. Radicular pain is sometimes present. Posterior column sensation is usually spared. Scoliosis is often present, and fasciculations and atrophy can be seen at the level of the lesion.

Congenital lesions. Congenital lesions are usually noted in childhood, particularly meningomyelocele and diastematomyelia. Occasionally lipomas associated with spina bifida can show up in adulthood. A cutaneous lesion (dimple, sinus tract, hair patch) is often noted on the overlying skin.

Familial spinal and spinocerebellar degenerations. Familial spinal and spinocerebellar degenerations are rare diseases that usually appear in childhood with gait abnormalities. Familial spastic paraplegia and Friedreich's ataxia are two examples. Onset of Friedreich's ataxia is usually in later childhood, with slurred speech, a high-arched instep, and scoliosis, as well as spinal cord and cerebellar findings.

Radiation myelopathy. Progressive cord symptoms can appear 6 to 12 months after irradiation that includes the spinal cord.

Vertebral junctional abnormalities. Vertebral junctional abnormalities (Arnold-Chiari malformations, foramen magnum meningiomas, and congenital bony abnormalities of the upper cervical vertebrae) produce bilateral limb findings and lower cranial nerve findings. MRI is certainly the first-choice procedure when these lesions are suspected.

Parasagittal meningioma. Occasional parasagittal tumors will produce bilateral leg spasticity with bladder symptoms. This should be considered when a routine spine evaluation is negative.

Evaluation Summary for Spinal Cord Disease can be seen in Box 19-8.

Spinal Trauma

Forceful extension, flexion, or rotation of the spine will often result in damage to the disks, vertebrae, or the muscular and ligamentous supporting soft tissues of the spinal column. The lumbar and cervical vertebrae are the most frequently affected, and the severity of the clinical symptoms is usually but not always related to the violence of the trauma. Lifting a piece of furniture can cause mild back pain from over-stretching the ligaments, whereas an accident on a motorcycle can cause tearing of ligaments, disloca-

---

 BOX 19-8

1 Vitamin B_{12} level and complete blood cell count

2 VDRL (serum and cerebrospinal fluid)

3 Plain spine roentgenograms often helpful

4 MRI scan of spine

5 Extensive cerebrospinal fluid analysis (cell count; protein; sugar; VDRL; cultures and staining for bacteria, fungus, *Mycobacterium tuberculosis* and *Cryptococcus;* quantitative immunoglobulin and oligoclonal bands; and one tube for special study) if infection or multiple sclerosis is suspected

6 Possibly electromyography if root symptoms are prominent or amyotrophic lateral sclerosis is suggested

7 Myelography with CT in selected cases after consultation with a neurosurgeon

8 Possibly CT brain scan

9 Bone scan

10 Spinal angiography if a vascular lesion is suggested

tion of the cervical vertebrae, rupture of the disks, and severe spinal cord injury.

Severe Cervical Injuries

Most neck injury is due to hyperextension or rotation of the neck. Hyperflexion is prevented by the chin hitting the chest, and excessive lateral motion is restricted by the shoulders. With rapid violent hyperextension the anterior spinal ligament is stretched and can tear. The posterior spinal ligament is weak, and pressure on the disk during hyperextension can cause the disk to herniate posteriorly in the midline thus impinging on the spinal cord. Facets can fracture and cause dislocation, hemorrhage can occur under either anterior or posterior ligaments and supporting ligaments, and muscles can be torn or stretched. Vertebral bodies can sublux (slide over each other—dislocate) and, particularly in children, return to normal position. In severe injury the spinal cord is damaged by pressure from an extruded disk, a blow to the actual cord during dislocation (this causes contusion or hemorrhage), and infarction secondary to damage to the cord vessels. In very violent cervical trauma, evulsion of the medullopontine junction can occur. If this occurs, death is instantaneous. Elderly persons are especially vulnerable to extension injuries because chronic disk degeneration and facet overgrowth have reduced the diameter of the spinal canal (spinal stenosis), leaving the cord very little room for displacement during neck movement. With trauma spinal cord compression can rapidly develop.

The acute cervical injury must be very carefully managed. Usually any spinal cord damage has occurred with the initial trauma, *but* 5% to 10% of the patients with cord damage from trauma have had neurologic symptoms appear or significantly worsen after the accident because of improper handling. In some cases facets have been fractured and the spine rendered unstable, but the cord remains intact. Delayed neurologic deficits are usually attributed to the failure to those handling the patient to appreciate and protect the unstable neck.

Steps in Acute Management are listed in Box 19-9.

The long-term management of spinal cord injury patients is a complex rehabilitation effort that can take many months or even years before the patient achieves his or her final functional level.

 BOX 19-9

1 Make sure that the neck is not allowed to move when the patient is moved. Tape the head to a board or sandbag the sides.

2 Perform a rapid physical examination to assess adequacy of respiration and extent of chest, abdominal, and other injuries. Quickly decide if major spinal cord damage is present based on motor, sensory, and autonomic deficit.

3 If respiratory distress is present, establish an airway. Tracheostomy or a nasal endotracheal tube is preferable to minimize neck extension. Respiratory problems are the most common cause of death in cervical cord injury. In cord injury below C4 the diaphragm will be the only respiratory muscle. In high cord injuries all respiratory muscles are paralyzed.

4 If cord damage is present, pass a nasogastric tube (paralytic ileus and abdominal distention are common).

5 Insert an indwelling urinary catheter.

6 Check vital signs and correct hypovolemic shock if present.

7 Perform a brief neurologic examination without unnecessary neck manipulation, which could potentially worsen a

BOX 19-9–cont'd

neurologic deficit. Any sign of retained function is a good sign prognostically. Assess for possible accompanying signs of head injury.

8 High-dose steroids can decrease cord swelling and minimize the damage.

Syndromes. In general, the motor defects in the acute stage of cord trauma (spinal shock) are characterized by flaccid paralysis and absent reflexes. In time, which is quite variable, tone and reflexes increase. In the chronic stage of quadriplegia, spasticity is often marked, and spontaneous flexor spasms are seen.

a *Complete cord transection.* No motor or sensory function remaining. Such patients can have hypotension, bradycardia, and paralytic ileus secondary to paralysis of the sympathetic outflow. They will not be cool and clammy like the patient with hypovolemic shock.

b *Central cord syndrome.* Arms much weaker than legs; this disparity occurs for two reasons: (1) the anterior horns in the cervical cord may be damaged thus destroying the motor neurons to the cervical roots, and/or (2) the corticospinal tracts to the legs are lateral and escaped damage from central cord trauma. Pain sensation to the sacral area is spared (sacral pain fibers lay laterally in the cord), and the posterior column sensations of proprioception and vibration are intact.

c *Hemicord, or Brown-Séquard syndrome.* With one half of the cord damaged, motor control and proprioception are absent ipsilateral to the lesion, and pain and temperature sensation are absent distal to the lesion on the side of the body contralateral to the lesion. This lesion has the best prognosis.

9 Neurosurgical consultation and spine roentgenograms are usually advisable. In patients with a spinal cord injury or possibly an unstable spine, it is advisable to have the neurosurgeon present before moving the patient to the radiology department. Roentgenograms should include adequate visualization of *all* cervical vertebrae.

10 Frequent reevaluation is necessary. A progressive deficit can indicate a developing hematoma within the spinal ligaments, and prompt surgical exploration can be necessary.

Benign Cervical Injury (Whiplash)

If no signs of spinal cord or root damage are present and cervical roentgenograms are negative, the cervical injury is diagnosed as a cervical strain or sprain. This is largely a soft tissue injury that is similar in many ways to sprain anywhere else in the body. Symptoms can be present directly after the injury or be delayed for several days. The principal symptom of a whiplash injury is posterior neck pain and spasm. The pain can radiate to the occiput and over the head or down into the shoulders and between the shoulder blades. This shoulder pain is usually referred pain from the spinal ligaments and is not a result of C5 nerve root impingement. Neck motion is painful. In the first week the anterior neck muscles will also be sore, but this usually heals quickly.

The examination of these patients should be guided toward identifying any root or subtle cord symptoms before instituting conservative management. Some false root signs, especially C8, can be seen with spasm of the anterior scalenus muscle, so it is important to assess the patient carefully before considering MRI. Listed below are nine management steps.

Management

- *Rest.* In severe injury 2 to 3 weeks rest can be necessary. If significant pain is present after 24 hours the patient should stay in bed at least 1 week.
- *Soft collar.* Wear a soft collar 24 hours per day for 2 to 3 weeks then intermittently for 4 to 6 weeks in serious injury. The collar should allow slight neck flexion and prevent extension.
- *Medications.* Muscle relaxants, sedation, analgesics, and antiinflammatory medicines are all useful in the first several weeks.

- *Heat and light massage.*
- *Activity Restrictions.*
  - Avoid neck extension (reaching above head and looking up).
  - Sleep on the side—*never on the face*—in bed at least 10 hours a day.
  - Avoid riding in a car as much as possible.
  - Avoid emotional tension; the symptoms of tension headache will markedly increase symptoms in the neck.
- *Cervical traction* (head slightly flexed). Traction can be used if it relieves symptoms.

Pain and neck stiffness can be prolonged for many months. Physical exercise or heavy work can exacerbate symptoms. If symptoms are present after 6 weeks, they will probably last 6 months or more; 10% to 15% of patients may be unable to do heavy work for several years.

Anxiety, depression, and anger (against those responsible for the injury) will all exacerbate symptoms. Disputes with employers and receipt of workers' compensation are definitely negative factors in recuperation. Repeated trauma or the effects of degenerative spine disease can result in chronic neck pain. This is best treated conservatively with rest, heat, and medication.

Lumbar Injuries

Low back trauma is quite common and is a major source of aggravation and disability yet does not hold the serious threat to neurologic function that is present with cervical trauma. Most low back injuries are the result of falls, improper or excessive lifting, or a sudden twisting motion. Often the initial insult can be as innocent as getting out of bed or mopping the floor.

The mechanism of low back injury involves three elements: (1) tearing or pulling ligaments and muscle insertions; (2) damage to the annulous fibrosus of disk with subsequent herniation of the nucleus pulposus (ruptured or "slipped" disk); and (3) strain on the posterior (facet) joints. The last mechanism is more common in older persons. Damage in the sacroiliac joint is very rare and usually is only seen with violent pelvic trauma.

The major symptom of a low back injury is pain; however, in disk herniation the major symptom can be that of root impingement. The most common disks to herniate are those between L4–L5 and L5–S1. The spinal cord ends at the L1 or L2 level so the cord is not involved. On occasion a disk will extrude centrally in the upper lumbar region and press on the cauda equina, thus producing bowel and bladder symptoms.

When taking a history from a patient with a low back injury, the symptoms listed in Box 19-10 should be explored.

The examination of the low back has many of the same aspects as that of any back examination: inspection—look for spasm, observe motion, perform a neurologic examination with careful examination for root lesion, and do a rectal examination.

The initial management of lumbosacral injury consists of lumbar spine films and then the following:

- Bed rest: Supine or on side with legs flexed, firm mattress, getting up only to go to the bathroom. *Never lie on the stomach!* The length of bed rest is determined by the severity of injury, and 2 weeks is usually necessary in serious cases.

- Sedation, analgesics, heat, antiinflammatory medications, and muscle relaxants as outlined under cervical injury previously. Pelvic traction is of little use except that it enforces bedrest.

BOX 19-10

1 *Location and character of the pain.*

2 *Radiation.* With acute root impingement, paresthesias or lightninglike pain will be present in individual root distributions. Constant aching pain only appears with time. This chronic steady pain is from the root irritation and inflammation that occurs as the nerve root is rubbed over the disk fragment or facet spur. An actual chemical irritation from the extruded disk material can be a factor in producing root pain.

Irritation of pain fibers in the lumbosacral *ligaments* will often cause radiating pain into sacroiliac region. On occasion, ligament pain can mimic root pain and radiate into hip (to stimulate primary hip joint disease) and, at times, down the sciatic distribution to the calf.

3 *Effect of motion or rest on the symptoms.* Sitting, getting up, and rapid movement usually aggravate the symptoms, whereas rest—and often standing—can relieve them. The most comfortable position is lying on the side with legs flexed (this is usually not the case in destructive disease of the vertebrae).

4 *Effect of cough or sneeze.* With a herniated disk these events will often produce radiating pain.

5 *Weakness.* The patient is asked about specific muscles or actions.

6 *Sensory symptoms.* Numbness, paresthesias, or other strange feelings in legs can be present without objective sensory loss.

7 *Bowel or bladder function.* The examiner should ask about subtle changes as well as gross features such as incontinence or retention.

- Surgery should be considered acutely in the following cases: bowel or bladder dysfunction, weakness of the muscle groups supplied by one or two nerve roots (10% of lumbar disk herniations involve two disks), a progressing neurologic deficit, and unrelenting root pain (several weeks).

A decreased reflex or dermatomal sensory signs or symptoms are not sufficient grounds for surgery. Of all acute lumbar disk lesions, 80% can be successfully managed conservatively. After the first 2 weeks of bed rest, medications are gradually reduced and ambulation is increased. A corset is often useful for 2 to 4 weeks in some patients, especially the obese or elderly. Chronic corseting is deleterious because it serves to weaken the back and abdominal muscles.

When fully ambulatory, the patient should follow the regimen described in Box 19-11 (most of these suggestions are designed to decrease the load on the lumbar spine).

Unfortunately reinjury and prolonged low back symptoms often produce a chronic condition. Conservative management with each attack is preferable, but if chronic root pain or root symptoms persist and are not relieved by rest and medication, electromyography (not abnormal until three weeks after acute lesions) and a spinal MRI scan should be obtained. Back pain alone is not reason enough to undertake surgery; root disease is. A significant percentage of patients with chronic root complaints are helped with surgery, but the selection of surgical candidates must be careful.

Chronic low back pain from repeated lumbosacral strain has many ramifications. Over time facet joints hypertrophy and degenerative disks develop spurs along their edges. This process of degeneration can lead to spinal (lumbar) stenosis. Such patients develop lumbar claudication (paresthesias and weakness when walking) and progressive often bilateral radiculopathy L4, L5, and S1. Plantar extension and flexion of the feet is decreased, reflexes are reduced, and distal sensory loss is seen.

BOX 19-11

1 If obese, lose weight. Excessive abdominal weight forces a lordotic posture that extends the spine and produces pain and root compromise.

2 Do not bend at the waist to lift; use the legs.

3 When standing, try to keep pelvis tilted slightly forward (putting one foot up will help).

4 When sitting, do not sit upright in military posture, sit partially forward on seat and slightly flex lumbar spine.

5 Sleep on side in firm bed with legs flexed.

6 Do regular exercise to strengthen abdominal muscles and stretch extensors of spine. Refer to Williams' textbook (see References) or discuss with a physical therapist or a physician in rehabilitation medicine. A sensible exercise program is the only proven regimen that will help prevent reoccurrence (Lahad et al., 1994).

7 Women should avoid wearing high heels.

Chronic low back pain can also be disabling to a person who does physical labor. Frequently the patient must change jobs to function. Disability claims and legal considerations also become a complicating aspect of the syndrome, and all too often the patient and his or her employer or insurance company enter into an adversary relationship rather than a sympathetic one.

Back pain, as with any chronic pain, can have a strong psychologic component from frank malingering to a minimal psychologic overlay on the real problem. Depression, reversals in personal life, financial hardship, and pending litigation all complicate the resolution of the problem. It is important to monitor pain medication carefully because of the potential for drug addiction. Occasionally a personality test such as the Minnesota Multiphasic Personality Inventory is useful in assessing this aspect of the problems, but it can only serve as a part of the overall evaluation. Each physician must learn to deal with this problem; there are no easy answers or dogmatic rules. Be sympathetic with the patient, but be aware of the multiple facets that can be present in each case.

 SUMMARY

Disease of the spine includes the spinal cord, nerve roots, and the supporting bony and soft tissues. Many clinical syndromes involve the spine, and most can be easily diagnosed by the history and physical examination. Judicious use of the newer imaging techniques, particularly MRI, have made it possible to diagnose such conditions as intervertebral disk disease and spinal cord tumor much more accurately and with less morbidity. Spine injury remains a common and frequently disabling symptom for which definitive treatment is lacking.

Suggested Readings

Lesions of Spine and Spinal Cord (Chapter 19)

Kelm HA, Kirkaldy-Willis WH: *Low back pain,* Ciba Found Symp, 1980.

Macnab I: *Backache,* Baltimore, 1977, Williams & Wilkins.

Rothman RH, Simeone FA: *The spine,* vols 1 and 2, Philadelphia, 1975, WB Saunders.

Van Gilder JC, Menezes AH, Dolan KO: *The craniovertebral junction and its abnormalities,* Mount Kisco, NY, 1987, Futura Publishing.

Vinken PJ, Bruyn GW: *Handbook of clinical neurology,* vols 25 and 26, Injuries of the Spine and Spinal Cord I and II, Amsterdam, 1976, North-Holland Publishing.

Williams PC: *The lumbosacral spine,* New York, 1965, McGraw-Hill.

Cervical Spine Conditions

Braakman R: Management of cervical spondylitic myelopathy and radiculopathy, *J Neur Neurosurg Psychiatry* 57:257, 1994.

Rowland LP: Surgical treatment of cervical spondylitic myelopathy: time for a controlled trial, *Neurology* 42:5, 1992.

Yoss RE, Corbin KB, Mac Carty CS: Significance of symptoms and signs in localization of involved root in cervical disc protrusion, *Neurology* 7:673, 1975.

Lumbar Abnormalities

Ellenberger C, Jr: MR imaging of the low back syndrome, *Neurology* 44:594, 1994.

Frymoyer JW: Back pain and sciatica, *N Engl J Med* 318:291, 1988.

Hall S, Bartelson JD, Onofrio BM: Lumbar spinal stenosis, *Ann Intern Med* 103:271, 1985.

Jensen MC, Brant-Zawadzki MN, Obuchowski N: Magnetic resonance imaging of lumbar spine in people without back pain, *N Engl J Med* 331:69, 1994.

Lahad A, et al: The effectiveness of four interventions for the prevention of low back pain, *JAMA* 272:1286, 1994.

Mixter WJ, Barr JS: Rupture of the intervertebral disc with involvement of the spinal canal, 211:210, 1934.

Spinal Injuries

Bracken MB: Randomized controlled study of methlyprednisolone or naloxone in treatment of acute spinal cord injury, *N Engl J Med* 322:1405, 1990.

Ditunno JF, Formal CS: Chronic spinal cord injury, *N Engl J Med* 330:550, 1994.

Spinal Cord Neoplasm

Bryne TN: Spinal cord compression from epidural metastases, *N Engl J Med* 327:614, 1992.

Koppel BS, Tuchman AJ, Mangiardi JR: Epidural spinal infection in intravenous drug abusers, *Arch Neurol* 45:1331, 1988.

Vermer EF, Musher DM: Spinal epidural abscess, *Med Clin North Am* 69:375, 1985.

Abnormal Involuntary Movement Disorders (Dyskinesias)

20

bnormal involuntary movement disorders are defined as orofacial, head, trunk, and extremity movements that can sometimes be modified but not abolished by the patient. These are superimposed on normal motor patterns and can interfere with coordinated voluntary motor activities and posture maintenance. The dyskinesias are usually classified as extrapyramidal. In certain disorders major biochemical and pathologic disturbances have been shown to occur in the basal ganglia; however, despite recent advances, the exact pathophysiology and neuropharmacology of the dyskinesias remain poorly understood.

The patient's motor function should be carefully characterized as he or she walks into the room, sits in the chair, and talks with the examiner. Special attention should be directed toward the following:

- Body and neck posture
- Gait
- Facial expression
- Speech

- Handwriting and ability to draw an Archimedes spiral (a circle of progressively increasing diameter)
- Muscle tone
- Posture of outstretched hands
- Performance of rapid successive and alternating movements

The dyskinesias are carefully analyzed for the following:

Occurrence. Resting state, posture maintenance, voluntary movements.

Morphology. Rhythmic or nonrhythmic, stereotyped or random, simple or complex, nonpurposeful or semipurposeful.

Distribution. Trunk, neck, face, extremities (proximal or distal, unilateral or bilateral).

Velocity and duration. Rapid or slow, brief or prolonged, spasmodic or persistent.

Relation to and possible interference with purposeful motor activities.

Modifying factors. Sleep, distraction, anxiety, alcohol, medications.

In assessing possible causes it is important to determine age at onset, rate of progression, family history, prior medication history, toxic exposure, and medical illnesses. Onset in infancy is suggestive of cerebral palsy, and those disorders initially developing in childhood or adolescence can be related to rheumatic fever, Wilson's disease, or dystonia musculorum deformans. Dyskinesias developing later in life can be of degenerative (Huntington's disease, Parkinson's disease), vascular, neoplastic, or drug-induced etiology. Movement disorders related to vascular disease, rheumatic fever, or medications develop rapidly, and those caused by degenerative disorders or neoplasms develop more slowly. Some disorders show a specific genetic pattern, for example, Huntington's disease. Because certain patients are not aware of the dyskinesias, clinical examination of the entire family is necessary before accepting a negative history. Patients should be questioned for use of medications that can induce dyskinesias (e.g., antipsychotics, phenytoin, oral contraceptives) or the possibility of toxic exposure (e.g., manganese). Certain medical conditions can be associated with dyskinesias (e.g., rheumatic fever, systemic lupus erythematosus, perinatal hypoxia, liver disease).

The characteristics of certain of the abnormal involuntary movements are listed. Although fasciculations are more completely discussed with motor neuron disease and myoclonus with epilepsy, both fasciculations and myoclonus clinically represent abnormal involuntary muscle activity and are described in this section.

▪ FASCICULATIONS

Occurrence. Observed at rest or following extended muscle contraction.

Modifying factors. Exacerbated by anxiety, caffeine, amphetamine, prolonged muscle activity; reduced by rest and sleep.

Characteristics. Rapid, brief, twitchlike muscle contractions of low amplitude and not sufficient to move the joint. No interference with purposeful activity.

Associated findings. "Benign" fasciculations are quite common in normal persons and are most common following extended muscle contraction or during rest. Those caused by motor neuron disease are more prolonged, spread across large portions of the muscle, and can involve the tongue; most important, muscle weakness and wasting accompany the fasciculations.

Etiologic conditions. Motor neuron disease or physiologic state caused by motor neuron fatigue in normal persons.

Biochemical abnormality. Metabolic imbalance of the motor neuron.

Treatment. None; allay anxiety that these disorders are benign and do not represent amyotrophic lateral sclerosis.

▨ MYOCLONUS

Occurrence. Random jerking movements observed in sleep and anxiety states; occur at rest or with voluntary activity in pathologic states including metabolic-electrolyte imbalances.

Modifying factors. Action myoclonus exacerbated by voluntary movement; can persist with sleep.

Characteristics. Rapid, coarse contraction of groups of muscles. There can be nonrhythmic isolated jerking or twitching of a portion of an extremity (finger, wrist, or shoulder), head, trunk, or neck. There can also be prolonged, continuous rhythmic contraction of isolated muscle groups (e.g., palatal myoclonus).

Associated findings. Can be seen in patients with epilepsy. Dementia develops in patients with Creutzfeldt-Jakob disease; spasticity and dementia develop in subacute sclerosing panencephalitis. In postanoxic myoclonus, cerebellar and corticospinal tract signs can be present.

Etiology. Metabolic and toxic encephalopathies (most frequently caused by cerebral hypoxia), Cruetzfeldt-Jakob disease, subacute sclerosing panencephalitis, and epilepsy.

Biochemical abnormality. Reduced cerebrospinal fluid levels of hydroxyindoleacetic acid (serotonin) has been reported in postanoxic myoclonus.

Treatment. Clonazapam, valproic acid (Depakene), and hydroxytryptophan (serotonin precursor).

TIC (HABIT SPASM)

Occurrence. Resting state causing no interference with voluntary movement.

Modifying factors. Exacerbated by anxiety; decreased by sleep and distraction; can be voluntarily stopped for short time periods.

Characteristics. Rapid, stereotyped, random, spasmodic, nonpurposeful movements. These include blinking, shoulder shrugging, facial grimacing, tongue darting or protrusion, coughing, or grunting.

Associated findings. Tics can be single or multiple. Coprolalia (obscene language) or echolalia occur in Tourette's syndrome.

Etiology. Can be of psychogenic origin; multiple tics characterize Tourette's syndrome.

Biochemical abnormality. None known.

Treatment. Good clinical response in Tourette's syndrome to haloperidol; isolated tic does not require treatment.

CHOREA

Occurrence. Resting state with no interference with voluntary activity; movements can appear to simulate semipurposeful activity.

Modifying factors. Exacerbated by anxiety; disappear in sleep.

Characteristics. Rapid coarse, semipurposeful, random, nonrhythmic movements of extremities, trunk, and face.

Associated findings. Dementia in Huntington's disease, carditis in Sydenham's chorea, facial rash in systemic lupus erythematosus, Kayser-Fleischer ring in Wilson's disease.

Etiology. Rheumatic fever, Huntington's disease, drug induced, aging, pregnancy, Wilson's disease, systemic lupus erythematosus.

Biochemical abnormality. In Huntington's disease, there is reduced glutamic acid decarboxylase and gamma-aminobutyric acid (GABA) in the neostriatum.

Treatment. Dopaminergic blocking agents (e.g., haloperidol).

BALLISM

Occurrence. Resting state; can interfere with voluntary movement.

Modifying factors. Same as chorea.

Characteristics. Irregular random and nonrhythmic violent flinging (flail-like) movements usually involving the arm, usually unilateral.

Associated findings. Can occur as isolated finding or as part of stroke syndrome.

Etiology. Focal lesion of the subthalamus (hemorrhage, tumor, infarction).

Biochemical abnormality. None known.

Treatment. Haloperidol and perphenazine; ventrolateral thalamotomy.

ATHETOSIS

Occurrence. Resting state or posture maintenance; can be severe enough to interfere with voluntary movements.

Modifying factors. Same as chorea.

Characteristics. Slow, coarse, irregular, and nonrhythmic writhing movements of the hands, feet, facial, and neck muscles.

Associated findings. Choreiform and dystonic movements.

Etiology. Usually results from peripheral hypoxic-ischemic injury or kernicterus.

Biochemical abnormality. Not known.

Treatment. Dopaminergic agents can be effective.

▨ DYSTONIA

Occurrence. At rest and posture maintenance.

Modifying factors. Exacerbated by anxiety states and disappears during sleep.

Characteristics. Usually slow, but can be more rapid. Coarse, sustained muscle contraction leads to abnormal turning or twisting postures including torticollis (wry neck), writer's cramp (contraction of muscles of fingers and forearm), blepharospasm, or inward turning of the foot (equinovarus deformity).

Associated findings. Contracture of the limb as a result of sustained muscle contraction.

Etiology. Drug induced (antipsychotics, dopaminergic agents), dystonia musculorum deformans, psychogenic conditions.

Biochemical abnormality. None known.

Treatment. Sedation with diazepam or haloperidol; dopaminergic agents have rarely been effective; high-dose anticholinergic agents, anterior cervical root or spinal accessory nerve denervation or local injection with botulinum toxin for spasmodic torticollis.

▨ AKATHISIA

Occurrence. At rest and posture maintenance.

Modifying factors. Exacerbated by anxiety or prolonged immobility.

Characteristics. Inability to sit still with constant body and limb motion.

Associated findings. Bradykinesia and rigidity can be present in parkinsonism. Part of restless leg syndrome in patients on neuroleptic therapy.

Etiology. Antipsychotic drugs.

Biochemical abnormality. Dopamine receptor blockade.

Treatment. Anticholinergics; clonazepam; benzodiazepines; beta-adrenergic antagonists.

■ TREMOR

Occurrence and characteristics. Rhythmic, stereotyped, nonpurposeful movement of group of muscles around a specific axis at fixed velocity and amplitude.

- Slow and coarse pill-rolling *resting* tremor of parkinsonism
- Rapid and fine amplitude *postural* tremor caused by anxiety, metabolic disorders (thyrotoxicosis, alcoholism), and benign essential tremor
- Coarse *intention* tremor of cerebellar disorders

Modifying factors. Exacerbated by anxiety and disappears in sleep; benign essential tremor reduced by alcohol.

Etiology. Resting tremor: parkinsonism. *Postural* tremor: anxiety, thyrotoxicosis, alcoholism, benign essential tremor, cerebellar disease. *Intention* tremor: Wilson's disease, cerebellar disease, medication effect (lithium, valproic acid).

Biochemical abnormality. Resting tremor: dopamine insufficiency in parkinsonism. Not known in other types.

Treatment. Resting tremor: anticholinergic and dopaminergic drugs. *Postural tremor:* diazepam, primidone, and propranolol. *Intention tremor:* No indication has been demonstrated to be effective. Use of weights on wrist may dampen amplitude of tremor.

■ CLINICAL SYNDROMES

Parkinson's Disease

The cardinal findings of parkinsonism include the following:

- Resting tremor, slow (3 to 5 cps) in velocity and coarse in amplitude; initially involves thumb, index, and middle fingers to cause pill-rolling movement

- Rigidity involving extremities, trunk, and neck; there can be superimposed cogwheel quality, which can represent superimposed tremor
- Bradykinesia or hypokinesia, which is most prominent on initiation of motor activity
- Impairment of postural reflexes
- Lack of facial animation or emotion (hypomimia)

This clinical constellation can be due to many different diseases; however, Parkinson's disease (PD) is the most common cause of parkinsonism. PD refers to a chronic progressive neurologic disorder caused by dopamine deficiency and associated with depigmentation within the zona compacta of substantia nigra.

Initial symptoms of PD include insidious onset of tremor, clumsiness, stiffness, or frequent falls. Motor dysfunction can initially be unilateral or asymmetrical. Rarely, patients show gait unsteadiness with no signs of parkinsonism in arms (lower-half syndrome). When only legs are involved and no tremor is present, this clinical pattern can cause diagnostic confusion with other neurologic disorders such as progressive supranuclear palsy.

Some patients seek treatment because of tremors. Tremor can be the source of embarrassment but not functional disability because it is maximal at rest and disappears with limb movement. Other symptoms include poor balance, frequent falls, weakness, aching pains and stiffness (especially in shoulder, neck, and extremities), seborrhea, and sialorrhea. Some PD patients have limb pain that simulates arthritis or peripheral vascular disease; however, careful examination of these patients can show other parkinsonism features.

When the PD patient is asked to arise from a chair, there is initial hesitation and delay. The patient walks stiffly, has stooped posture, and takes small shuffling steps that progressively accelerate to a running pace (festinating gait). Associated swinging arm movements that accompany normal gait are decreased in PD patients. Impaired postural reflexes can be demonstrated by asking the patient to stand with feet together, then applying sudden force to the sternum; patient falls backward en bloc (retropulsion) rather than having the normal response of broadening the base to regain balance. When the trunk or extremities are passively moved, increased resistance (rigidity) is detected. This can be accentuated by having the patient perform rapid successive movements (e.g., opening and closing fists) with one extremity while the physician tests the tone in trunk or other limbs. Handwriting shows tremor, is small in size (micrographia), and is performed slowly. The face lacks animated emotional expression, and drooling is common. Skin is oily as a result of seborrhea. Tapping over the glabella (bridge of nose) produces sustained blinking (Myerson's sign). Impairment of intellectual capabilities or dementia are uncommon in PD; however, mental disturbances simulating frontal lobe dysfunction (slowness to initiate mental tasks) are common.

If parkinsonism occurs in a young patient, Wilson's disease or drug use can be considered although a juvenile form exists. Manganese and N-methyl-4-phenyltetrahydropyridine (MPTP), which is a synthetic meperidine produced by "street chemists" and is toxic to striatal dopaminergic cells, can cause parkinsonian syndrome. Parkinsonism can start unilaterally then later generalize, but in unilateral cases tumors or vascular lesions must be excluded. Patients with benign essential tremor are sometimes initially diagnosed as having parkinsonism; however, the tremor is postural, and there is no rigidity or bradykinesia. Not all patients who shake as a result of tremor suffer from parkinsonism; conversely, not all PD patients have tremor.

Neurologic deficit as a result of PD can remain stable for many years or progress rapidly; most frequently there is slow deterioration over several years to one decade. The initial symptoms are usually unilateral hand tremor with difficulty using limbs as a result of rigidity and bradykinesia. Later these symptoms become generalized. Rigidity and hypokinesia with loss of postural reflexes are major causes of functional disability, whereas tremor causes minimal interference with daily living activities. Symptoms can be ameliorated with medication, but eventually the condition worsens as medication becomes less effective.

Treatment strategies for PD are directed at correcting striatal dopamine insufficiency. It is important to obtain a careful medical history, such as prior use of antipsychotic or antiemetic phenothiazine drugs, possible exposure to neurotoxins (MPTP), or prior viral encephalitis. The neurologic examination is directed toward excluding findings that suggest a multisystem degenerative process such as olivopontocerebellar degeneration, progressive supranuclear palsy, striatonigral degeneration. The CT/MRI excludes normal pressure hydrocephalus, cerebral infarct(s), basal ganglia neoplasm, or subdural hematoma as the cause of parkinsonian syndrome. If the diagnosis of PD is most likely, it should next be determined if the patient shows functional neurologic impairment. For example, a moderate resting hand tremor can be embarrassing to patient but not interfere with hand dexterity, whereas mildly impaired postural reflexes and bradykinesia can cause the patient to fall and be afraid to go out of the house. If there is functional impairment, treatment of PD should be initiated. Eighty to 90% of patients with PD respond to dopaminergic drugs; failure to respond should suggest an alternative diagnosis.

Dopaminergic medication is the most effective treatment. Levodopa in combination with a decarboxylase inhibitor (Sinemet) is usually preferred because the side effect incidence is low. Medication should be taken with food to avoid gastric irritation, nausea, and vomiting. The dosage is increased slowly, for example, every 5 days. When levodopa alone is used, some patients show good clinical response at 2 g daily; others require 8 to 12 g daily. The goal of therapy is to use the lowest possible dosage of levopoda; therefore levodopa alone is rarely used and dopamine–dopamine decarboxylase preparations are preferred.

Because a significant proportion of levodopa is enzymatically decarboxylated peripherally to dopamine (which does not effectively cross the blood-brain barrier) before it reaches the CNS, it is possible to potentiate the effect using a peripheral dopa decarboxylase inhibitor. The addition of a dopa decarboxylase inhibitor has reduced the incidence of nausea and vomiting and orthostatic hypotension, which were much more common with levodopa. Available preparations of decarboxylase inhibitors with levodopa (Sinemet) include doses of 10/100, 25/100, or 25/250. Some patients require 1 to 3 g of levodopa with 100 to 200 mg of decarboxylase inhibitor; however, the dose of levodopa should be kept to 500 to 700 mg to minimize and delay the onset of motor fluctuations that can complicate therapy. Sinemet 25/100 causes minimal nausea and vomiting. If gastrointestinal symptoms persist, hydroxyzine (Vistaril) or trimethobenzamide (Tigan) can be used, but prochlorperazine (Compazine) should be avoided because of its potential to cause parkinsonian side effects. Sinemet is initiated at a low dosage and is increased rapidly; it is initially administered twice per day and can later be increased to four or five times daily. Sinemet is considerably more expensive than levodopa alone; however, less medication is needed. When patients get into difficulty with dyskinesias, a smaller and more frequent dose administration schedule can help.

Potential complications of dopaminergic agents are listed in Box 20-1.

Although peripheral untoward effects are reduced by Sinemet, central untoward effects are not modified. Dyskinesias are initially dose dependent and can be avoided by low doses. With chronic dopaminergic therapy, dyskinesias occur at progressively lower doses. Delirium, confusion, and hallucinations can develop acutely, and their occurrence can require medication discontinuation; thioridazine (Mellaril) or clozapine (Clozaril) should be used because other antipsychotic agents can worsen parkinsonism. The on-off phenomenon is characterized by an abrupt change from good control, alternating with a sudden unexpected return of maximal symptoms, then a return to good control—all within a several-minute interval. It occurs in PD patients receiving longstanding Sinemet therapy who have rapidly fluctuating levodopa blood levels. Motor fluctuations can become more frequent and incapacitating as a result of the medication effect or disease progression. Several strategies have been used to reduce motor fluctuations. These include a low-protein diet (especially limiting protein eaten early in day), use of controlled

BOX 20-1

1 Nausea and vomiting

2 Orthostatic hypotension

3 Cardiac arrhythmias

4 Mental change (e.g., confusion, psychoses, hallucinations, depression)

5 Dyskinesias (chorea, dystonia, buccal-lingual-facial movements)

6 Clinical fluctuations (e.g., early wearing off effect, early morning akinesia, freezing episodes in which the patient suddenly becomes immobile, on-off phenomena that are random, sudden, and unexpected motor fluctuations of good control alternating with sudden development of an inadequate effect)

or sustained release dopaminergic medication (Sinemet CR), shortening the interval between Sinemet doses, and the use of dopamine receptor agonists (bromocriptine [Parlodel], pergolide [Permax]).

Anticholinergic drugs are effective in treating parkinsonism by reducing the striatal cholinergic effect or increasing dopaminergic concentration. Benztropine mesylate (Cogentin) is supplied as 0.5-, 1-, or 2-mg tablets. It has a long half-life and is administered once or twice daily. The starting dosage is 0.5 mg daily; this can be increased to a maximal dosage of 4 mg twice daily. Biperiden (Akineton) is supplied in 2-mg tablets; it has a shorter half-life, and therapy is usually started at 1 mg and increased to 2 mg three times daily. Trihexyphenidyl (Artane) is supplied in 2- and 5-mg tablets; the therapeutic range is quite variable, with the dosage ranging from 1 to

5 mg three times daily. These agents are initiated at low dosages and gradually increased. Anticholinergic drugs are frequently the initial medication for PD patients if symptoms are mild or tremor and mild rigidity are the only abnormalities. These drugs do not improve akinesia or impaired postural reflexes. Side effects include dry mouth, visual blurring, glaucoma, constipation, urinary retention, delirium, and hallucinations. These drugs have been reported to decrease tremor with less effect on rigidity or bradykinesia. Treatment can be initiated with anticholinergic drugs alone or in combination with dopaminergic drugs. If used as combination therapy, the dosage should be lower than if used alone.

Amantadine (Symmetrel) is usually used in combination with dopaminergic drugs to potentiate their effect, but it has little activity when used alone. It appears to enhance dopamine production and release. Toxicity includes depression, delirium, congestive heart failure, orthostatic hypotension, and skin lesions (livedo reticularis). The dosage is usually 100 mg, two or three times daily. It may initially be effective, but with time it becomes less effective.

Initiate treatment with Sinemet using 100 mg of levodopa and 25 mg of decarboxylase inhibitor once daily. The dose is increased slowly every 5 days by one-half tablet. Increases are continued until adequate functional improvement occurs or signs of toxicity develop. Maximal improvement with minimal toxicity occurs within the initial years; however, with increasing time of treatment, drug effectiveness diminishes and drug toxicity increases. As the drug becomes less effective, there are clinical fluctuations in motor function. These include akinetic periods alternating with dyskinesias. Certain fluctuations are related to less degree of effect obtained with same drug amount. These include end-of-dose, morning time akinesia, and wearing-off effect; these can be managed by more frequent administration of the drug. Increasing sensitivity to the dopaminergic medication can cause peak-dose dyskinesia or dystonia. Less predictable and more dangerous to the patient are the "on-off" effect and paroxysmal dyskinesia; these have no relation to the drug administration schedule. These effects can occur without warning and are managed by a lower dose that is administered at more frequent intervals or by the addition of dopamine agonists. Recently controlled-release (CR) levodopa preparations have been introduced. It is believed that more evenly distributed (less fluctuating) dopamine levels are achieved with Sinemet CR and this reduces frequency or severity of motor fluctuations. Sinemet CR (50/200) is usually initiated at a dosage of one-half tablet twice per day. There is less bioavailable levodopa in a controlled-released tablet, and if a patient is switched from regular to Sinemet CR the levodopa amount should be increased by 33%. Also with Sinemet CR it takes longer time for the patient to achieve mobility in the morning and sometimes regular Sinemet is given as morning dose supplementing the CR tablet.

Dopamine agonists directly act on dopamine receptor. Bromocriptine and pergolide are dopamine receptor agonists available for clinical use. These drugs produce fewer dyskinesias than levodopa and have a more prolonged therapeutic effect than Sinemet. The latter effect is useful in combating wearing-off effects; however, neurobehavioral side effects are more common with the dopamine agonist than with Sinemet. Dopamine agonists have prominent vascular (vasoconstrictive) effects. There is controversy as to whether they should be used early in course of PD; however, it is best to use Sinemet initially. Later it is feasible to combine Sinemet with dopamine agonists or use these agents only when clinical fluctuations occur. Initial treatment with bromocriptine is one 1.25-mg tablet twice daily with a gradual increase until clinical effect or toxicity occurs (usually 15 to 30 mg). With pergolide the initial dose can be 0.05 mg, and this is increased to 2 to 6 mg daily.

Treatment with anticholinergic, dopaminergic, or dopamine receptor agonist medication provides symptomatic improvement. Selegiline (Deprenyl, Eldepryl) is a selective monoamine oxidase (MAO) inhibitor that can act as a neuroprotective agent to slow the actual pathologic progression of PD by reducing oxidative stress (antioxidant therapy) within the central nervous system (CNS). Selegiline can reduce levodopa metabolism, increase synaptic dopamine, and prevent free radical formation in brain. The initial dosage is 2.5 mg daily, and this is usually increased to a maximum dosage of 5 mg twice daily. Untoward effects include sleep disturbances, dyskinesias, and behavioral disorders. Because dopamine levels are reduced by 80% when PD patients become initially symptomatic, the dopamine system has already suffered severe damage; therefore Deprenyl can be more effective if preclinical (before motor dysfunction occurs) diagnosis is possible. Unfortunately it is not possible to identify these asymptomatic patients at risk for PD at the present time. Deprenyl should be maximally effective in patients with early parkinsonism. There is some evidence that Deprenyl not only slows disease progression but also can have a symptomatic effect on motor dysfunction. Certain surgical procedures for PD (adrenal medullary transplantation, fetal nigral transplantation) have been tried in medically intractable PD, but effectiveness has not been established. In addition, pallidotomy has been utilized in certain medically refractory PD patients.

Progressive Supranuclear Palsy

This disorder resembles PD; however, there are additional features. The diagnosis of progressive supranuclear palsy (PSP) is established by these features: parkinsonian signs including impaired postural reflexes causing frequent falls, bradykinesia, rigidity; resting tremor is *not* usually present; slow vertical rapid eye-movements especially with impaired downward but intact (oculocephalic) reflex; rigidity affecting axial more than appendicular muscles; dysarthria; dysphagia; dysphonia; blepharospasm; eyelid opening apraxia; dementia; and bilateral corticobulbar and corticospinal signs (Babinski signs). Compared with PD, PSP patients have no tremor; impaired balance is prominent, and this leads to sudden frequent falls. The course of PSP is relentless progression. Treatment with dopaminergic medication is less effective than in PD patients, and much higher doses of levodopa have been used in PSP patients, but usually with minimal success. The lack of response to dopaminergic agents differentiates PD from PSP.

Benign Essential Tremor

Benign essential tremor is often familial and transmitted as an autosomal-dominant trait with variable penetrance. Tremor usually develops in childhood and adolescence but becomes clinically evident and functionally disabling in adult life. Tremor incidence increases with age (e.g., senile tremor). Tremor is postural. Initially it involves the hands; it causes difficulty writing and shaving. Also, the patient is clumsy holding a drinking cup, combing hair, or using food utensils. Later, head or voice tremors can develop. There is no gait disturbance, mental change, rigidity, or hypokinesia; absence of these findings permits differentiation from parkinsonism. The condition is defined as "benign"; however, the tremor can be very disabling by interfering with writing, shaving, grooming, dressing, and feeding. If the tremor develops late in life, it is called "senile tremor."

The condition remains relatively unchanged throughout life. Tremor is ameliorated by alcohol and exacerbated by anxiety, caffeine, fatigue, and exercise. It can be precipitated by theophylline, lithium, valproic acid, or hyperthyroidism. Frequency and amplitude of tremors are reduced by diazepam (Valium), primidone (Mysoline), or propranolol (Inderal). Because the tremor may not interfere with activities of daily living, risks of drug addiction (diazepam) and cardiorespiratory (propranolol) complications must be considered relative to potential benefits of treatment. The patient can use drugs as indicated by lifestyle pattern. For example, a professor with voice tremor may use medication only when giving speech in public. The most effective drugs are primidone and propranolol. Initiate treatment with primidone in the smallest possible dose (50 mg daily) and gradually increase until tremor reduction is achieved or side effects occur. Other beta-adrenergic antagonists such as metroprolol may be used in patients with asthma or cardiovascular disease, in which cases propranolol is contraindicated.

Huntington's Disease

The cardinal features of Huntington's disease (HD) are choreiform movements and progressive cognitive and behavioral deterioration. The disorder usually becomes evident in third or fourth decade. It is transmitted as an autosomal dominant trait with complete penetrance such that each patient likely has an affected parent. There are areas of high prevalence (western Scotland, Lake Maracaibo region of Venezuela). This disorder results from genetic expression (DNA expansion syndrome) involving chromosome 4. With improving DNA technology it is becoming possible to predict which family members will become symptomatic.

The earliest symptoms are usually stereotyped tics (shoulder or face), generalized motor restlessness, clumsiness, awkwardness, or frequent falls. The patient can be unaware of dyskinesias, which can be initially reported by family members or friends; however, certain families go to fantastic extremes to hide family evidence of HD. Onset can be quite insidious with initial psychiatric symptoms including affective disorder, obsessions and compulsions, irritability, and aggressive behavior. Some patients have dementia or acute psychoses; more commonly these symptoms develop after the onset of dykinesias. In later stages of HD, dementia becomes prominent, and speech is slurred almost to becoming incomprehensible. There is a juvenile form of HD characterized by dystonia, rigidity, dementia, and seizures as well as chorea.

Certain potentially treatable conditions should be considered in suspected HD patients. In children and young adults chorea can appear as a major manifestation of rheumatic fever or postencephalitic syndrome. In Sydenham's chorea dyskinesia develops acutely. It usually persists for 2 to 6 months and spontaneously remits but can subsequently recur. Chorea can develop in women during pregnancy or with oral contraceptive agent use. Other etiologic considerations for chorea include systemic lupus erythematosus, Wilson's disease, neurosyphilis, thyroid disorders, and parathyroid disorders.

Biochemical analysis of brains of patients who have died of HD show abnormalities of several neurotransmitter types; however, most striking is the decreased level of gamma-aminobutyric acid and enzyme glutamic acid decarboxylase in the caudate nucleus, putamen, and cerebral cortex (especially frontal lobes). The CT/MRI can show the characteristic "squared-out" appearance of anterior frontal horns of lateral ventricles as a result of caudate atrophy. Positron emission tomography can show decreased oxygen and glucose utilization within the striatum; this can be even detected in asymptomatic HD patients. No treatment halts the progressive nature of HD. Although dopamine antagonist drugs can treat psychoses and chorea, no abnormalities of dopamine metabolism have been reported. Dopaminergic blocking agents (e.g., haloperidol, perphenazine) are used to reduce choreiform movements but do not alter the progression of cognitive-intellectual (dementia) symptoms. If active rheumatic fever or systemic lupus erythematosus is the cause of chorea (Sydenham's chorea), antibiotics or corticosteroids are also administered.

Gilles de la Tourette Syndrome

Gilles de la Tourette syndrome (TS) begins in childhood or adolescence and is more common in boys. Initial symptoms include hyperactive motor behavior (face and eye twitching or facial grimacing). Tics spread to neck and shoulder and later involve extremities. Repetitive stereotyped vocal involuntary movements (grunting, coughing, spitting) can develop several years later; this is followed by involuntary vocalization of obscene language in 50% of patients. Tics disappear with sleep and decrease with distraction; they are worsened by anxiety. They can be suppressed for short periods of time but then recur. Tics can change in pattern and location, and they frequently undergo remissions, but later tics can exacerbate. TS is a chronic disorder with maximal frequency in adolescence and early adulthood, then tics diminish as the patient gets older. Tic occurrence can cause psychologic problems and social isolation.

In TS, behavioral features include obsessive-compulsive disorder and attention deficit–hyperactivity syndrome. TS is a hereditary condition with the following diagnostic criteria: multiple motor tics, the presence of one or more vocal tics, initial presentation of symptoms before 21 years of age, and symptom duration exceeding 1 year. Chronic tic disorder that is *not* TS has motor or vocal tics, but *not* both disorders. Transient tic disorder differs from TS in that symptoms last less than one year.

Treatment consists of haloperidol, but this can require extremely high doses (30 to 100 mg/day). Haloperidol has benefited certain patients; however, the sedative effect limits the maximal dosage. The physician should be concerned about tardive dyskinesias with prolonged haloperidol use, and there should be drug-free periods. Clonazepam (Clonopin) or pimozide (Orap) are alternative drugs that are less likely to cause side effects. Pimozide is as effective as Haldol in tic suppression, has less sedative effect, and is less likely to cause dyskinesias; however, electrocardiogram monitoring is warranted because of the risk of cardio-vascular complications. If tics are mild, they need not always be treated.

Wilson's Disease (Hepatolenticular Degeneration)

This is an autosomal recessive genetic disorder of copper metabolism that causes pigmentation of the cornea with pathologic damage of liver and brain and effects on the kidney tubular system and red blood cells (hemolytic anemia). The majority of copper in the body is bound to plasma protein (ceruloplasmin). The major abnormality in Wilson's disease is low ceruloplasmin level, but this is not the primary abnor-mality. Because copper is not bound to ceruloplas-min, it is free in plasma, and copper urinary excretion is increased. Copper is deposited in brain, liver, kid-ney, and red blood cells to cause pathologic damage to these organs. Major neuropathologic disturbances are located in the putamen and globus pallidus.

Tremor (resting, postural, and intention) is the major dyskinesia; however, choreoathetosis and par-kinsonism symptoms can develop. Postural tremor is most characteristic; if it is present at the shoulders, this tremor can have a "wing-beating" quality. Tremor is brought out by having patient hold out the arms in abducted position and bend the elbows to touch fingertips. The patient is uncoordinated using the hands and frequently falls because of ataxia. The face has a fixed smile and constant drooling. In chil-dren initial symptoms can be deterioration in school performance and behavioral changes with character-istic rapid outbursts of anger or crying. An examina-tion shows muscular rigidity, bradykinesia, poor pos-tural control, dysarthria, and ataxia. The eyes must be examined with a slit lamp for the presence of green-yellow corneal rim (Kayser-Fleischer ring); this feature is invariably seen in patients with CNS manifestations. Wilson's disease should be suspected in children and young adults with unexplained hepatic disease or hemolytic anemia.

Laboratory studies are necessary to confirm the diagnosis (Box 20-2).

Wilson's disease is a chronic and progressive disorder, and without treatment there is severe disability. The goal of therapy is to remove copper from tissues by reducing copper intake and increasing excretion. Treatment strategies include reducing dietary copper, potassium sulfide to reduce copper absorption, and penicillamine. Penicillamine (250 to 500 mg four times daily) is a chelating agent; it rapidly binds copper, removes it from tissues, and facilitates excretion. Untoward effects of penicillamine include leukopenia, optic neuritis, myasthenic syndrome, aplastic anemia, and thrombocytopenia. If the patient cannot tolerate penicillamine, use trientine (triethylene tetramine) dihydrochloride (Syprine), which is a chelating agent used for removal of excessive copper from the body, or metallic zinc acetate.

 BOX 20-2

1 Decreased serum ceruloplasmin levels (less than 20 mg/dl)
2 Serum copper levels decreased to 100 µg/ml
3 Urine copper excretion is markedly elevated (most reliable parameter to establish diagnosis)
4 Impaired hepatic function
5 Elevated liver copper content

Myoclonus

Myoclonus refers to sudden, brief, shocklike muscular contractions (single or multiple) confined to individual muscle groups (face, tongue, extremity) or widespread in distribution. The movements are rapid and irregular in rate and amplitude. They cannot be controlled voluntarily in contrast with tics. Brief rapid irregular muscle contractions of myoclonus are different from dystonic movements, which consist of more sustained muscular contractions. Rhythmic myoclonus (as seen in palatal myoclonus) can resemble intention tremor. In myoclonus there is repetitive character to movements in contrast with chorea in which movements are random and unpredictable in distribution. Myoclonus is due to abnormal neuronal excitability at cerebral cortex, brain stem, or spinal cord levels.

Myoclonus can be seen in normal persons (physiologic) as manifested by sleep jerks and anxiety- or exercise-induced movements and can be suppressed by alcohol. Hypnagogic myoclonus are single or bursts of jerks experienced by patients as they fall asleep or can occur when patients are in a light sleep stage. Other patients develop rapid and frequent myoclonic jerks during sleep; these are noted by a bed partner and can prevent sleep. Myoclonus caused by abnormal cerebral neuronal excitability can be associated with seizures and EEG abnormalities. Myoclonic jerks can be triggered by stimulus-sensitive conditions (lights flashing, limb movement). Palatal myoclonus is rhythmic rapid movement of the palate and pharynx, facial, neck, and diaphragmatic muscles. This condition is due to lesions interrupting the central tegmental tract, inferior olivary nucleus, brachium conjunctivum, and dentate nucleus. Intention (action) myoclonus is myoclonus resulting from hypoxic-ischemic brain injury. In action myoclonus, jerks can be so frequent and of such high amplitude as to interfere with purposeful limb movements. There are usually associated gait ataxia, dysarthria, and intention tremor. Also immediately after cardiopulmonary arrest, transient myoclonus can occur as a result of cortical irritability, and these are usually self-limited.

Myoclonus can be one manifestation of generalized encephalopathy. When it occurs in young patients, complete evaluation for metabolic storage disease is indicated (see Chapter 13) as well as an EEG to exclude epileptic myoclonus or Creutzfeldt-Jakob disease. In adult patients structural CNS (cerebral cortex, brainstem, spinal cord) disease should be excluded, and metabolic studies including investigation for toxic substances (bismuth, heavy metals, methyl bromide) should be performed. Viral encephalitis can cause myoclonus, and CSF examination should be performed. Treatment of myoclonus includes valproic acid (Depakene), clonazepam, or 5-hydroxytryptophan. The prognosis depends on the underlying cause.

Blepharospasm and Hemifacial Spasm

This results in constant blinking and closing of the eyes. It can occur so frequently that it interferes with the patient's ability to read or drive. There can be ocular discomfort and photophobia caused by repeated blinking. Because of ocular symptoms, patients may be initially seen by ophthalmologist. Blepharospasm can be an isolated finding or can be associated with oral, jaw, or neck spasms (Meige syndrome). It is believed that blepharospasm is due to hyperirritability of the facial nucleus in the pons of the brainstem. An underlying structural lesion is almost never identified as the cause of blepharospasm. This should be contrasted with hemifacial spasm in which the patient reports difficulty in opening the eyes and has frontalis muscle spasm with elevated eyebrows. For patients with hemifacial spasm an MRI is warranted to exclude cerebellopontine or posterior fossa lesion. Treatment of blepharospasm and hemifacial spasm should be botulinum toxin injection.

Dystonia Musculorum Deformans

Dystonia musculorum deformans occurs in children and adolescents. It is characterized by slow inversion and plantar flexion of foot (equinovarus). It can later involve the upper extremities (writer's cramp, athetoid writhing of hands). If head, neck, and axial muscles are involved, this can result in torticollis, retrocollis, or spinal deformity (e.g., kyphoscoliosis). Dystonic movements are initially intermittent and nonpurposeful and interfere with voluntary motor activities. They are frequently painful. Postures subsequently become fixed. This can lead to development of contractures, muscular hypertrophy, skeletal deformities, and osteoarthritic changes. There is progressive impairment of gait, speech, and extremity movements. The patient becomes disabled and bedridden because of skeletal and joint deformities.

This disorder has two forms. The autosomal recessive type most commonly occurs in patients of Jewish origin, has onset between 4 and 15 years of age, and initially involves extremities. The disorder rapidly progresses, and the patient is soon reduced to a bedridden state with deforming contractures. There is no disorder of mentation, and patients are frequently of superior intelligence. In the autosomal dominant form there is no racial or ethnic predilection; it can affect several members in one generation of a family. Onset is variable and can occur as late as age 40, Axial muscles (torticollis, retrocollis) are most frequently initially involved. The course is static or slowly progressive. No drug has been proved beneficial to control dystonia and slow the disease progression. No characteristic pathologic substrate has been identified by autopsy examination of these patients.

Spasmodic Torticollis

Torticollis (wry neck) is characterized by sustained contraction of trapezius and sternocleidomastoid muscles. This results in lateral deviation of neck. Other patients have neck flexion (anterocollis), extension (retrocollis), and head tilt (laterocollis). Movements can be sustained and *not* always spasmodic. Dystonia can result from acute phenothiazine or dopaminergic toxicity. If drug induced, treatment with 50 mg of diphenhydramine (Benadryl) causes immediate and dramatic reversal. Multiple therapies (e.g., dopaminergic agents, anticholinergic medication, muscle relaxant medication, haloperidol, cervical rhizotomy, and biofeedback techniques) have been tried in chronic disorders but are of questionable value. The high doses of medication used to control dystonia usually cause unacceptable side effects. Recently local injection of botulinum toxin (Botox) into spasmodic contracted dystonic muscles has been used successfully. This is relatively safe procedure, and almost no botulinum toxin enters systemic circulation. Rarely, weakness may result from toxicity relating to impaired neuromuscular transmission.

With repeated use, antibodies may develop, and this reduces effectiveness of Botox therapy.

Drug-Induced Dyskinesias

Several types of disorders result from antipsychotic and antiemetic medications. Four dyskinetic patterns have been described. They are more common with high-potency antipsychotics (e.g., fluphenazine [Prolixin], haloperidol [Haldol]). These include acute dyskinesias, akathisia, parkinsonism, and tardive dyskinesias. Acute dyskinesias include dystonic neck posturing, oral-facial-tongue spasms or grimacing, and oculogyric crisis (sustained upward eye deviation). These usually occur in children and young adults. They can appear within several hours after the initial dose. Resolution can be spontaneous, or patients respond to diphenhydramine (Benadryl) in a dose of 50 mg (intravenously or intramuscularly) or benztropine (Cogentin) (one mg intravenously). Once acute reaction is controlled, antipsychotic medication can be restarted, preferably on a different antipsychotic medication and if the patient is concurrently treated with anticholinergic medication.

Akathisia (motor restlessness) is characterized by the patient being in constant motion. The patient feels unable to stay in one place and carries out motor activities to satisfy inner feeling of motor restlessness. Patterns include tapping of feet, leg shifting, body rocking or swaying, aimless pacing, and airplanelike swinging arm movements. It is important to differentiate akathisia caused by antipsychotic medication from behavior related to worsening of psychoses. Akathisia is sometimes associated with parkinsonian features (e.g., bradykinesia, rigidity). Akathisia does not usually remit spontaneously but can disappear after discontinuation of the antipsychotic drug. Akathisia is due to a dopamine receptor blockade. Treatment consists of lowering the medication dose or switching to a lower-potency neuroleptic drug. Medications that have been used include clonazepam, benzodiazepine, and beta-adrenergic antagonists.

Parkinsonism that is drug induced (e.g., antipsychotics, reserpine) most commonly affects elderly patients, but it can also be seen in young adults. Rigidity and hypokinesia are the most common clinical abnormalities; resting tremor occurs in only 50% of cases and develops several weeks to months after initiation of antipsychotic medication. Parkinsonism rarely causes significant functional disability. It is usually self-limited, and findings can disappear within several months even without treatment. Resolution occurs after antipsychotic medication is discontinued; however, switching the patient to another antipsychotic drug does not usually avoid recurrence of parkinsonism. It is therefore usually necessary to treat these patients with anticholinergic drugs or amantadine (Symmetrel) if symptoms are severe enough to interfere with motor function.

Tardive dyskinesia consists of a stereotyped pattern of oral-facial-lingual movements. These include tongue darting, lip smacking, lip pursing, eye blinking, and rhythmic jaw opening and closing. Movements resemble chorea. They can become severe enough to interfere with speaking, swallowing, and breathing (as a result of diaphragmatic involvement). Also, tardive dystonia and tardive myoclonus can be manifestations of neuroleptic-induced movement disorders. Fine, rhythmic lip and oral movements (rabbit syndrome) can develop. It is most important to differentiate parkinsonian syndrome from tardive dyskinesia because the latter condition requires changes in the neuroleptic drugs. Tardive dyskinesias are caused by high-potency antipsychotics. There is increased risk of this complication in certain patient populations (e.g., schizophrenics, women, and elderly patients, and those with preexisting organic brain damage). There is evidence that prophylactic treatment with anticholinergic drugs increases risk of tardive dyskinesia. Dyskinesias usually occur after years of treatment, although they can be precipitated by drug withdrawal.

If tardive dyskinesia is detected at a early stage, immediate reduction and discontinuation of antipsychotic drug causes movements to disappear; however, dyskinesia is not usually reversible if the disorder has been present for prolonged time. It is believed that early detection with rapid reduction in the drug dose can be the most important preventive measure. Dyskinesia can be initially detected or exacerbated when the antipsychotic drug is discontinued for a drug holiday. Dyskinesia can be suppressed by reinstituting the drug at the previous dosage. If the patient is kept off the drug, there is a gradual decrease in dyskinesia over several months. If tardive dyskinesia persists, drug treatment is unrewarding in most cases. Treatment strategies include antidopaminergic agents (e.g., haloperidol, reserpine), cholinomimetic drugs (e.g., choline [deanol], lecithin, physostigmine, or gamma-aminobutyric acid blocking agents, such as benzodiazepines [diazepam, clonazepam]). Reserpine (1 to 5 mg/day) is believed the most effective treatment.

The link between increased dopamine blockage reduces psychotic symptoms but leads to a state of denervation hypersensitivity. Dopaminergic hyperactivity predisposes patients to the development of tardive dyskinesias. By increasing the dosage of anti-psychotic drugs it is possible to abolish movements temporarily, but this strategy eventually worsens dyskinesias. The best treatment is judicious and limited use of antipsychotics with appropriate drug-free intervals. It is a tragic situation in which tardive dyskinesia disables the patient who has received antipsychotic medication inappropriately (e.g., anxiety states, neurosis).

Neuroleptic Malignant Syndrome

This disorder is precipitated by dopamine blocking medication, for example, haloperidol. It can occur at any point of time during therapy. Findings include severe hyperthermia, muscular rigidity, autonomic instability (tachycardia, hypertension, diaphoresis), and elevation of creatine phosphokinase. Because of intense muscularr rigidity, rhabdomyolysis can occur to cause renal dysfunction. Treatment includes immediate cessation of the neuroleptic drug, hydration of the patient, reduction of elevated temperature, and cardiopulmonary support. Bromocriptine, which is specific dopamine receptor agonist, and dantrolene, which is a muscle relaxant, can be used to reverse the condition.

▨ SUMMARY

Dyskinesias are abnormal movements that are not under voluntary control. On the basis of observation of the patient with dyskinesias, clinical classification is usually possible. By specifically classifying the dyskinesia, the potential causes and appropriate treatment are determined. Observation of the dyskinesia is crucial to establish the correct diagnosis, and neuro-imaging studies are not usually helpful in assessing dyskinesia patients. Hypokinetic movement disorders such as parkinsonism can be treated with dopaminergic medication, whereas hyperkinetic movement disorders such as chorea are treated with dopamine receptor blocking agents. The most common dyskinesia is tremor. The tremor that occurs with parkinsonism develops at rest and disappears with voluntary activity and is therefore not disabling. It is important to remember that shaking or trembling is not always due to parkinsonism. The most common and disabling dyskinesia is essential tremor in which the shaking movements interfere with activities of daily living, for example, holding a cup, using utensils, writing, shaving, and using a comb or toothbrush.

Suggested Readings

General

Calne DB, Eisler T: The pathogenesis and medical treatment of extrapyramidal disease, *Med Clin North Am* 63:715, 1979.

Campanella G, Roy M, Barbeau A: Drugs affecting movement disorders, *Ann Rev Pharmacol Toxicol* 27:113, 1987.

Duvoisin RC: Clinical diagnosis of the dyskinesias, *Med Clin North Am* 56:1321, 1972.

Parkinson's Disease

Calne DB, Kebabian J, Silbergeld E: Advances in the neuropharmacology of parkinsonism, *Ann Intern Med* 90:219, 1979.

Hoehn MM, Yahr MD: Parkinsonism: onset, progression and mortality, *Neurology* 17:427, 1967.

Quinn NL: The modern management of Parkinson's disease, *J Neurol Neurosurg Psychiatry* 53:93, 1990.

Koller WC, Giron LT: Selegiline: selective MAO-type B inhibitor, *Neurology* 40(Supp 3):61, 1990.

Scigliano G: Mortality associated with early and late levo-dopa therapy initiation in Parkinson's disease, *Neurology* 40:265, 1990.

Klawans HL, ed: Emerging strategies in Parkinson's disease, *Neurology* 40(Suppl 3):1, 1990.

Progressive Supranuclear Palsy

Maher ER, Lees AJ: The clinical features and natural history of Steele-Richardson-Olszewski syndrome (progressive supranuclear palsy), *Neurology* 36:1005, 1986.

Huntington's Disease

Shoulson I: Huntington's disease: a decade of progress, *Neurol Clin North Am* 3:515, 1984.

Folstein SE, Leigh RJ, Parhad IM: The diagnosis of Huntington's disease, *Neurology* 36:1279, 1986.

Duvoison RC: Chorea, *Semin Neurol* 2:351, 1982.

Dewy RB, Jankovic J:P Hemiballism-hemichorea, *Arch Neurol* 46:862, 1989.

Martin JB, Gusella JF: Huntington's disease; pathogenesis and management, *N Engl J Med* 315:1267, 1986.

Dystonia

Fahn S, Eldridge R: Definition of dystonia and classification of the dystonic states, *Adv Neurol* 14:1, 1976.

Fahn S: Torsion dystonia: clinical spectrum and treatment, *Semin Neurol* 2:316, 1982.

Tics

Butler IJ: Tourette's syndrome, *Neurol Clin North Am* 2: 571, 1984.

Kurlan R: Tourette's syndrome: current concepts, *Neurology* 39:1625, 1989.

Wilson's Disease

Dabyns WB, Goldstein NP, Gordon H: Clinical spectrum of Wilson's disease, *Mayo Clin Proc* 54:35, 1979.

Strickland GT, Leu ML: Wilson's disease: clinical and laboratory manifestations in 40 patients, *Medicine* 54:113, 1972.

Drug-Induced Dyskinesia

Jeste OV, Wyatt RJ: In search of treatment for tardive dyskinesia, *Schizophr Bull* 5:251, 1979.

Rosenberg MR, Green M: Neuroleptic malignant syndrome, *Arch Intern Med* 149:1927, 1989.

Burke RE: Tardive dyskinesias: current clinical issues, *Neurology* 34:1348, 1984.

Myoclonus

Chadwick D: Clinical, biochemical, and physiological features distinguishing myoclonus responsive to 5-hydroxytryptophan, tryptophan with monamine oxidase inhibitor and clonazepam, *Brain* 100:455, 1977.

Tremor

Fahn S: Differential diagnosis of tremors, *Med Clin North Am* 56:1363, 1972.

Hern JC: Tremor, *Br Med J* 288:1072, 1984.

Koller WC: Diagnosis and treatment of tremors, *Neurol Clin North Am* 2:499, 1984.

Findlay LJ, Koller WC: Essential tremor: a review, *Neurology* 37:1194, 1987.

CHAPTER

Demyelinating Disease

21

Demyelinating diseases are disorders of unknown cause characterized by the focal breakdown of previously normal central nervous system (CNS) myelin with relative preservation of axons. By this definition, hypoxia, leukodystrophies, toxic-metabolic conditions—such as subacute combined degeneration and central pontine myelinolysis—and other secondary lesions of CNS myelin are excluded.

◼ MULTIPLE SCLEROSIS

Multiple sclerosis (MS, disseminated sclerosis, or sclerose en plaque) is characterized by the disseminated multifocal deterioration of CNS myelin. Its clinical presentation consists of impairment of various motor, sensory, cerebellar, visual, and other systems. The disease usually starts in early adulthood and is "the great crippler of young adults." It can have a relapsing-remitting course with progressive neurologic impairment. The clinical manifestations vary from patient to patient and from attack to attack without a predetermined pattern; however, initial symptoms recur rather than new symptoms developing. Motor deficit in one or more extremities occurs in 50% of patients; it is either isolated or associated with the sensation of numbness or tingling in one extremity or a bandlike numbness or pressure around the trunk. In 25% of patients the initial symptom is monocular blindness as a result of retrobulbar neuritis or papillitis. Other symptoms include unsteadiness of gait as a result of cerebellum or cerebellar tract lesions and brain stem deficits, including impaired ocular motility (internuclear ophthalmoplegia and horizontal or vertical nystagmus), vertigo, or crossed sensorimotor findings. A tingling or electric shocklike feeling that radiates down the back or thighs and is triggered by passive neck flexion (Lhermitte's sign) can be seen in patients who have spinal cord lesions. The lower extremities are affected earlier and more frequently than the upper extremities and consist of spasticity, flexor spasms, and hyperreflexia. Two thirds of the patients show disturbance of sphincter control. Seizures can occur rarely.

Cognitive impairment occurs in longstanding progressive disease and is manifested by euphoria, denial of illness, or depression. Fatigue is a complaint in 65% of the patients. Precipitating factors in relapses of the disease include infections, trauma, lumbar puncture, emotional illness, and pregnancy. The variable clinical features and lack of a specific marker make the diagnosis difficult and create a problem for the selection of patients to participate in therapeutic trials. Assessing neurologic impairment is also difficult but was standardized by the Kurtzke Expanded Disability Status Scale. The reader is advised to look at the reference listed. There are two degrees of confidence in the clinical diagnosis of MS: clinically definite and clinically probable (Box 21-1).

These degrees were described during a workshop held to establish new diagnostic criteria for MS. (See Posner for further explanation of Box 21-1.)

The natural history of the disease is unpredictable, but a benign course with few attacks and complete or nearly complete remission occurs in at least 20% of the MS population. An exacerbating remitting course is the most frequent form, but a progressive course can also occur.

Etiology

The cause of MS is not known. Environmental factors may explain why the disease is more prevalent in

---

 BOX 21-1

Clinically definite MS (CDMS)

Two attacks and clinical evidence of two separate lesions

Two attacks; clinical evidence of one lesion and paraclinical evidence of another, separate lesion

Laboratory-supported definite MS (LSDMS)

Two attacks; either clinical or paraclinical evidence of one lesion; and CSF oligoclonal bands (OB) or increased CNS synthesis of IgG

One attack; clinical evidence of two separate lesions; and CSF OB/IgG

One attack; clinical evidence of one lesion and paraclinical evidence of another, separate lesion; and CSF OB/IgG

Clinically probable MS (CPMS)

Two attacks and clinical evidence of one lesion

One attack and clinical evidence of two separate lesions

One attack; clinical evidence of one lesion and paraclinical evidence of another, separate lesion

Laboratory-supported probable MS (LSPMS)

Two attacks and CSF OB/IgG

temperate than in tropical areas. High risk persists if migration from high-risk areas to low-risk areas occurs after the fifteenth birthday, implying that risk factors have their effect during childhood. Prevalence of the disease is higher in upper socioeconomic groups in which sanitation is generally better. Although dairy products in the diet and exposure to pets and other environmental factors have been suspected, there is no established proof of these relationships.

In Japan, where prevalence of the disease is influenced by place of residence rather than geoclimatic conditions, genetic factors are suspected. About 10% of patients with MS have an affected relative. The concordance rate in monozygotic twins is 20% to 40% and in dizygotic twins 15%. Genetic factors are related to the human lymphocyte antigen (HLA) complex, primarily HLA-A3 and B7.

Elevation of antibodies against measles, rubella, mumps, and herpes viruses has been found in the serum and CSF of some MS patients; however, the significance of these findings has not been established. Although the role of environmental factors is not certain, there may be an infective agent acquired in childhood, which after years of latency evokes or contributes to the causation of the disease. This infective agent can be a modified or partial virus infecting genetically susceptible persons. Finally immunocytochemical studies indicate that the inflammatory cells found in the acute lesions are T4 (helper-inducer) and T8 (suppressor-cytotoxic) lymphocytes, suggesting a strong immunologic mechanism of myelin destruction. There is also extensive literature suggesting that abnormalities in the immune system have an important role in mediating MS attacks. There is also evidence of good therapeutic response to immunomodulatory therapies.

Pathology

The lesions of MS consist of scattered, multiple, sharply delineated areas of demyelination found anywhere in the CNS white matter but predominantly in the periventricular areas, spinal cord, brain stem, optic nerves, and optic chiasm. Under the microscope there is loss of myelin with relative preservation of axons and degeneration and absence of myelin producing cells (oligodendroglia). The amount of mononuclear perivascular cell reaction and edema (acute lesions) and glial proliferation (chronic lesions) varies with the age of the lesion. Lesions can occur in major pathways without recognizable clinical symptoms. These lesions can be found incidentally on imaging studies or at autopsy.

Laboratory Tests

Although the diagnosis is usually established on a clinical basis, confirmatory laboratory tests can assist in some MS cases. *CSF studies:* In fewer than one third of the patients there can be some modest mononuclear pleocytosis in the CSF, usually fewer than 50 cells/mm^3 in the acute phase of the illness. One third of the patients have a mild increase in CSF protein content, usually not more than 100mg/dI. In 60% of patients quantitation of gammaglobulin by radioimmunodiffusion shows an increase in the percentage of total CSF protein (normal 12%). Electroimmunodiffusion shows that IgG is elevated out of proportion to the albumin in CSF in 90% of MS patients. High-resolution agarose electroimmunodiffusion shows that migration patterns of IgG segregate into discrete bands, known as oligoclonal IgG bands, very early in the disease in 85% to 95% of patients with definite MS. Although elevation of CSF gammaglobulin with

normal CSF protein content is not specific for MS
and can be seen in systemic lupus erythematosus, sarcoidosis, subacute sclerosing panencephalitis, neurosyphilis, and chronic CNS infections, it can be
helpful in establishing the diagnosis when found in a
patient who has a normal serum protein electroimmunodiffusion and clinical evidence of the disease.
Viral antibodies (mainly to measles but also to
rubella, herpes simplex, vaccinia, and varicella
zoster) have been found to be elevated in the CSF of
MS patients. Myelin basic protein has been detected
in the CSF of MS patients during acute attacks. *Electrophysiologic studies* are helpful in the diagnosis of

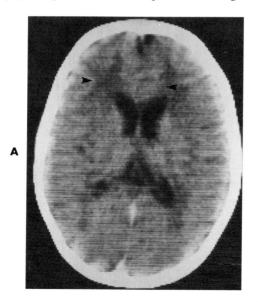

FIGURE 21-1. CT scan shows bilateral periventricular (**A**) and
subcortical white matter (**B**) hyperdense lesions (*arrows*)
consistent with demyelination of the MS type.

MS and include pattern shift visual (PSVER), brainstem auditory (BAER), and short latency somatosensory (SER) evoked potentials. All these tests measure impulse conduction times in the white matter tracts, which are prolonged or delayed in 60% of MS patients. These tests can also detect subclinical lesions and can provide additional evidence for diagnosis of multiple lesions. *Imaging studies:* Computerized tomography (CT) scans (Figure 21-1) in acute MS can reveal periventricular and deep white matter contrast-enhanced lesions that evolve into low density "old" lesions or resolve to normal white matter density. The CT can also show clinically silent

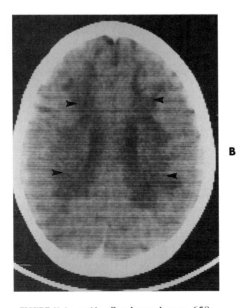

B

FIGURE 21-1, cont'd.   See legend on p. 658.

lesions. Magnetic resonance imaging (MRI) can also show white matter lesions and is more sensitive and specific than the CT scan (Figure 21-2). Although none of the tests described above is specific for the diagnosis of MS, one or several abnormal results along with the clinical features can help in reaching an accurate diagnosis.

Differential Diagnosis

In the differential diagnosis spinal cord lesions, including tumors, myelopathy caused by cervical spondylosis, and spinocerebellar degeneration, have

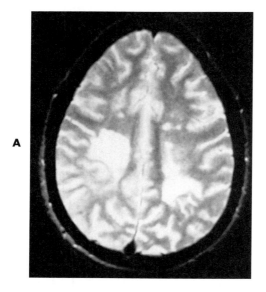

FIGURE 21-2. MRI scan shows multiple high-signal intensity periventricular (**A**) and subcortical white matter (**B**) lesions consistent with MS. There is also a right pontine lesion (*arrow*) (**C**) not seen on the CT scan.

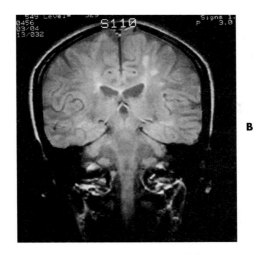

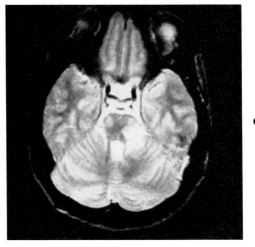

FIGURE 21-2, cont'd. See legend on p. 660.

to be considered. Chiari malformation type I and platybasia with basilar impression of the skull with compression of the brain stem and upper spinal cord can also be confused with MS. All of these diseases can be diagnosed by the clinical findings and ancillary laboratory tests.

Probably one of the most important diseases that is difficult to differentiate from MS is lupus erythematosus of the CNS. Cerebral, spinal cord, or optic nerve microinfarcts caused by arteriolar fibrinoid necrosis can be transient and can also be the first manifestation of lupus. Ancillary laboratory tests including erythrocyte sedimentation rate and antinuclear antibodies may be needed to differentiate lupus from MS.

Treatment

The exact cause of MS has not been established; therefore there is no specific treatment. The spontaneous remitting nature of the disease makes evaluation of therapy difficult. However, the important role that the immune system has mediating relapses of the disease has prompted several immunosuppressive therapy trials. Only two scientifically well-designed trials have shown efficacy in controlling the progression of the disease. In the first study patients with the relapsing-remitting form of the disease received alternate-day subcutaneous injection of eight million international units of interferon-beta-1b (Betaseron). This dose was found to lessen the frequency of MS attacks by one third and of serious attacks by one half and also reduce new MRI lesions for a period of 2 years or more. The high cost of the treatment restricts its use. The Quality Standards Subcommittee of the American Academy of Neurology has made recommendations to help the clinician who is considering the use of Betaseron in MS patients (see reference). The second study used intravenous methylprednisolone 250 mg four times daily for 3 days, followed by oral prednisone 1 mg/kg for 11 days, which was then tapered off over 3 days. This treatment, done in patients with optic neuritis without definite or probable MS, clearly delayed the development of definite MS. Other less convincing studies reported that long-term (15 months) immunosuppressive therapy consisting of antilymphocyte globulin, prednisolone, cyclophosphamide (Cytoxan), and azathioprine (Imuran) reduced the number of relapses and retarded the clinical course of the disease. Symptomatic treatment must include consideration of bladder dysfunction, spasticity, and the psychosocial needs of the patients and their families. Symptomatic treatment should be individualized for each patient and can require special consultations with occupational and physical therapists.

NEUROMYELITIS OPTICA (DEVIC'S DISEASE)

Neuromyelitis optica is a transverse or ascending myelitis followed or preceded by acute or subacute blindness in one or both eyes. It is a rare form of demyelination usually seen in young patients. The spinal cord, most often at the upper thoracic level, is usually necrotic, with nerve cell and axon destruction. The necrosis is probably produced by a demyelinating process with edema and circulatory impairment. Identical lesions have been found in typical cases of MS, and the optic nerve demyelination is indistinguishable from that in MS. Typical MS plaques have been found outside the spinal cord and optic nerves in typical cases of neuromyelitis optica, and some patients have clinical manifestations and autopsy findings of chronic relapsing MS. All these features suggest that neuromyelitis optica is an acute form of MS. The treatment consists of high dose methylprednisolone as delineated earlier.

OPTIC NEURITIS

In optic neuritis there is diminution of vision, scotomata, or complete blindness that is usually sudden and unilateral. Rarely both optic nerves are involved at different time. It usually affects young patients. Frequently there is ocular or retroocular pain. If the demyelinating lesion is limited to the optic nerve and the optic disk and retina appears normal, the process is known as retrobulbar neuropathy or, less appropriately, retrobulbar neuritis. If the demyelinating lesion is near the nerve head, the disc margins can be blurred and surrounded by hemorrhage so-called papillitis. Decreased visual acuity differentiates this lesion from papilledema. Papillitis and retrobulbar neuropathy are frequently associated with painful eye movements. Resolution of the lesion occurs in most patients. In 40% of patients there is progression to MS; conversely, most patients with established MS have optic nerve involvement. It is difficult to predict which patients who have optic neuritis will develop MS, but it seems that certain histocompatibility groups carry higher risks. Most optic neuritis patients do not have the CNS changes seen in definite MS patients. Evoked potentials or CT/MRI scanning that reveals multiple lesions can show the presence of MS. CSF oligocional bands and myelin basic protein are also diagnostic of MS. Simultaneous occurrence of bilateral optic neuritis usually suggests a toxic-nutritional cause rather than MS.

Treatment

The Longitudinal Optic Neuritis Study showed that 250 mg of intravenous methylprednisolone four times daily for 3 days, followed by oral prednisone 1 mg/kg for 11 days and tapered over 3 days gives a 57% reduction of new clinical neurologic attacks. The study also showed that oral prednisone alone was of no benefit. Certain cases of optic neuritis are associated with corticosteroid-responsive autoimmune disorders including systemic lupus erythematosus.

◼ ACUTE DISSEMINATED ENCEPHALOMYELITIS

Acute disseminated encephalomyelitis is a rare demyelinating disease that is usually monophasic and self-limiting and preceded or accompanied by some viral exanthematous infection such as chickenpox, measles, smallpox, rubella, or a nonspecific respiratory infection (so-called postinfectious or parainfectious encephalomyelitis). The same type of disease can be precipitated by vaccination against rabies or smallpox (so-called postvaccinal or allergic encephalomyelitis). Although a viral infection precedes or is associated with the disease, no virus has been isolated from the CSF or brain tissue, and the histopathologic changes are different from those in viral encephalomyelitis and most closely resemble the central nervous system lesions seen in experimental allergic encephalomyelitis. An immune-mediated complication of infection seems most likely. Foci of demyelination around veins, which are cuffed by lymphoreticular cells, are disseminated throughout the cerebrum, brain stem, cerebellum, and spinal cord. Clinically there is an acute onset of somnolence, confusion, and meningeal signs followed by ataxia, involuntary movements, convulsions, or coma. Paraplegia or quadriplegia can occur when the spinal cord is involved. The mortality varies from 10% to 50%. Complete recovery occurs in some patients; others can have permanent sequelae such as epilepsy, behavioral problems, or permanent motor deficit. Treatment with corticosteroids (see earlier protocol) seems to reduce the severity of the disease. Anticonvulsants should be used when needed. Atypical cases that are "transitional" between acute disseminated encephalomyelitis and MS have been observed, probably implying some common immune mechanism. It is impossible to differentiate clinically between acute MS and acute disseminated encephalomyelitis.

SUMMARY

Demyelinating diseases are a group of acquired disorders of unknown cause that affect the CNS myelin. They should be differentiated from other disorders that also affect the myelin as a secondary phenomenon, such as some genetic metabolic disorders (leukodystrophies), toxic-metabolic conditions (subacute combined degeneration and central pontine myelinolysis), hypoxia, and so on. The acute forms include acute disseminated encephalomyelitis, optic neuritis, and neuromyelitis optica. Some patients with the acute forms respond to high dose steroid treatment. The chronic form, or MS, has a relapsing-remitting course with progressive neurologic impairment and poor response to treatment. The important role that the immune system has mediating relapses of the disease has prompted several immunosuppressive therapy trials that have lessened the frequency of MS attacks.

Suggested Readings

Multiple Sclerosis—General

Constant CF: Pathogenesis of multiple sclerosis, *Lancet* 343:271, 1994.

Multiple sclerosis update, *Neurology* 30(7):1, 1980.

Rudick RA, Herdon RH: Disorders of myelin, *Semin Neurol* 5:85, 1985.

Sobel RA: The pathology of multiple sclerosis, *Neurol Clin North Am* 13:1, 1995.

The etiology of multiple sclerosis (Editorial). *Lancet* 1: 1347, 1981.

Optic Neuritis

Beck RB, Cleary PA, Anderson MN: A randomized controlled trial of corticosteroids in treatment of optic neuritis, *N Engl J Med* 326:581, 1992.

Beck RW: The effect of corticosteroids for acute optic neuritis on the subsequent development of multiple sclerosis, *N Engl J Med* 329:176, 1993.

Transverse Myelitis

Ropper AH, Poskanzer DC: The prognosis of acute and subacute transverse myelopathy, *Ann Neurol* 4:51, 1978.

Multiple Sclerosis—Clinical

Birk K: The clinical course of MS during pregnancy and puerperium, *Arch Neurol* 47:738, 1990.

Joffe RT, Lippert E: Mood disorders and MS, *Arch Neurol* 44:376, 1987.

Kurtzke JF: Rating neurologic impairment in multiple sclerosis: an Expanded Disability Status Scale (EDSS), *Neurology* 33:1444, 1983.

McAlpine D, Lumsden CE, Acheson ED: *Multiple sclerosis: a reappraisal,* London, 1968, E & S Livingstone Ltd.

Posner CM: New diagnostic criteria for multiple sclerosis: guidelines for research protocols, *Ann Neurol* 13:227, 1983.

Reisner T, Maida E: Computerized tomography in multiple sclerosis, *Arch Neurol* 37:475, 1980.

Multiple Sclerosis—Treatment

Brown JR: The design of clinical studies to assess therapeutic efficacy in multiple sclerosis, *Neurology* 29(9):1, 1979.

Ebers GC: Treatment of multiple sclerosis, *Lancet* 343:275, 1994.

Kupersmith MJ: Megadose corticosteroids in multiple sclerosis, *Neurology* 44:1, 1994.

Mertin J: Double-blind controlled trial of immunosuppression in the treatment of multiple sclerosis, *Lancet* 2:949, 1980.

Report of the Quality Standards Subcommittee of the American Academy of Neurology: Practice advisory on selection of patients with multiple sclerosis for treatment with Betaseron, *Neurology* 44:1537, 1994.

Silverberg DH: Multiple sclerosis: approaches to management, *Ann Neurol* 36(suppl):1, 1994.

The IFNB MS Study Group: Interferon beta-1b is effective in relapsing-remitting MS, *Neurology* 43:655, 1993.

C H A P T E R

Neurologic Complications of Systemic Diseases

22

▨ RENAL DISORDERS

Neurologic complications can be related directly to renal impairment or can result from dialysis or kidney transplant. Central nervous system (CNS) dysfunction occurs when the glomerular filtration rate declines below 10% of normal; however, no relationship exists between encephalopathy and blood urea nitrogen or serum creatinine level. Early encephalopathy symptoms include anorexia, nausea, hyperactivity, sleep disruption, and inattention. As the renal function worsens, symptoms include vomiting, lethargy, impaired cognition, paranoia, and abnormal fatigue. In severe encephalopathy, symptoms can include confusion, abnormal behavior, dysarthria, myoclonus, asterixis, seizures, and coma. The electroencephalogram (EEG) shows a diffuse slow pattern. Renal encephalopathy can be exacerbated by other metabolic abnormalities, for example, acidosis, hyperosmolarity, hyponatremia, and hypocalcemia. Seizures develop late in renal encephalopathy. Treatment of seizures with phenytoin and phenobarbital requires careful monitoring because blood phenytoin levels are usually low in uremic patients, but free drug levels can be high, low, or normal depending on protein binding changes.

Polyneuropathy occurs in two thirds of chronic renal failure patients. This can not be distinguished from neuropathy caused by other metabolic conditions, for example, alcohol or diabetes mellitus. In chronic renal failure patients, "restless legs" syndrome, characterized by burning, prickling, crawling, and aching sensations in the legs, can develop. Following dialysis there is usually improvement in neuropathy, but this can worsen, especially in diabetic patients undergoing dialysis; however, renal transplant causes predictable neuropathy remission.

Because of fluid and electrolyte shifts, neurologic disturbances develop in patients undergoing dialysis. The "dysequilibrium syndrome" is characterized by headaches, nausea, cramps, altered mentation, and seizures. This develops within 24 hours postdialysis and usually spontaneously resolves; therefore treatment of a single seizure immediately after dialysis is probably not warranted. Because renal failure patients have bleeding disorders, dialysis can precipitate intracranial bleeding such as subdural or intracerebral hematomas. If neurologic findings do not clear rapidly following dialysis, neurodiagnostic studies (EEG, cerebrospinal fluid [CSF], computed tomography/magnetic resonance imaging [CT/MRI]) are indicated; however, in most cases they are not necessary because clinical improvement develops within 48 hours.

In renal failure patients who have undergone chronic hemodialysis, "dialysis dementia" can occur. This is characterized by speech disorders (dysarthria, dyspraxia, stuttering, mutism), seizures, or motor disturbances. EEG findings consist of bilateral spike and wave complexes and bursts of diffuse slow waves. Epileptic causes of these EEG abnormalities are possible and rarely improve with anticonvulsants; the clinical course is usually progressive deterioration. Aluminum, contained in the dialysate, has been found in high levels in gray matter of these patients and has been suggested as a possible etiologic agent; however, other trace elements have also been implicated. By deionization of dialysate water, trace elements are removed, and the incidence of "dialysis dementia" lowered. It is important to exclude other metabolic conditions (hypercalcemia, Wernicke's syndrome with thiamine deficiency, hyponatremia, drug effect) or structural neurologic conditions (subdural hematoma, stroke, infectious-inflammatory disorders, lymphomas) as the cause of the dementia. Neurologic complications of renal transplantation can occur (p. 713).

DIABETES MELLITUS

Neurologic complications of diabetes mellitus include accelerated atherosclerotic disease involving large or small blood vessels to cause strokes; encephalopathy as a result of metabolic abnormalities such as hypoglycemia, ketoacidosis, and hyperosmolarity; retinopathy and visual loss; neuropathy; amyotrophy; and thoracoabdominal radiculopathy.

In nerve conduction velocity studies performed on neurologically asymptomatic diabetics, many show nerve slowing. Early slowing of nerve conduction velocity, which is subsequently reversed by the initiation of insulin therapy, has been reported. Polyneuropathy usually develops slowly, with initial sensory disturbances in distal extremities. Patients report aching or cramping pain and paresthesias, which are most severe nocturnally. Clinical findings in diabetic neuropathy include absent ankle jerks and impaired vibration sense on the soles of the feet; distal motor weakness is less frequent. If there is proprioceptive dysfunction, neuropathic ulcers and joint deformity (Charcot joints) develop. It is important to differentiate vascular from neuropathic ulcers because treatment differs. The course of neuropathy is variable; some patients spontaneously improve and others show progressive impairment. It is not clear whether rigorous blood sugar control improves peripheral nerve dysfunction.

Diabetic mononeuropathy can involve any nerve(s). Onset is sudden. Frequently pain is the initial symptom, followed by motor dysfunction. Functional recovery develops several weeks to months later, consistent with vascular causes with pathologic evidence of infarction in the vasa nervorum of peripheral nerve. The most frequently involved nerves are the femoral and sciatic in lower extremities and the median and ulnar in upper extremities. Sudden onset of paresthesias in the lateral thigh (lateral femoral cutaneous nerve) is characteristic of meralgia paresthetica. Cranial nerves (especially facial and extraocular) are frequently involved. If there is sudden onset of painful unilateral oculomotor paresis, diagnosis of a ruptured posterior communicating artery aneurysm should be suspected; however, in diabetic oculomotor paresis, the pupil is spared and clinical recovery occurs spontaneously.

Diabetic amyotrophy is characterized by asymmetrical proximal pelvic girdle weakness. There are dysesthesias in the anterior thigh without objective sensory loss. These patients appear cachectic (wasted). The electromyogram and muscle biopsy findings are consistent with neuropathic process. Diabetic amyotrophy patients frequently improve with rigorous blood sugar control. Autonomic dysfunction usually occurs in diabetic polyneuropathy. Clinical findings include orthostatic hypotension, impotence, intermittent nocturnal diarrhea, delayed gastric emptying, and atonic bladder causing urinary incontinence.

CNS disorders such as impaired consciousness, seizures, or focal neurologic deficit can complicate hyperglycemia. In patients with ketoacidosis, encephalopathy and generalized seizures can develop; however, in nonketotic, hyperosmolar, hyperglycemic states, focal seizures and lateralized neurologic deficit can occur frequently. Potential mechanisms for this dysfunction in diabetic, nonketotic, hyperosmolar, hyperglycemic states include acidosis, ketosis, systemic hypotension, cerebral hypoxia, hyperosmolar condition, dehydration, and intravascular coagulation. Despite the presence of strokelike syndromes, diagnostic and pathologic findings do not show vascular ischemia.

ALCOHOLISM

Alcoholism is a chronic disease. The patient drinks despite medical, neurologic (Box 22-1), psychiatric, social, economic, and legal contraindications. Alcohol has a specific effect on excitatory (glutamate) receptors and alters neuronal membrane lipids and proteins.

In acute intoxication patients demonstrate impaired judgment, euphoria, poor coordination, slurring of speech, and socially inappropriate behavior. Brief episodes of memory "blackouts" can occur. Certain patients become agitated and combative and cause property or personal damage (pathologic intoxication); this can occur independently of the amount of alcohol ingested. Stupor, coma, respiratory depression, and death can be precipitated by the direct neurotoxic effect of alcohol or by other alcohol-related

BOX 22-1   Neurologic Complications of Alcohol

Acute intoxication

Euphoria
Impaired judgment and coordination deficit
Decreased inhibition
Memory lapses (blackouts)
Nystagmus, ataxia, dysarthria, diplopia
Pathologic intoxication (acute agitated excited state with violent behavior)
Acute auditory hallucinosis
Stupor and coma
Hypothermia, hypotension, hypoventilation
Death caused by respiratory or cardiovascular collapse

Withdrawal syndrome

Tremulousness
Seizures
Hallucinosis
Delirium tremens

Nutritional-related alcoholic

Wernicke-Korsakoff syndrome
Toxic amblyopia (optic neuropathy)
Peripheral neuropathy

Disorder of unknown pathogenesis

Cerebellar degeneration
Myopathy
Dementia and cerebral atrophy
Marchiafava-Bignami disease
Central pontine myelinolysis

Disorders related to hepatic failure

Asterixis
Non-Wilsonian hepatolenticular degeneration
Coma
Spastic paraparesis
Subdural and intracerebral hematoma related to coagulopathy

complications, for example, hypoglycemia, metabolic acidosis, hepatic encephalopathy, and subdural hematoma. Respiratory depression can occur when mixing alcohol with sedatives. The correlation between blood alcohol level and intoxication severity is a function of alcohol tolerance and duration of alcohol exposure. For example, chronic alcoholics can tolerate blood alcohol levels of 400 mg/dl, whereas nonalcoholics can be severely affected by this blood alcohol level.

Symptoms of alcohol withdrawal occur in patients who have been drinking constantly and suddenly stop as a result of lack of money or intercurrent illness. Initial symptoms include tremulousness, nervousness, insomnia, hyperirritability, hypervigilance, nightmares, auditory, visual, or tactile hallucinations; these improve after patients have a drink. If patients remain abstinent, symptoms can persist for 7 to 14 days. Seizures can develop 6 to 48 hours after the last drink; in fact, seizures or hallucinosis can occur during drinking. Seizures can be more delayed after cessation of alcohol intake if other CNS depressant medications are used. Seizures are generalized major motor in type. They are usually single or can consist of brief seizure clusters. The EEG is usually normal, with the exception of spikes in postictal period. The EEG can show photomyoclonic or photoconvulsive response. Not all alcohol withdrawal seizures are benign! Five percent are status epilepticus. Because most alcohol withdrawal seizures are self-limited, anticonvulsant treatment is not always needed. Prophylactic anticonvulsant treatment is not indicated after acute hospitalization episode; alcoholic patients frequently discontinue their medications especially when drinking heavily. The toxic effect of alcohol and abrupt anticonvulsant cessation would lower the seizure threshold to cause clinical seizures.

Acute delirium tremens develop 3 to 5 days following cessation of drinking. It is characterized by acute confusion, tremulousness, motor restlessness, and autonomic hyperactivity (tachycardia, hypertension, sweating, fever, pupillary dilatation). This is usually self-limited, lasting several days; however, it is sometimes more prolonged (as long as 2 weeks) and associated with mortality if complicated by infection, Wernicke's syndrome, or cardiomyopathy. Treatment of acute delirium tremens include four vital components (Box 22-2).

Nutrition-related neurologic disorders include Wernicke-Korsakoff syndrome. Patient with this syndrome have altered mentation, unsteady ataxic gait, and eye movement disorders. Because these patients are confused and inattentive, memory function cannot be adequately tested. The patient's stumbling gait is related to neuropathy in association with vestibular and cerebellar dysfunction. Abnormal eye findings include abducens paresis, lateral gaze palsy, and horizontal or vertical nystagmus. Pathologic lesions char-

---

 BOX 22-2

1 Adequate fluid replacement to prevent dehydration resulting from fever, motor activity, and inadequate fluid intake except for alcohol

2 Parenteral glucose and multivitamins, including high-dose thiamine

3 Sedative medication (chlordiazepoxide, paraldehyde) and avoidance of drugs impairing cardiac function (diazepam or chlorpromazine)

4 Investigation for systemic infection, hepatic or hematologic dysfunction, and intracranial (traumatic or infectious) lesions

acterized by petechial hemorrhagic and diffuse microscopic necrotic lesions are seen in mammillary bodies, the hypothalamus, and the thalamus.

As the confusional state resolves, Wernicke's syndrome patients can show amnestic (Korsakoff's) syndrome. There is an inability to learn new information (anterograde amnesia) and an inability to retain and retrieve previously learned facts (retrograde amnesia). These patients appear apathetic and dull but can demonstrate entertaining (confabulation) response to mental questioning. Treatment of Wernicke-Korsakoff's syndrome includes thiamine (100 mg parenterally initially with daily oral multivitamins). Administration of glucose-containing fluids without thiamine can exacerbate the neurologic deficit and precipitate cardiovascular collapse in Wernicke's syndrome patients.

Alcoholic-related cerebellar degeneration develops frequently in poorly nourished patients. Pathologic findings are cerebellar cortex and anterior vermis degeneration. These patients have broad-based ataxic gait with impaired heel-to-shin movements and relatively intact finger-to-nose movements. The clinical course can show progressive worsening or stabilization; deterioration usually occurs during a subsequent drinking period. If patients become abstinent and maintain good nutritional status, improvement occurs. In alcoholics neuropathy frequently develops. In some cases paresthesias are intense, and patients cannot tolerate the pressure of bed sheets on the feet. Amblyopia with centrocecal scotoma is frequently caused by nutritional optic atrophy.

Other neurologic conditions of undetermined cause include myopathy, characterized by muscle pain, tenderness, and proximal weakness; central pontine myelinolysis, characterized by quadriplegia, mutism, bulbar involvement, and eye movement abnormalities with pathologic evidence of focal brainstem demyelination visualized by CT or MRI; Marchiafava-Bignami syndrome, characterized by dementia, seizures, rigidity, aphasia, and urinary incontinence and demyelination involving anterior corpus callosum; and cerebral atrophy and dementia with ventricular and subarachnoid space dilatation. The brain atrophy can normalize (reverse) with abstinence, hydration, and protein repletion.

▨ HEPATIC DISORDERS

Hepatic encephalopathy characterized by altered mentation and abnormal motor function (e.g., tremor, asterixis, myoclonus) that is not necessarily caused by hepatitis or cirrhosis develops in patients with hepatic dysfunction. The most characteristic finding is "liver flap" or asterixis. There is sudden wrist flexion when the wrist is dorsiflexed and the fingers are extended. There is a sudden, rapid palmar flapping movement followed by a slow return to original dorsiflexed wrist position. The EMG shows an absence of muscle activity as wrist flaps downward followed by bursts of action potentials as the wrist returns to dorsiflexed position. Asterixis is best stimulated by the examiner pushing against the patient's outstretched wrist. Asterixis can spread to the feet or tongue. It is seen in awake patients but disappears as consciousness deteriorates. Asterixis is seen most commonly in hepatic disease but also in renal or pulmonary encephalopathies. Patients with hepatic encephalopathy can be mildly confused or more severely impaired (coma). Some hepatic encephalopathy patients are delirious with asterixis and tremor to simulate delirium tremens. The severity of hepatic encephalopathy correlates with elevated blood (arterial) ammonia level, although the role of other brain neurotransmitters (glutamate, gamma-aminobutyric acid, organic thio-alcohols, short-chain fatty acids) must be considered. The EEG shows a diffuse slowing with superimposed paroxysmal triphasic delta waves. Because patients with hepatic impairment are predisposed to trauma-related and infectious-inflammatory neurologic conditions, CT, MRI, and CSF examinations can be indicated. In rare instances patients with hepatic dysfunction develop a neurologic deficit including dyskinesias caused by non-Wilsonian hepatolenticular degeneration and spastic paraparesis caused by cortical or spinal cord degeneration. Pathologic findings in patients who had hepatic encephalopathy include abnormal astrocytes (Alzheimer type II) visualized in the cerebral cortex, putamen, globus pallidus, thalamus, and cerebellum. Treatment of hepatic encephalopathy includes correction of the underlying hepatic disorder and metabolic abnormalities, oral lactulose (to reduce ammonia levels) in doses of 20 to 30 g four times daily, and protein restriction. Neomycin treatment (2 to 3 g daily) has been replaced by lactulose because neomycin has auditory-vestibular and renal toxicity.

▪ FLUID AND ELECTROLYTE DISORDERS

Water Intoxication and Hyponatremia

Hyponatremia can occur if water intake exceeds urinary excretion; this results in decreased plasma osmolality, increased intracellular and extracellular water, and possibly cerebral edema, herniation syndromes, and ultimately death. In water intoxication, there can be brain swelling with expansion and flattening of the cerebral gyral pattern and narrowing of sulcal spaces. There is swelling of astrocytes, especially in white matter. This condition can result from excess secretion of vasopressin (syndrome of inappropriate antidiuretic hormone [SIADH]). It can also occur in patients with CNS diseases including head trauma, meningitis, and postoperative neurosurgical (hypothalamic-pituitary) procedures. Other causes for hyponatremia include compulsive (psychogenic) water drinking, Addison's disease, and renal disease with defective water excretion.

In hyponatremic patients the diagnosis of SIADH is established when serum osmolality is paradoxically low compared with urine osmolality. Neurologic manifestations of hyponatremia include mental confusion, muscle cramps, weakness, and seizures. Certain patients are asymptomatic despite marked hyponatremia if hyponatremia developed gradually; others are comatose with recurrent seizures if hyponatremia and low serum osmolality develops rapidly. Some patients with symptomatic hyponatremia are rapidly corrected with hypertonic saline, and this can cause central pontine myelinolysis. Because of this potential risk, never overcorrect hyponatremia rapidly.

Treatment of hyponatremia consists of fluid restriction or administration of hypertonic saline. If status epilepticus develops as a result of hyponatremia, treatment with intravenous hypertonic saline infusion may be necessary. Hyponatremic patients who are volume expanded (congestive heart failure, nephrotic syndrome) should be fluid restricted. If hyponatremia is caused by endocrine disorders such as adrenal insufficiency or hypothyroidism, treatment of these conditions should correct hyponatremia. Certain medications can cause hyponatremia by interfering with the patient's ability to excrete water (oral hypoglycemics, antipsychotics, narcotics, sedatives, antineoplastic drugs). Withdrawal of causal medication is necessary. Certain patients develop SIADH insidiously, and hyponatremia can be asymptomatic. These patients can have an underlying neoplasm or chronic respiratory disease. Hyponatremia caused by SIADH can also be corrected with lithium or demeclocycline.

Hypernatremia

Hypernatremia most commonly occurs in infants and elderly patients. Hypernatremia results from water loss producing sodium excess, such as sweating and vomiting. This usually occurs in patients with an impaired thirst mechanism, decreased fluid intake, diabetes insipidus, or as consequence of osmotic diuresis. It is most common in dehydrated infants or elderly patients who do not receive adequate fluid replacement. Neurologic findings include altered mentation, an increase in muscle tone (rigidity and opisthotonos), and seizures. There is extracellular hyperosmolarity and intracellular dehydration with brain shrinking. In hypernatremic infants rapid fluid shifts can cause intracranial hemorrhage or a hypercoagulable condition predisposing to cerebral infarction. Treatment includes rehydration with plasma expanders. This must be performed carefully to avoid intracellular edema and signs of water intoxication. During treatment of hypernatremia prevent severe hypotension by using isotonic colloid solutions, monitoring blood pH to avoid acidosis, replacing fluids using hypotonic fluid, and treating the underlying cause of hypernatremia.

Hypocalcemia

Hypocalcemia results from low oral intake, high intestinal loss, malabsorption, vitamin D deficiency, high urinary loss, or hypoparathyroidism. Calcium is necessary for neuronal membrane stability. Hypocalcemia results in hyperexcitability in CNS (seizures, mental change), peripheral and cranial nerves (tetany, laryngeal stridor, paresthesia, muscle cramps, spasms), and the cardiac conduction system (prolonged Q-T interval). Clinical features are exacerbated by hyperventilation, hypomagnesemia, and alkalosis. The cardinal finding of acute hypocalcemia is tetany (intermittent tonic muscle contractions). This is manifested by twitching of face and mouth muscles in response to tapping over the facial nerve (Chvostek's sign) and carpopedal spasm that is spontaneous or develops in response to inflating a blood pressure cuff between systolic and diastolic levels for three minutes (Trousseau's sign). Neurologic findings caused by chronic hypocalcemia include papilledema, cataracts, parkinsonism, mental retardation, and basal ganglia calcification. For acute hypocalcemia, parenteral therapy consists of 1 or 2 ampules (containing 90 mg calcium/ampule) administered intravenously in 15-minute intervals to prevent seizures, laryngospasm, and death. Treatment of chronic hypocalcemia includes oral calcium gluconate and vitamin D.

Hypercalcemia

Primary hyperparathyroidism with production and release of excess parathyroid hormone can result from parathyroid hyperplasia, adenoma, or carcinoma. Other causes of hypercalcemia include sarcoidosis, metastatic carcinoma, multiple myeloma, and prolonged immobilization. Muscle weakness is a very early complaint. Other clinical manifestations include headache, irritability, depression, anxiety, abdominal pain, constipation, polydipsia, polyuria, encephalopathy (ranging from mania with hallucinations to stupor), myopathy, and polyneuropathy. Treatment depends on the specific cause of hypercalcemia.

Hypokalemia

Hypokalemia can result from renal tubular necrosis or adrenal (hyperaldosteronism) dysfunction, mineralocorticoid drugs, diuretic therapy, vomiting, or diarrhea. Neurologic symptoms include weakness, which can be episodic and does not occur until the potassium concentration falls below 3 mEq/L. Findings include hyporeflexia and proximal muscle weakness; this can cause bulbar and respiratory dysfunction. Episodic (lasting 30 minutes to several days) paralysis can occur with minor changes in extracellular potassium content and no loss of potassium from the body (shift from extracellular to intracellular fluid); this is characteristic of familial periodic paralysis (FPP). Episodic weakness can develop with either hypokalemia or hyperkalemia. FPP is transmitted as an autosomal dominant traits. In hypokalemic FPP attacks can be precipitated by high carbohydrate diet, sodium intake, diuretics, diarrhea, and rest after vigorous exercise.

Hypophosphatemia

This disorder develops in patients receiving hyperalimentation, malnourished hospitalized patients, alcoholics, and patients with respiratory alkalosis and diabetic ketoacidosis. The neurologic dysfunction includes encephalopathy, ataxia, seizures, asterixis, dyskinesias, ptosis, dysphagia, dysphonia, and respiratory dysfunction caused by muscle weakness. Also neuropathy simulating Guillain-Barré's syndrome can develop. Patients at risk for hypophosphatemia should receive phosphorus-containing food (skim or low-fat milk) or phosphorus supplementation. Phosphorus deficiency can increase magnesium excretion to cause hypomagnesemia. This can exacerbate muscle weakness with reduced deep tendon reflexes.

▨ ENDOCRINE CONDITIONS

Hyperthyroidism

Patients with hyperthyroidism have CNS dysfunction (hyperkinesia, anxiety, insomnia, mood swings, and postural tremor), ophthalmoplegia, myelopathy, or muscle disorders (myopathy or myasthenia gravis). Some disturbances are caused by sympathetic (adrenergic) hypersensitivity and respond to treatment with β-adrenergic blocking agents (propranolol). Myopathy improves when patients become euthyroid. Myasthenia gravis can exacerbate or remit when patients become euthyroid. Hypokalemic periodic paralysis can exacerbate in thyrotoxic patients and resolve in the euthyroid state. Hyperthyroidism can be associated with pernicious anemia (B_{12} deficiency) and adrenal insufficiency (p. 686).

Ophthalmologic findings as a result of adrenergic hypersensitivity include upper lid retraction, lid lag, widened palpebral fissures, and infrequent blinking. These resolve following restoration of the euthyroid condition and respond to treatment with β-blocking agents. Other eye findings caused by infiltrative ophthalmopathy include muscle restriction (especially on superior or lateral gaze), exophthalmos, corneal ulceration, and decreased visual acuity. Exophthalmos is usually bilateral; however, if findings are asymmetrical, this can simulate the orbital mass. Radiologic studies (orbital ultrasound, CT/MRI) may be necessary in this situation. The relationship of thyroid hormone abnormalities to infiltrative ophthalmopathy is not clearly established. Ocular findings can develop in patients after successful medical thyroid treatment or surgical thyroidectomy. Ophthalmopathy can progress such that the eyeball becomes immobile, vision is impaired, and corneal ulceration occurs. Corticosteroids are indicated if vision is threatened; orbital surgical decompression may be required to preserve vision.

Hypothroidism

In adults myxedema can cause psychomotor retardation, confusion, dementia, psychoses (myxedema madness), peripheral neuropathy, myopathy, myasthenia gravis, cerebellar ataxia, abnormal reflexes with delayed relaxation phase and myoedema (mounding of muscles when directly percussed), or auditory-vestibular nerve impairment.

In myxedema patients coma with severe hypothermia can be precipitated by sedative drugs (which depress respiration to cause carbon dioxide retention), infection, or trauma. Treatment consists of measures to control temperature regulation, corticosteroids (because of associated adrenal insufficiency), and gradual restoration of the thyroid hormone. Myxedema coma is a medical emergency. This requires treatment with intravenous triiodothyronine, which is biologically active thyroid hormone.

Excess Corticosteroid States

The most common cause is iatrogenic or endogenous (Cushing's syndrome of adrenal or hypothalamic origin). Hypercortisol states can cause behavioral effects (depression, euphoria, insomnia, mania) but also psychoses with suicidal ideation. Cognitive impairment and confusional states are less common. The incidence of psychoses can be less than 1% in patients receiving less than 40 mg of prednisone, but 20% in patients receiving 80 mg of prednisone. Daily corticosteroid treatment is more likely to cause psychoses than alternate-day therapy. Other adverse effects of corticosteroid excess include papilledema caused by idiopathic intracranial hypertension, weakness because of myopathy, spinal cord or nerve root dysfunction relating to spinal compression by epidural fat, spinal compression fracture as a result of osteoporosis, visual impairment as a result of glaucoma or cataract formation, proptosis, and impaired ocular motility disorder caused by enlarged retro-orbital fat. Systemic side effects include peptic ulceration, hypertension, enhanced fat production, enhanced capillary fragility, lymphopenia, impaired immunologic response, and protein catabolism.

Corticosteroid Insufficiency

Primary adrenal gland insufficiency (Addison's disease) is the most common cause of corticosteroid insufficiency. Neurologic manifestations include behavioral effects such as abnormal fatigue, lethargy, apathy, or cognitive inefficiency. These patients are extremely sensitive to low doses of CNS drugs (hypnotics, sedatives, anticonvulsants, analgesics, narcotics), which can cause encephalopathy. In patients with adrenal insufficiency, consider adrenoleukodystrophy, especially in boys (see Chapter 13).

Hypoglycemia

Neurologic symptoms do not usually develop unless the blood sugar concentration is less than 40 mg/dl. The most common causes of hypoglycemia are insulin therapy for diabetes mellitus and alcoholism with acute fatty liver and reduced hepatic glycogen.

Hypoglycemic symptoms include hunger, abdominal cramps, irritability, headache, diaphoresis, tachycardia, palpitations, pallor, and lightheadedness. Neurologic symptoms include paresthesias, blurred vision, diplopia, slurred speech, and confusion; with severe hypoglycemia, syncope, Babinski signs, seizures, and even coma with impaired brainstem reflexes (absent caloric response with preserved pupillary reactivity) can occur. Consider hypoglycemia as a possible cause in patients with anxiety neurosis of recent onset, episodic unresponsiveness, or status epilepticus. Blood glucose measurement should be obtained when patients are symptomatic. Treatment includes intravenous administration of 1 or 2 ampules of glucose (50 g/ampule).

▦ NEUROLOGIC CONDITIONS ASSOCIATED WITH SYSTEMIC VASCULITIS

Systemic Lupus Erythematosus

CNS involvement usually occurs late in course of systemic lupus erythematosus (SLE), although rarely it can be the initial symptom. Pathologic features include multiple small infarctions caused by arteriolar and capillary occlusions, large vessel nonvasculitic infarctions, and rare instances of multifocal necrotizing angiitis with fibrinoid degeneration. It should be noted that despite "vasculitis" being seen pathologically, the exact mechanism of neuropsychiatric manifestations of SLE are not known and can be multiple, including nonbacterial thrombotic endocarditis and valvular inflammatory disorder, which causes cardiogenic cerebral embolism, thrombotic thrombocytopenic purpura, infectious-inflammatory disorders or thrombotic coagulation states. Neurologic findings of SLE are listed in Box 22-3.

BOX 22-3

1 "Lupus cerebritis" with symptoms including confusion, dementia, psychoses, seizures, cortical blindness

2 Stroke syndromes including subarachnoid and parenchymal hemorrhage or ischemic stroke

3 Migrainelike headaches, which occur in more than 50% of SLE patients and respond to conventional migraine treatment

4 Papilledema

5 Myelopathy

6 Dyskinesias, especially chorea

7 Cranial neuropathies involving facial, oculomotor, trigeminal, acoustic nerves

Less commonly patients with SLE have clinical evidence of peripheral nervous system involvement including polyneuropathy, mononeuritis multiplex, or myopathy. Contrasted with CNS pathologic findings the peripheral nervous system is affected by systemic vasculitis as demonstrated by nerve or muscle biopsy findings. Intracerebral hemorrhage causes death in 25% of SLE patients.

CSF findings in lupus cerebritis can include pleocytosis, elevated protein content with increased gamma-globulin component, and decreased complement level. Most patients with neurologic abnormalities have evidence of renal impairment and decreased serum complement level. Consistent with pathologic findings with minimal evidence of vasculitis, angiography usually shows no evidence of angitis.

Improvement of neurologic function in SLE usually follows treatment with corticosteroids (prednisone, 60 to 120 mg/day), but the ultimate prognosis is determined by the severity of systemic SLE. In SLE patients receiving corticosteroids, the onset of neuropsychiatric symptomatology suggests several diagnostic possibilities: lupus cerebritis, corticosteroid-induced psychoses, single or multiple stroke episodes, infectious-inflammatory disorders caused by immunologic abnormalities secondary to SLE or immunosuppressive medication effect.

Periarteritis Nodosa

Periarteritis nodosa (PN) is a systemic necrotizing inflammatory arteritis that affects medium and small vessels. Arteritis predisposes patients to thrombosis with ischemia and infarction; aneurysms can develop in involved vessels. Patients with PN have gastrointestinal, renal, or cardiac symptoms; neural involvement occurs in 50%. CNS manifestations include stroke syndromes as a result of thromboembolism or intracranial hemorrhage caused by ruptured inflammatory aneurysms. Peripheral nervous system involvement consists of mononeuritis multiplex, polyneuropathy, or myopathy. The diagnosis of PN is established by nerve or muscle biopsy, showing pathologic evidence of vasculitis. Corticosteroids combined with cyclophosphamide have been efficacious in PN.

Giant Cell Arteritis and Polymyalgia Rheumatica

An arteritis with giant cell formation involving large and medium-size vessels can occur, most commonly involving the temporal artery. The majority of patients are over 60 years old; a few are in their 50s; and even fewer are in their 40s. The initial clinical manifestations include fever, myalgia, headache, jaw claudication, and arthralgias. Polymyalgia rheumatica is characterized by joint pains, myalgias, and stiffness, but without arthritis. This disorder can represent the prodromal phase of giant cell arteritis. If headache is present, it is usually boring rather than throbbing. Headache precedes visual symptoms by several months.

In patients with temporal arteritis, the examination can show palpable and nodular temporal artery. Patients can have impaired visual acuity, and funduscopic findings include optic disc pallor with narrowing of retinal arterioles consistent with arteritic anterior ischemic optic neuropathy (see Chapter 7). Arteritis can involve other cranial nerves, for example, the third, fifth, sixth, and seventh. The erythrocyte sedimentation rate is markedly elevated in TA. The diagnosis is established by a temporal artery biopsy; a characteristic finding is segmental arteritis with giant cell and granuloma formation. It is important to obtain an adequate sample of the temporal artery because "skip lesions" with granulomas and arteritic changes separated by normal regions can exist. Treatment consists of corticosteroids (prednisone, 60 mg/day) for 2 to 3 months. Prednisone should be tapered slowly over 6 to 12 months while ESR and visual function are monitored. If symptoms or laboratory studies show signs of recurrence, increase the prednisone dose immediately and continue the corticosteroids for a more prolonged course. This is effective in relieving headaches and preventing further visual loss; however, visual impairment that developed before treatment is not usually reversible.

Antiphospholipid Antibody Syndrome

These include lupus anticoagulant (LA) and anticardiolipin (ACL) antibodies. They represent polyclonal immunoglobulins that bind negatively charged phospholipids. They can cause recurrent thrombotic events in both arterial and venous circulations. These patients can have ischemic stroke syndrome, retinal artery occlusion, seizures, chorea, multiinfarct dementia, or migraine. These patients often have a history of prior deep vein thrombosis, multiple spontaneous abortions, and skin lesions classified as livedo reticularis. A stroke in a young person should initiate an investigation for antiphospholipid antibody syndrome (APL). Laboratory findings can include false positive VDRL (syphilis) serology, low platelet count, prolonged prothrombin and activated partial thromboplastin time, positive lupus erythematosus preparation and positive antinuclear antibody, and LA and ACL antibodies. The echocardiogram can show thrombotic vegetations on heart valves. The cerebral angiogram shows single or multiple intracranial arterial occlusions without evidence of vasculitis. Treatment is controversial and includes suppression of immune mediated thrombotic response using steroids or immunosuppressive medication (azathioprine, methotrexate, cyclophosphamide); plasmapheresis to reduce thrombotic-producing antibodies; and reducing the arterial thrombotic state with anticoagulant or antiplatelet medication.

▪ HEMATOLOGIC DISORDERS

Vitamin B$_{12}$ Deficiency (Subacute Combined System Disease)

Pernicious anemia is the most common cause of B$_{12}$ deficiency; other causes include gastrointestinal disorders (blind loop syndromes, tapeworm, celiac disease, vegetarian diet). B$_{12}$ deficiency can develop in dentists and anesthesia personnel who abuse nitrous oxide; this inactivates B$_{12}$. Most patients are usually anemic (macrocytic) with megaloblastic bone marrow. They have a low serum B_{12} level and decreased hydrochloric acid secretion. Neurologic symptoms can develop in patients who are not anemic but who have low B_{12} levels (less than 200 pg per ml). The definitive diagnosis is established by serum determination of methylamalonic acid and homocystine levels; these accumulate when B_{12}–dependent reactions are blocked.

The earliest pathologic change is myelin sheath swelling. This involves the largest diameter fibers; later the myelin is destroyed and the axon affected. Sensory disturbances are the initial neurologic manifestation. Clinical findings are sensory ataxia, impaired position and vibration sense, areflexia, and bilateral Babinski signs. Onset is subacute; peripheral neuropathy, not myelopathy, represents the initial finding of neurologic B_{12} deficiency. Neurologic findings include myelopathy, peripheral neuropathy, and neuropsychiatric disorders (irritability, hallucination, confusion, dementia). Despite pathologic findings of diffuse CNS demyelination, the relationship of mental aberrations to B_{12} deficiency is not clear. Treatment consists of intramuscular B_{12} injection. The prognosis is best in patients who have a short duration of symptoms. In patients with folate and B_{12} deficiency it is a long-believed but inconclusively proved myth that treatment with folate only can precipitate neurologic symptoms of B_{12} deficiency. Cyanocobalamin or hydroxocobalamin can be administered intramuscularly or subcutaneously; however, oral preparations are not effective.

Hemolytic Anemias

Disorders characterized by shortened red blood cell survival time can be broadly classified into two groups: intrinsic defect in red cell composition including hemoglobinopathies (sickle cell disease) and extrinsic abnormal factors in plasma (autoimmune disorders).

Hemoglobinopathies

Inherited disorders of hemoglobin synthesis that cause abnormal neurologic features include hemoglobin SS and sickling cell disease. Neurologic disorders are rare in patients with the sickle cell trait (hemoglobin SA). The pathophysiologic mechanism of cerebrovascular complications is vascular occlusion caused by sickling. This causes increased blood viscosity, endothelial capillary damage, and activation of the coagulation mechanism to cause thrombosis. Precipitating factors for sickling include hypoxia, dehydration, and metabolic acidosis. These can cause the formation of deoxyhemoglobin. This causes the Hgb S molecule to become insoluble and polymerize to deform the red blood cell. If the patient is dehydrated, this increases the Hgb S concentration as a result of reduced water content, and the blood has increased viscosity, which results in vascular thrombosis. This is initially seen in small vessels and later in larger vessels. Vascular thrombosis leads to cellular hypoxia, which increases vascular sickling. There can be involvement of large and small intracranial vessels. This especially involves the border zone between major arteries such as anterior and middle cerebral arteries or middle and posterior cerebral arteries. Spinal cord infarction can be caused by sickle cell disease. This diagnosis should be suspected in young black patients who develop paraparesis. Diagnosis of SS disease is established by blood smear (showing sickling) and hemoglobin electrophoresis. Common neurologic manifestations include ischemic stroke syndromes, which are frequently recurrent. Visual disturbances result from retinal circulation occlusive disease. The diagnosis of cerebral infarction can be established by CT/MRI scan. Angiography demonstrates site of vascular occlusion; it should be performed with caution because iodinated contrast can precipitate sickling. Treatment of sickle cell patients with acute stroke includes hydration, correction of metabolic abnormalities including acidosis (use bicarbonate), oxygen administration, and treatment of the identified intercurrent infection. Indications for treatment with antisickling agents (urea, sodium cyanate, vasodilators) and exchange transfusion remain controversial.

Polycythemia Vera

Neurologic disorders in polycythemia vera are caused by occlusive thrombotic (hyperviscosity, platelet clumping, thrombocytosis) and hemorrhagic (abnormal thromboplastin formation) stroke. Other clinical disturbances include headache, lethargy, dizziness, vertigo, and papilledema. Polycythemia occurs in association with cerebellar hemangioblastoma, hepatic and renal disease, uterine fibroids, and hypoxia. Treatment of neurologic symptomatology resulting from hyperviscosity includes phlebotomy.

Hemorrhagic Disorders

Hemorrhagic disorders occur in congenital (e.g., hemophilia) or acquired disorders (e.g., hepatic disease, leukemia, anticoagulant therapy). In hemophilia bleeding can cause peripheral (nerve or plexus) or intracranial (subdural, subarachnoid, intracerebral) lesions. Peripheral nerve compression lesions are the most common neurologic complication of hemophilia; these are usually secondary to intramuscular bleeding (spontaneous or traumatic). In hemophilia patients, sudden development of neurologic abnormalities is evidence of recent bleeding; blood replacement therapy is initiated, and surgery is usually avoided. In anticoagulated patients the effects of heparin can be reversed rapidly by intravenous protamine (2 mg/ml). The effects of warfarin are reversed rapidly by infusing fresh frozen plasma or more slowly (within 6 to 12 hours) with intravenous vitamin K (50 mg). Intracranial hemorrhage can also occur in patients treated with thrombolytic agents (urokinase, streptokinase, tissue plasminogen activator).

Thrombotic Thrombocytopenic Purpura

The diagnosis of thrombotic thrombocytopenic purpura (TTP) is established by these criteria:

- Neurologic disturbances
- Thrombocytopenia
- Hemolytic anemia
- Fever
- Renal impairment

Neurologic manifestations include altered consciousness, focal neurologic deficit, seizures, retinal hemorrhages, papilledema. Pathologic findings include platelet-rich thrombi and endothelial hyperplasia; these thrombi are associated with necrotic and petechial hemorrhagic lesions. Most patients die within several weeks. Treatment with heparin, corticosteroids, plasma exchange, or plasma infusion have been unsuccessful; however, remission following exchange plasmapheresis and antiplatelet agents (aspirin and dipyridamole) can occur.

Disseminated Intravascular Coagulopathy

Diffuse intracranial thrombotic lesions are caused by activation of a coagulation mechanism with fibrin deposition on the endothelial wall with fibrinolytic response. Pathologic findings are fibrin thrombi in small intracranial vessels. These can result in infarction or multifocal hemorrhages. Hemorrhagic lesions result from consumption of coagulation factors and platelets in addition to the coagulant effect of fibrin-split products. Conditions causing tissue damage such as surgery, sepsis, or trauma can result in the release of tissue thromboplastin and coagulation system activation. Neurologic manifestations depend on number, distribution, and type of lesion(s). Multifocal microvascular thrombotic lesions cause encephalopathy, and large intracerebral hematoma cause altered consciousness and focal neurologic deficit.

Oral Contraceptive Pills

Neurologic complications of oral contraceptive pills (OCP) are due to hypercoagulability (effect on platelets, protein S, protein C, antithrombin III factor). These effects can be correlated with OCP estrogen content. There is increased risk of thromboembolic phenomena in patients who have used OCP containing estrogen with excess of 50 μg per tablet, and laboratory studies can demonstrate hypercoagulability. Neurologic complications include cerebral arterial thromboembolism, venous sinus thrombosis, benign intracranial hypertension, retinal vascular disease, and migraines.

The incidence of stroke syndrome in young women has increased in the four decades since the introduction of OCP; however, it is important to know that pregnancy is also associated with the increased risk of stroke. Migraine is sometimes exacerbated in both frequency and intensity by these drugs, but it is not known if the development of migraine increases stroke risk. Those patients who use OCP, smoke cigarettes, are hypertensive or have family history of hypertension, and are older than 35 years old have the highest stroke risk.

ANOXIC-ISCHEMIC BRAIN DISORDERS

Subacute and Chronic Hypoxic Encephalopathy

Subacute and chronic hypoxic encephalopathy occurs in patients who have inadequate brain oxygen content as a result of certain disorders including pulmonary dysfunction, anemia, and low cardiac output (congestive heart failure and aortic stenosis). Neurologic symptomatology can develop if oxygen content is less than 55 mm Hg. Neurologic manifestations include irritability, agitation, impaired judgment, confusion, and myoclonus. This condition can persist for several weeks to months if the underlying cause is not corrected; however, if another acute event (rapid decrease in cerebral blood flow and perfusion, febrile illness, anesthesia) is superimposed, acute anoxic-ischemic brain damage can worsen neurologic function.

Acute Anoxic-Ischemic Encephalopathy

In patients who require cardiopulmonary resuscitation inadequate support of the brain function can cause neurologic sequelae. If cerebral circulation is terminated for more than 10 seconds, brain oxygen reserves are depleted, and neurologic dysfunction (lightheadedness, blindness, altered consciousness, myoclonus, decerebration, pupillary dilatation, Babinski signs) can develop. After successful resuscitation from any shock state, (e.g., sepsis, smoke inhalation, carbon monoxide poisoning, strangulation, cardiac arrest) complete recovery can occur or the patient can develop a mild amnestic syndrome.

In certain cases a hypoxic episode causes cerebral edema and ischemia. Postanoxic ischemia is most commonly encountered after cardiac arrest in which there has been cessation of cerebral blood flow. Cerebral ischemia can be diffuse (global) or focal. In these cases ischemic changes occur in border zone regions (the territory between anterior and middle cerebral arteries or between posterior and middle cerebral arteries). Swelling of capillaries is postulated to decrease blood flow, and this can persist even if cerebral circulation is adequately restored. Decreased tissue perfusion can cause permanent neurologic deficit including amnesia, dementia, blindness, weakness (bibrachial paresis, quadriparesis), myoclonus, ataxia, seizures, or extrapyramidal (parkinsonism, hemiballism) disorders. In certain cases of hypoxic-ischemic injury there is severe neocortical brain damage with intact brain stem and spinal cord reflexes. These patients are severely neurologically impaired but can survive for prolonged periods in vegetative states. In cases of irreversible coma (brain death) cortical function and brain stem reflexes are absent. Anoxia affects the myocardium and brain; therefore there is also myocardial ischemia with anoxic brain damage. This is manifested by electrocardiographic changes and elevated serum enzymes (creatine phosphokinase, CPK). Because a portion of CPK originates from brain, isoenzyme patterns can be required to determine the exact enzyme source (e.g., skeletal or myocardial muscle, brain).

Following initial stabilization or recovery from anoxic injury, certain patients subsequently deteriorate one to three weeks later. Findings include altered consciousness, rigidity, spasticity, and Babinski signs.

Pathologic findings are diffuse demyelination involving cerebral white matter; however, the cause of delayed postanoxic encephalopathy is unknown.

Pulmonary Encephalopathy

In patients with carbon dioxide retention and respiratory acidosis caused by acute respiratory disorders, neurologic symptomatology (altered mentation, generalized seizures, myoclonus, asterixis) can develop. Headache that occurs at night or immediately upon awakening is due to nocturnal hypoventilation and CO_2 retention. Other conditions such as emphysema, bronchitis, and massive obesity (pickwickian syndrome) cause chronic hypercapnia. Neurologic dysfunction can develop as a result of elevated arterial carbon dioxide levels, decreased arterial oxygen levels, or decreased arterial bicarbonate levels (respiratory acidosis); these disturbances result in cerebral vasodilation. Neurologic manifestations include intracranial hypertension; encephalopathy with altered consciousness, asterixis, or myoclonus; and diffuse EEG slowing. Narcosis developing in patients with chronic hypercapnia is quite different from an agitated confusional state caused by hypoxia. Treatment of carbon dioxide retention should initially include assisted ventilatory support because the brain stem respiratory centers are depressed and treatment with oxygen alone may not be effective. Sleep apnea syndromes are associated with cardiovascular and respiratory disturbances (see Chapter 23).

Hyperventilation can occur in anxiety states and can cause paresthesias involving extremities or the perioral region, light-headedness, muscle cramps, carpopedal spasms, and occasionally brief periods of unconsciousness.

█ IDIOPATHIC INTRACRANIAL HYPERTENSION

Patients with idiopathic intracranial hypertension (IIH) (also referred to as pseudotumor cerebri) develop symptoms of increased intracranial pressure without altered consciousness or focal neurologic deficit. IIH most commonly occurs in young obese females. It has been associated with endocrine conditions (menarche, menorrhagia, metrorrhagia), Addison's disease, corticosteroid excess or withdrawal, thyroid or parathyroid dysfunction), vitamin A intoxication, drugs (tetracycline, nalidixic acid), and other conditions including anemia and SLE.

Symptoms include headache, vomiting, dizziness, diplopia, and transient visual blurring. A funduscopic examination shows bilateral papilledema; some patients have lateral rectus muscle palsy or visual impairment. The visual field examination shows enlarged blind spots. The major complication of IIH is irreversible visual loss.

A CT or MRI scan is necessary to exclude expanding mass or hydrocephalus; these are expected to be normal in IIH. If intracranial hypertension is chronic, a skull radiogram can show sella turcica enlargement and erosion. Angiography or magnetic resonance angiography can be necessary to exclude venous sinus thrombosis. Lumbar puncture is performed to exclude infectious-inflammatory causes; the CSF should be normal except for elevated pressure.

In most patients there is spontaneous clinical remission. This occurs immediately following the initial lumbar puncture. Weight reduction in obese patients and treatment of specific etiologic conditions are usually effective. Other treatment modalities include lumbar puncture with removal of 30 to 50 ml of CSF three times weekly; however, this is theoretically irrational because the CSF turns over five times each day. There is inconclusive evidence that diuretics (chlorothiazide [Diuril], acetazolamide [Diamox]) or glycerol are effective treatments. In refractory cases corticosteroids are used; however, their systemic toxicity is high, especially in obese young women and if used for prolonged time intervals. If intracranial hypertension persists despite medical therapy, lumboperitoneal shunt or surgical decompression of the optic nerve sheath is required to prevent visual loss and relieve headache. The major threat in IIH is visual loss; visual function (including tests of contrast sensitivity) studies monitoring optic nerve function must be carefully performed.

SARCOIDOSIS

Sarcoidosis is a systemic granulomatous disorder of unknown cause. It can involve the nervous system in the minority of cases, and in some patients neurologic manifestations are the initial signs. Pathologic CNS findings are basilar meningitis with thickening of meninges and diffuse noncaseating granulomatous nodules; rarely granulomas extend into the brain parenchyma and spinal cord. Sarcoid granulomas can be seen peripherally (nerve, muscle). Neurologic manifestations in sarcoidosis, except when caused by hypercalcemia, are secondary to granulomas and basilar meningitis.

Neurologic features of sarcoidosis are listed in Box 22-4.

In sarcoid meningitis CSF findings can include sterile pleocytosis with lymphocyte predominance, decreased sugar content, elevated protein content, and

BOX 22-4

1 Cranial nerve palsies of which facial nerve involvement is most frequent, but pupillary abnormalities are usually secondary to uveitis, not oculomotor involvement

2 Chronic or subacute meningoencephalitis

3 Mass effect caused by intracranial granuloma

4 Symptoms of hydrocephalus caused by obstruction of fourth ventricle or basal cisterns

5 Juxtasellar syndrome (visual defects, diabetes insipidus, hypopituitarism) caused by hypothalamic-pituitary granuloma

6 Seizures caused by cortical granulomas or vasculopathy

7 Peripheral neuropathy, mononeuritis multiplex

negative studies for infectious causes. To establish the diagnosis of sarcoidosis biopsy evidence is necessary (lymph nodes, liver, skin, conjunctiva, muscle), but confirmation of CNS involvement can require dural or brain biopsy.

Treatment of neurologic symptoms with corticosteroids (prednisone, 60 to 120 mg/day) is usually efficacious, but this must be continued for several months to years. If lesions do not respond to prednisone, consider high-dose intravenous methylprednisolone. For refractory cases of neurosarcoidosis, radiation therapy can be used. Spontaneous remission and recurrence can characterize the course of neurosarcoidosis. Hydrocephalus can require a shunting procedure, and hormonal replacement may be needed if there is hypothalamic-pituitary dysfunction. Intracranial granulomas rarely require surgical removal.

PORPHYRIA

Several disorders of porphyrin metabolism are associated with neurologic symptomatology including acute intermittent porphyria (AIP), hereditary coproporphyria, and variegate prophyria. AIP is inherited as an autosomal dominant trait and is characterized by increased production of delta-aminoevulinic acid and porphobilinogen (PBG). These are porphyrin precursors and are excreted in urine. Urine contains increased amounts of coproporphyrin and uroporphyrin. AIP is believed to result from uroporphyrin synthetase deficiency. Pathologic findings include neuronal degeneration with central and peripheral white matter demyelination. Patients have abdominal symptoms (pain, nausea, vomiting, distention, constipation, diarrhea) that simulate acute abdominal crisis; these features are believed caused by autonomic dysfunction. Other symptoms are due to central (mental changes with confusion, delirium, psychoses with hallucinations, mania or depression, seizures, hyponatremia, water intoxication) or peripheral (acute or subacute ascending paralysis) nervous system involvement. In rare instances symptoms and signs caused by brainstem dysfunction including dysarthria, dysphagia, diplopia, ophthalmoplegia, respiratory depression, and hypertensive vascular crisis develop.

Acute attacks of AIP can be precipitated by drugs (barbiturates, sulfonamides, oral contraceptives, estrogens, alcohol), a fasting state, or hormonal shifts (menstruation). It is possible that these induce delta-aminolevulinic acid dehydrase and that during attacks this enzyme can be hyperactive. During acute attacks urine appears burgundy red and darkens in the test tube; it contains no red blood cells and gives a negative hemoglobin reaction. The Watson-Schwartz test for PBG is usually positive during attacks, but a negative test does not exclude AIP. During acute episodes avoidance of exacerbating drugs, monitoring of respiratory function, careful fluid replacement, opiates to control pain, and phenothiazines for psychoses are effective treatments. Barbiturates and phenytoin should not be used to treat seizures because they aggravate the disorder; diazepam, lorazepam, carbamazepine, or paraldehyde are more effective and safer. Fluid management is necessary as SIADH can occur to cause hyponatremia. Pain should be managed carefully using low dose phenothiazines or meperidine only if absolutely necessary. There has been a report of improvement in neural symptoms following a high-carbohydrate diet or intravenous administration of hematin; both act to lower hepatic delta-aminolevulinic acid synthetase activity. The role of chelating agents in AIP is controversial.

▨ NEUROLOGIC COMPLICATIONS OF PREGNANCY

Cerebrovascular Disease

The incidence of stroke in pregnant women is higher than in nonpregnant women including those using oral contraceptives. Potential mechanisms of stroke in pregnancy include disseminated intravascular coagulation caused by abruptio placentae, venous sinus, and cortical vein thrombosis; and hemorrhage caused by metastatic choriocarcinoma, eclampsia, and ischemic arterial cerebrovascular disease. Berry aneurysms can rupture during pregnancy, most commonly during the last trimester. Arteriovenous malformations can also enlarge and hemorrhage during pregnancy. If rupture of an aneurysm or arteriovenous malformation occurs during pregnancy, surgery may be necessary. The mechanism of ischemic arterial stroke in the pregnant patient is not known; however, a search for cardiac embolic source or vasculitis should be performed.

Eclampsia

Eclampsia is hypertensive disease that occurs in pregnant women and terminates after childbirth. Neurologic manifestations include headache, visual symptoms (blurring, visual field defect, cortical blindness), hyperreflexia, Babinski signs, seizures, and altered consciousness. If focal deficit occurs, this suggests intracerebral hemorrhage or infarction. In eclampsia pathologic findings include brain swelling with edema, small infarctions, hemorrhage, and vasopasm. There is a predilection for pathologic changes in the parieto-occipital cortex. Management of eclampsia includes rapid lowering of blood pressure and pregnancy termination. Seizures usually stop with blood pressure control; however, anticonvulsants (diazepam, lorazepam, phenytoin) may be needed. Magnesium sulfate can be used as anticonvulsant for eclampsia. This drug blocks autonomic and neuromuscular transmission; therefore it can cause respiratory depression and arrhythmias and must be used with caution. It is not established whether magnesium sulfate or conventional anticonvulsants should be utilized for control of eclamptic seizures.

Seizures

For a discussion of those seizures not caused by eclampsia, see Chapter 11.

Headache

Migraine usually improves during pregnancy. If a migraine does occur, ergots should be avoided because they stimulate uterine contractions. New onset of headaches in pregnant women must be assessed carefully neurologically. The need for diagnostic studies is determined by the presence of abnormal neurologic findings. Brain neoplasms can expand in size as a result of increased tumor vascularity, and symptoms can progress during later pregnancy stages.

Multiple Sclerosis

There is little evidence to support the belief that pregnancy exacerbates multiple sclerosis. It is important for patients with multiple sclerosis to avoid fatigue in the postpartum period when MS exacerbates.

Neuromuscular Disease

Mononeuropathies (e.g., facial paralysis, median nerve compression at carpal tunnel, lateral femoral cutaneous nerve involvement) are common in pregnancy. Nutritional neuropathy and Wernicke-Korsakoff syndrome can occur in patients with hyperemesis gravidarum. Lumbosacral joint laxity and the weight of the fetus in the abdomen can cause mechanical back strain symptoms. Obstetrical complications include peroneal, femoral, and sciatic neuropathy. Transient myasthenia gravis occurs in newborns of myasthenic mothers (see Chapter 17).

SUBSTANCE ABUSE

Narcotics

Narcotics include morphine, heroin, hydromorphone (Dilaudid), oxycodone (Percodan), and methadone. Major neurologic complications are due to overdoses and include coma, respiratory depression, miotic pupils, and death. Treatment includes respiratory and cardiac support. Naloxone is administered in doses of 0.4 mg every 5 minutes to reverse narcotic effects. If recovery from an acute overdose occurs, neurologic sequelae can develop. These include seizures, dementia, delayed postanoxic encephalopathy, stroke, and dyskinesias. Toxic optic neuropathy can result from quinine, used as a diluent for "street-made" illicit narcotics. Transverse myelitis can occur in patients who use intravenous heroin once again after there has been a period of abstinence, for example, after release from prison. Compressive neuropathies can result from injection into a nerve or from tourniquet-induced nerve ischemia. After a prolonged narcotic coma myoglobinuria can result. Infections occurring commonly in narcotic addicts include tetanus, local abscesses, osteomyelitis, endocarditis, and hepatitis. Withdrawal symptoms include marked signs of sympathetic overdischarge and agitated delirious state.

Stimulants

Cocaine and amphetamine (Dexedrine, methylphenidate [Ritalin], Benzedrine) are the most commonly used stimulant drugs. Cocaine causes heightened awareness and perception, agitation and anxiety, and an increased sympathomimetic discharge (tachycardia, hypertension). Seizures and cardiac arrest (because of arrhythmias) can also result. An acute hypertensive crisis severe enough to cause intracranial hemorrhage can result from the reuptake block of sympathomimetic neurotransmitters by cocaine. Amphetamines can produce an acute agitated delirious state, paranoia, hallucinations, and seizures. Following the use of methamphetamine, cerebral vasculitis can cause stroke. Methylphenidate hydrochloride (Ritalin) can be mixed with certain substances (starch) and injected intravenously. The particulate matter can embolize to the brain to cause stroke.

Hallucinogens

Hallucinogens include lysergic acid diethylamide (LSD), phencyclidine (PCP), and mescaline. LSD causes prominent behavioral manifestations (psychoses, acute anxiety, panic states, hallucinations). PCP causes psychoses, autonomic overdischarge (with cardiovascular effect and dilated pupils), and seizures. Fatal status epilepticus has been reported with PCP use.

Pentazocine and Pyribenzamine

Pentazocine (Talwin) and an antihistamine Pyribenzamine tablet are usually crushed and mixed with water (T's and blues) and injected intravenously. They can produce embolic particles, which cause stroke.

GASTROINTESTINAL DISORDERS

Pancreatic Disease

It is believed that some patients with chronic pancreatitis develop "pancreatic encephalopathy." This disorder is characterized by an agitated confusional state with hallucinations, speech disturbances, muscular rigidity, and quadriplegia. Pathologic findings include petechial hemorrhages and demyelination seen in subcortical and brain stem regions. It is important to consider pancreatic disorders in adult patients with otherwise unexplained neurobehavioral symptoms of recent onset. Pancreas tumors (insulinomas) can cause intermittent hypoglycemia with a perplexing array of neurobehavioral manifestations.

Celiac Disease

Celiac disease is an idiopathic steatorrhea with malabsorption caused by small intestinal disease. The condition remits when a gluten-free diet is instituted. Neurologic features occur in 10% of patients and include myopathy, neuropathy, cerebellar ataxia, myoclonus, seizures, encephalopathy. Myopathy is associated with osteomalacia as a result of abnormal calcium and vitamin D metabolism. Neuropathy and ataxia can be due to vitamin E deficiency. Seizures can be due to calcium, magnesium, or pyridoxine deficiency.

Whipple's Disease

Whipple's disease is relapsing-remitting multisystem disease (diarrhea, steatorrhea, weight loss, abdominal pain, arthralgias) with CNS manifestations (dementia, ataxia, myoclonus, seizures, focal deficit) occurring uncommonly. Neurologic manifestations can occur without evidence of clinically apparent intestinal disease. The diagnosis is established by intestinal biopsy; this shows periodic acid-Schiff-positive macrophages. The disease is believed to be infectious and responds to antibiotic therapy.

ACQUIRED IMMUNE DEFICIENCY SYNDROME

Neurologic disorders affecting the central or peripheral nervous system occur in more than 80% of patients. The human immunodeficiency virus (HIV) has neurotrophic features. Patients infected with HIV develop opportunistic infections and unusual CNS neoplasms. Neurologic manifestations of acquired immune deficiency syndrome (AIDS) can be due to the direct or indirect effects of HIV. Neurologic manifestation in asymptomatic seropositive patients or those who have the AIDS-related complex are uncommon; the majority of neurologic complications occur in AIDS patients.

Direct Effect of HIV on Nervous System

AIDS-Dementia Complex

The earliest signs of the AIDS-dementia complex are usually neurobehavioral (impaired memory, difficulty concentrating, psychomotor retardation, apathy, depression). Motor signs include impaired coordination and ataxia. CSF findings are lymphocytic pleocytosis with elevated protein content; studies for opportunistic infections are negative. The CT and MRI are usually negative in early stages; later a generalized cerebral atrophic pattern with hypodense lesions in periventricular white matter, subcortical regions (basal ganglia, thalamus), and brain stem regions can be seen. The clinical course is characterized by rapid progression with development of dementia, myoclonus, seizures, motor impairment, and incontinence. Zidovudine (azidothymidine, AZT) blocks retrovirus replication in CNS; this drug slows the progression of AIDS. Occurrence of AIDS-dementia complex is less common since the introduction of AZT. Other antiviral drugs used to treat HIV infection include didanosine and dideoxycytidine. The major adverse effects of these two medications are neuropathy and pancreatitis. In AIDS-dementia patients, autopsy findings include necrotic and vacuolated brain lesions containing multinucleated macrophages. The lesions are located predominantly in white matter and the brain stem, with the cerebral cortex relatively spared.

Myelitis-Myelopathy

The spinal cord can also show vacuolar necrotizing lesions, believed caused by HIV. Myelography is necessary to exclude spinal cord lesions caused by opportunistic infection or neoplasm. CSF should be performed to exclude herpes zoster, which can cause meylitis, and to exclude neurosyphilis.

Radiculopathy

Involvement of lumbar and sacral roots by HIV can cause leg weakness and paresthesias with autonomic (bladder, bowel) dysfunction. Radiculopathy is frequently caused by cytomegalovirus (CMV). There is usually also evidence of retinitis. The CSF can show polymorphonuclear pleocytosis with a positive CSF culture for CMV. Ganciclovir is used to treat CMV.

Muscle Disease

Severe inflammatory myositis in which muscles show profound muscle necrosis with lymphocytic infiltrates can develop in AIDS patients. Viral conditions and toxoplasmosis can precipitate polymyositis. AZT can cause mitochondrial myopathy. Differentiation of HIV-induced or toxoplasmosis myopathy from AZT-induced myopathy can be established by muscle biopsy findings in which drug-related muscle damage shows marked mitochondrial abnormalities.

Neuropathy

Acute inflammatory demyelinating polyneuropathy (similar to Guillain-Barré syndrome) can cause ascending or descending motor weakness. The initial feature of demyelinating neuropathy can be bilateral facial paresis. This can occur in early stages of HIV infection. The CSF can show pleocytosis. This disorders responds to plasmapheresis or immunoglobulin G treatment. In AIDS patients painful sensormotor neuropathy of axonal type can develop. This can be due to direct HIV effects, complications of AZT, or a complicating metabolic-toxic disorder. Sensory symptoms are more prominent than motor weakness in AIDS neuropathy; treatment with amitriptyline or use of pain medication administered at bedtime can be effective in controlling the neuropathic pain.

Indirect Effects of HIV on Nervous System

The indirect effects of HIV result from immunodysfunction. It is not uncommon for patients to have multiple infections.

Opportunistic Infections

Toxoplasmosis. This is an intracellular protozoan (Toxoplasma gondii) that is transmitted by human secretions or through blood transfusions. Pathologically, multiple diffuse necrotizing intracranial lesions with minimal cellular inflammatory response develop. The CSF can show lymphocytic pleocytosis. The CT/MRI shows multiple ring-enhancing intracranial lesions; however, these findings are not specific enough to establish the diagnosis of toxoplasmosis. Serologic toxoplasmosis tests can have false-positive and false-negative results. Because this is the most common CNS lesion in AIDS patients, empiric anti-toxoplasmosis therapy is initiated if the CT/MRI show intracranial lesion(s). Treatment includes sulfadiazine and pyrimethamine. If the patient is allergic to sulfa, substitute clindamycin. If there is improvement evident clinically and with the CT/MRI, this supports the presumptive diagnosis; however, if the condition progresses with empiric treatment, a brain biopsy is needed. Life-long suppressive treatment for toxoplasmosis is necessary. Corticosteroids are used to supplement antibiotics in the acute stage only if edema and mass effect occur.

Fungal disease. Cryptococcosis is the most common (see chapter 18).

Neurosyphilis. See chapter 18.

Myobacteria. See chapter 18.

Viral infections. "Subacute meningitis" is most common neurologic disorder affecting patients with AIDS. The CSF shows lymphocytic pleocytosis and elevated protein and gamma globulin content. Meningitis can be the initial response to HIV and can be seen in 33% of neurologically asymptomatic seropositive patients even in the early stages of the illness.

Progressive multifocal leukoencephalopathy. See Chapter 18.

Central nervous system neoplasms. Primary CNS lymphomas may be present with dementia, seizures, motor disturbances, and cranial nerve dysfunction. These tumors are located in basal ganglia, thalamus, cerebellum, and periventricular white matter. The diagnosis is established by CT/MRI. Brain lymphomas are highly radiosensitive and also respond to corticosteroids but can recur. Kaposi's sarcoma also occurs in AIDS patients and can metastasize to the brain and undergo hemorrhagic degeneration. These lesions are radiosensitive but also rapidly recur.

▣ NEUROLOGIC COMPLICATIONS OF ORGAN TRANSPLANTATION

These can include the neurologic effect of underlying condition for which organ transplantation was performed, for example, diabetes, hypertension, and SLE; immunosuppressive therapy can cause nervous system toxicity and impair immunologic response to result in opportunistic infections, for example, Cryptococcus and Listeria monocytogenes or neoplasms, such as lymphomas.

In patients undergoing renal transplants cerebrovascular disorders (ischemic, hemorrhage) are the most common complication. Following cardiac transplantation, perioperative hypoxic-ischemic complications are most common. Other complications of heart transplants include cardiogenic cerebral embolism, opportunistic infections, lymphoma. Of patients undergoing liver transplants, neurologic complications including encephalopathy, seizures, and focal neurologic deficit are common. Intracranial hemorrhage and opportunistic infection are common causes of these liver transplant complications.

The outcome of transplants is highly dependent upon the prevention of host rejection. This must be prevented by suppressing the recipient immune system. The following drugs have neurotoxicity: cyclosporine, methotrexate, cytarabine, corticosteroids, OKT-3 monoclonal antibody. Cyclosporine has hepatic, renal, and neurologic toxicity. It is lipophilic and can cause adverse CNS effects, including encephalopathy, seizures, tremor, ataxia, leukoencephalopathy, and burning extremity dysesthesias. Cyclosporine-induced seizures should be treated with valproic acid because other anticonvulsants lower the cyclosporine blood levels by enzymatic-induction. Cyclosporine-induced leukoencephalopathy—characterized by confusional state, ataxia, cortical blindness, motor deficit (paraparesis, quadriparesis)—may simulate clinical features of progressive multifocal leukoencephalopathy (see Chapter 18). Sustention and intention tremor is the most common neurologic adverse effect of cyclosporine. Methotrexate can cause neurotoxic syndrome consisting of aseptic meningitis or transverse meylitis, especially if administered intrathecally. Strokelike syndromes and leukoencephalopathy have also been reported (espe-

cially when combined with cranial irradiation). Monoclonal antibody OKT-3 can cause fever, chills, shaking spells, tremor, and headache as well as aseptic
meningitis. Cytarabine can cause peripheral neuropathy and myelopathy. Corticosteroids effects are
described elsewhere (p. 685).

◼ NEUROLOGIC ADVERSE EFFECTS OF NEOPLASTIC THERAPY

The agents shown in Box 22-5 have proven especially
effective in treating leukemia, lymphoma, Hodgkin's
disease, choriocarcinoma, and testicular, lung, and
breast carcinoma. They can have central or peripheral
nervous system toxicity.

◼ INFECTIVE ENDOCARDITIS

Thirty percent of patients with infective endocarditis
develop neurologic complications. Most commonly
there is septic embolic stroke with vegetations (consisting of microorganisms with platelet-fibrin material) embolizing to cerebral vessels. If an embolus
contains microorganisms, these can infect the arterial
wall. There is necrosis and weakening of the arterial
wall leading to mycotic aneurysm formation. A
mycotic aneurysm forms at a distal arterial branch (as
contrasted with the proximal site of berry aneurysm).
This mycotic aneurysm can rupture to cause intracranial hemorrhage. If microorganisms migrate into the
brain parenchyma, cerebritis or abscess may form.
The mycotic aneurysm can be single or multiple.
These are detected by angiography. Antibiotics treat
endocarditis, and mycotic aneurysm can heal with
medical (antibiotic) therapy. Those that do not
resolve with antibiotics can require surgery to avoid
the risk of hemorrhage. Heparin should not be used to
prevent embolic stroke in patients with endocarditis.

BOX 22-5

1 Methotrexate. When this drug is administered intrathecally, acute neurotoxicity includes aseptic meningitis and transverse myelopathy. Following high-dose intravenous methotrexate, strokelike syndrome and leukoencephalopathy (which may be delayed or chronic effect) can develop, especially when methotrexate is combined with cranial irradiation.

2 Cisplatin is antineoplastic drug that has a heavy metal base; therefore, it is not surprising that it can cause peripheral neuropathy. Neuropathy involves large sensory fibers, and findings are absent deep tendon reflexes, reduced vibration and position sensation, and sensory ataxia. Cisplatin can also cause ototoxicity and vestibular dysfunction. Carboplatin has similar antineoplastic effects but minimal neurotoxicity.

3 Vincristine and vinblastine are vinca alkaloids and frequently cause peripheral or cranial neuropathy. It is rare for the vincristine-treated leukemic patient to have intact ankle jerks and normal vibration sensation in the feet.

4 Asparaginase. This interferes with coagulation mechanism (interfering with anti-thrombin III) to cause venous thrombosis (see Chapter 10).

5 Procarbazine can act as a monoamine oxidase inhibitor and cause encephalopathy or manic psychotic episodes. Patients must be advised to avoid tyramine-containing food or sympathomimetic medications.

6 5-fluorouracil can cause cerebellar disorders such as ataxia, dysmetria, and tremor.

7 Cytosine arabinoside can cause aseptic meningitis or transverse myelopathy if administered intrathecally or cerebellar syndrome if administered intravenously.

8 Taxol is a naturally occurring antineoplastic agent that causes peripheral neuropathy.

9 Tamoxifen is a hormonal agent (synthetic anti-estrogen) used in breast cancer treatment that can cause encephalopathy, cerebellar syndrome, retinopathy, or optic neuropathy.

10 Doxorubicin. After parenteral use, it may cause cardiac thrombus, which results in stroke syndrome.

11 Suramin. This may cause demyelinating (rapidly progressing) motor neuropathy that is reversible after drug is discontinued.

BOX 22-5—cont'd

---

12 Cranial irradiation can cause acute, early delayed (1 to 3 months later) or late delayed (after 3 months) syndrome. Acute encephalopathy most commonly develops in patients treated with high-dose irradiation for primary or metastatic brain neoplasms. Symptoms include headache, vomiting, altered mental state, and worsening of pre-existing neurologic dysfunction. This syndrome is due to increased intracranial pressure. It can be treated with high-dose corticosteroids, which are frequently administered before initiating radiation therapy. Early delayed syndrome consists of gradual development of encephalopathy or other signs that can simulate neoplasm progression; however, this can resolve spontaneously. Late delayed radiation-induced syndrome occurs months or years after completion of radiation therapy. This is due to radiation-induced necrosis. The CT/MRI can show findings simulating recurrent neoplasm; differentiation of radiation necrosis from recurrent neoplasm can only be established by pathologic findings obtained from surgery or autopsy.

NEUROLOGIC EFFECTS OF CARDIAC SURGERY

Neurologic sequelae are stroke, hypoxic-ischemic encephalopathy, and diffuse encephalopathy as results of multiple surgical, medical, and anesthetic factors. With extracorporeal circulation there are coagulation factor abnormalities and blood pressure fluctuations that can result in microembolization. Following surgery patients may report memory, cognitive, and behavioral abnormalities. With improved extracorporeal systems that use microfilters, neuropsychologic sequela is less common now than in the past. Ischemic (carotid and vertebral-basilar) thromboembolic and cardiogenic cerebral embolic stroke can result from cardiac surgery, and intracranial hemorrhage can result from anticoagulant and thrombolytic medication. Focal neuropathies or brachial plexus dysfunction can complicate cardiac surgery because of stretch injuries secondary to patient positioning. In patients undergoing cardiac transplantation, immunosuppression is common cause of neurologic complications, for example, aspergillosis, toxoplasmosis.

▨ CHRONIC FATIGUE SYNDROME

Fatigue is a state of discomfort and decreased mental and motor efficiency resulting from excessive exertion. This is relieved by rest and avoided by conditioning efforts. Chronic persistent fatigue that develops without the exertion necessary to cause exhaustion in normal people represents a perplexing and poorly defined disorder. In one study 21% of patients who came to primary care physicians had chronic fatigue as their chief complaint. The definition of chronic fatigue syndrome (CFS) includes persistent and recurrent fatigue lasting at least 6 months, fatigue not improving with bed rest, activities of daily living reduced by 50%, and other medical, neurologic, rheumatologic, infectious, and psychiatric illnesses causing fatigue have been excluded. Other symptoms of CFS include low-grade fever, pharyngitis, lymphadenopathy, myalgia, postexertional malaise, arthralgia, memory and cognitive disturbances, headache, and sleep disturbances. CFS frequently follows viral infections such as infectious mononucleosis, and an antigen of Epstein-Barr virus can be demonstrated by serological studies.

Fatigue symptoms can be a prominent feature of multiple sclerosis, parkinsonism, myasthenia gravis, postpolio syndrome, and postconcussion syndrome, and these disorders should be excluded by careful neurologic examination before establishing the diagnosis of CFS. Fatigue can be seen in psychiatric disorders including affective and somatization disorders however, psychogenic fatigue is characterized by fatigue present upon awakening in morning and is constantly present throughout day. In CFS neurodiagnostic studies show no abnormalities; however, certain inconsistent immunologic abnormalities have been reported (lymphocytosis, hypo- or hypergammaglobulinemia, antinuclear antibodies, serologic evidence of Epstein-Barr virus infection). It is believed that multiple triggering events (infection, trauma, physical or emotional stress) can trigger immunologic response with elaboration of cytokineses and trigger CFS. Symptomatic treatment using amantadine, stimulants, and antidepressants have variable success. Many patients who develop CFS after clearcut viral illness recover slowly; however, other patients with CFS remain permanently disabled.

Suggested Readings

Sarcoid

Stern BJ, Krumholz A, Johns C: Sarcoidosis and its neurological manifestations, *Arch Neurol* 42:909, 1985.

Stern BJ: Neurosarcoidosis, *Neurol Chron* 2:1, 1992.

Peyton D: Neurologic manifestations in sarcoidosis, *Ann Intern Med* 87:336, 1977.

Luke RA, Stern BJ: Neurosarcoidosis, Neurology 37:461, 1987.

Calcium and Phosphate Abnormalities

Knochel JP: The pathophysiology and clinic characteristics of severe hypophosphatemia, *Arch Intern Med* 137:203, 1977.

Dimich A, Bedrossian PB, Wallach S: Hypoparathyroidism, *Arch Intern Med* 120:449, 1967.

Mallette IE: Primary hyperparathyroidism: clinical and biochemical features, *Medicine* 53:127, 1974.

Pattern BM: Neuromuscular disease in primary hyper-parathyroidism, *Ann Intern Med* 80:182, 1974.

Adrenal Disorders

Rimsza ME: Complications of corticosteroid therapy, *Am J Dis Childhood* 132:806, 1978.

Seale JP, Comptom MR: Side effects of corticosteriod agents, *Med J Aust* 144:139, 1986.

HIV Infection

McArthur JC: Neurologic disease associated with HIV infection. In Johnson RT, Griffin JW, eds: *Current therapy in neurologic disease*, Philadelphia, 1993, BC Decker.

Levy RM, Bredesen DE, Rosenblum ML: Neurologic manifestations of the acquired immunodeficiency syndrome, *J Neurosurg* 62:475, 1985.

Navia BA, Jordan BD, Price RW: The AIDS-dementia complex, *Ann Neurol* 19:517, 1986.

Snider WD, et al: Neurological complications of AIDS, *Ann Neurol* 14:403, 1983.

McArthur JC: Neurologic manifestations of AIDS, *Medicine* 66:407, 1987.

Infective Endocarditis

Lerner PI: Neurological complications of infective endo-carditis, *Med Clin North Am* 69:385, 1985.

Idiopathic Intracranial Hypertension

Wall M: Idiopathic intracranial hypertension, *Neurol Clin North Am* 9:73, 1991.

Weisberg LA: Benign intracranial hypertension, *Medicine* 54:197, 1975.

Wall M, George D: Idiopathic intracranial hypertension, *Brain* 114:155, 1991.

Hematological Disorders

Adams R: Cerebral infarction in sickle cell anemia, *Neurology* 38:1012, 1988.

Mishra SK: Thrombotic thrombocytopenic purpura, *Semin Neurol* 5:317, 1985.

Merkel KH, et al: Cerebrovascular disease in sickle cell anemia, *Stroke* 9:45, 1978.

Amorosi FS, Ultmann JE: Thrombotic thrombocytopenic purpura: report of 10 cases and review of literature, *Medicine* 45:139, 1966.

Hypoglycemia

Malouf R, Brust JCM: Hypoglycemia causes neurological manifestations and outcome, *Ann Neurol* 17:421, 1985.

Service FJ, Dale AJD, Elveback LR: Insulinoma: clinical and diagnostic features of 60 consecutive cases, *Mayo Clin Proc* 51:417, 1976.

Diabetes Mellitus

Colby AD: Neurologic disorders of diabetes mellitus, *Diabetes* 14:516, 1965.

Thomas PK: Metabolic neuropathy, *J R Coll Phys* 7:154, 1973.

Brown MJ, Asbury AK: Diabetic neuropathy, *Ann Neurol* 15:2, 1984.

Harati Y: Diabetic peripheral neuorpathies, *Ann Intern Med* 107:546, 1987.

Johnson PC, Doll SC, Cromey DW: Pathogenesis of diabetic neuropathy, *Ann Neurol* 19:450, 1986.

Pregnancy and Oral Contraceptive Medication

Aminoff MJ: Neurologic disorders and pregnancy, *Am J Obstet Gynecol* 132:325, 1978.

Heyman A, Hurtig H: Clinical complications of oral contraceptives, *Dis Month* 1:3, 1975.

Donaldson JO: Neurology of pregnancy. In *Major Problems in Neurology Series,* ed 2, Philadelphia, 1990, WB Saunders.

Sodium Abnormalities

Arieff AI: Hyponatremia, convulsions, respiratory arrest and permanent brain damage after elective surgery in healthy women, *N Engl J Med* 314:1529, 1986.

Ayus JC, Krothapelli RK, Arieff AI: Treatment of symptomatic hyponatremia and its relation to brain damage, *N Engl J Med* 317:1190, 1987.

Addleman M, Pollard A, Grossman RI: Survival after severe hypernatremia due to salt ingestion by an adult, *Am J Med* 78:176, 1985.

Morris-Jones PH, Houston IB, Evans RC: Prognosis of neurologic complications of acute hypernatremia, *Lancet* 2:1385, 1967.

Arieff AI, Llach F, Massry SG: Neurological manifestations of hyponatremia, *Medicine* 55:121, 1976.

Drugs and Ethanol Effects on Nervous System

Charness ME, Simon RP, Greenberg DA: Ethanol and the nervous system, *N Engl J Med* 321:442, 1989.

Caplan LR, Hier DB, Banks G: Current concepts of cerebrovascular disease: stroke and drug abuse, *Stroke* 13:869, 1982.

Cregler LL, Mark H: Medical complications of cocaine abuse, *N Engl J Med* 315:1495, 1987.

Vasculitis

Devinsky O, Petito CK, Alonso DR: Clinical and neuropathological findings in SLE, *Ann Neurol* 23:380, 1988.

Feinglass EJ, Arnett FC, Dorsch LA: Neuropsychiatric manifestations of systemic lupus erythematosus: diagnosis, clinical spectrum and relationship to other features of the disease, *Medicine* 55:323, 1976.

Christian CL Sergent JS: Vasculitis syndromes: Clinical and experimental models, *Am J Med* 61:511, 1976.

Sergent JS, Lochshin MD, Klempner MS: Central nervous system disease in systemic lupus erythematosus, *Am J Med* 58:654, 1975.

Moore PM, Cupps TR: Neurological complications of vasculitis, *Ann Neurol* 14:155, 1983.

Levine SR: Cerebrovascular and neurologic disease associated with antiphospholipid antibodies, *Neurology* 40:1181, 1990.

Antiphospholipid antibodies in stroke study group: Clinical and laboratory findings in patients with antiphospholipid antibodies and cerebral ischemia, *Stroke* 21:1268, 1990.

Gastrointestinal Disorders

Comer GM, Brandt LJ, Abissi CJ: Whipple's disease: a review, *Am J Gastroenterol* 78:107, 1983.

Carpenter D: Celiac disease, *Semin Neurol* 5:271, 1985.

Sharf B, Bental E: Pancreatic encephalopathy, *J Neurol Neurosurg Psychiatry* 34:357, 1971.

Thyroid Disorders

Blum M: Myxedema coma, *Am J Sci* 264:432, 1972.

Sanders V: Neurological manifestations of myxedema, *N Engl J Med* 266:547; 599, 1962.

Teng CS, Yeo PPB: Opthalmic Graves' disease, *Br Med J* 1:273, 1977.

Bulens C: Neurologic complications of hyperthyroidism, *Arch Neurol* 38:669, 1981.

Swanson JW, Kelly JJ, McConahay WM: Neurologic aspects of thyroid dysfunction, *Mayo Clin Proc* 56:504, 1981.

Wall JR, Henderson J, Stakosch CR: Graves' ophthalmopathy, *Can Med Assoc J* 124:855, 1981.

Pulmonary Disorders
Jozefowicz RF: Neurologic manifestations of pulmonary disease, *Neurol Clin North Am* 7:605, 1989.

Renal Disorders
Fraser CL, Arieff AI: Nervous system complications in uremia, *Ann Intern Med* 109:143, 1988.

Raskin NH, Fishman RA: Neurologic disorders in renal failure, *N Engl J Med* 294:143, 1976.

Vitamin B_{12}
Lindenbaum J, Healton EB, Savage DG: Neuropsychiatric disorders caused by cobalamin deficiency in the absence of anemia or macrocytosis, *N Engl J Med* 318:1720, 1988.

Healton EB, Savage DG, Brust JCM: Neurologic aspects of cobalamin deficiency, *Medicine* 79:229, 1991.

Hepatic Disorders
Fraser CL, Arieff AI: Hepatic encephalopathy, *N Engl J Med* 313:865, 1985.

Victor M, Adams RD, Cole M: The acquired (non-Wilsonian) type of chronic hepatocerebral degeneration, *Medicine* 44:345, 1965.

Sherlock S: Hepatic coma, *Gastroenterology* 54:754, 1968.

Temporal Arteritis
Hamilton CR, Shelley WM, Tumulty PA: Giant cell arteritis including temporal arteritis and polymyalgia rheumatica, *Medicine* 50:1, 1971.

Rosenfeld SI, Kosmorsky GS, Klingle TG: Treatment of temporal arteritis with ocular involvement, *Am J Med* 80:143, 1986.

Porphyria
Goldberg A: Diagnosis and treatment of the porphyrias, *Proc R Soc Med* 61:193, 1968.

Tschudy DP: Acute intermittent porphyria, *Ann Intern Med* 83:851, 1975.

Potassium Abnormalities

Knochel JP: Neuromuscular manifestations of electrolyte disorders, *Am J Med* 72:525, 1982.

Comi G, Testa D, Cornelio F: Potassium depletion myopathy, *Muscle Nerve* 8:17, 1985.

Transplantation Nervous System Complications

Walker RW, Brochstein JA: Neurologic complications of immunosuppressive agents, *Neurol Clin North Am* 6:261, 1988.

Brun A, Adams HP: Neurologic problems in renal transplant recipients, *Neurol Clin North Am* 6:305, 1988.

Adams HP, Dawson D, Coffman TJ: Stroke in renal transplant recipients, *Arch Neurol* 43:113, 1986.

Neurologic Adverse Effects of Antineoplastic Treatment

Weiss HD, Walker MD, Wiernik PH: Neurotoxicity of commonly used antineoplastic agents, *N Engl J Med* 291:127, 1974.

Gilbert HA, Kagan AR: *Radiation damage to the nervous system,* New York, 1980, Raven Press.

Pluss JL, Dibella NJ: Reversible CNS dysfunction due to tamoxifen in patients with breast cancer, *Ann Intern Med* 101:652, 1984.

Neurological Effects of Cardiac Surgery

Gilman S: Cerebral disorders after open-heart operations, *N Engl J Med* 272:489, 1965.

Breuer AC, Furlan AJ, Hanson MR: CNS complications of coronary artery bypass graft surgery, *Stroke* 14:682, 1983.

Chronic Fatigue Syndrome

Shafran SD: The chronic fatigue syndrome, *Am J Med* 90:730, 1991.

Holmes GP, Kaplan JE, Gantz NM: Chronic fatigue syndrome: a working case definition, *Ann Intern Med* 108:387, 1988.

Sleep Disorders

23

A significant number of people suffer with either problems sleeping at night or difficulty staying awake during the day. An estimated 15% of the general population have serious sleep disorders, and an additional 35% have transient but frequently recurrent sleep difficulties. Although often viewed as a mundane complaint, sleep disorders can have serious medical, social, occupational, and personal ramifications. The problem of sleep disorders has been systematically studied in specialized sleep laboratories. This research, which includes carefully monitored all-night electroencephalographic (EEG) recordings (polysomnography), has led to a tremendous increase in the knowledge of normal and abnormal sleep patterns. In the laboratory EEG electrodes and physiologic sensors are used (electrodes over the outer canthi of the eyes to record eye movements, electrodes over the chin to measure mentalis muscle tone, sensors to measure respiratory rate and air flow, and an electrocardiogram). The polysomnogram allows a careful minute-to-minute analysis of sleep-wake pattern, respiratory function, and muscle activity.

▨ PHYSIOLOGY OF SLEEP

Sleep is a normal periodic interruption of consciousness that is necessary for restoration of mental and, quite possibly, other body functions. Sleep onset occurs when there is a decrease in activity in the reticular activating system (largely from a decrease in environmental stimulation). As drowsiness occurs, certain ascending sleep-inducing neurons are activated, that maintain sleep. Sleep is not a unified event; it has been divided into five stages:

Stage I. This represents the transition between full wakefulness and sleep. During this stage, reactivity to external stimuli is reduced. Patients may feel awake, but memory and thinking are impaired. The EEG shows a low amplitude, slower voltage pattern than is seen in full wakefulness. Muscle tone is slightly reduced in stage I sleep. This stage lasts 1 to 7 minutes.

Stage II. This is the first definite sleep stage (light sleep). Muscle tone is reduced compared with stage I, and eye movements are absent. The EEG shows a low-amplitude, mixed-frequency pattern with the predominant pattern being 4 to 8 cps (theta wave) activity. In this stage, sleep spindles (bursts of 12 to 14 cps rhythmical activity) and K-complexes (high-voltage, mixed slow and sharp waves) are seen. The onset of stage II is usually within 7 to 30 minutes.

Stages III and IV. These stages represent deep sleep and are usually entered within 30 to 40 minutes. Muscle tone is reduced, and eye movements are absent. The EEG shows high-amplitude slow (delta) waves, which are less than 4 cps.

Stage V. This state is characterized by a marked reduction in muscle tone (hypotonus), although facial and occasional limb twitching can occur. Rapid eye movements (REMs) are the most characteristic of this stage. The EEG is similar to stage I with a low-amplitude, mixed-frequency pattern. Active dreaming takes place during this stage. During REM sleep the following physiological changes occur: (1) all autonomic function cycles irregularly as a result of changes in the balance between sympathetic and parasympathetic tone, and blood pressure, heart rate, and cardiac output increase; (2) respiratory activity changes (it can become irregular, and increase or decrease in frequency); (3) thermoregulation is impaired; (4) cerebral blood flow and brain metabolism increase (at times even exceeding waking levels); and (5) penile erection occurs. The production of growth hormone is most active early in the night when slow-wave sleep predominates.

Stages I, II, III, and IV collectively are called non-rapid eye movement (NREM) sleep. During these stages the EEG slows and the amplitude of waves progressively increase. During stage V or REM sleep an EEG shows increased rhythm and reduced waveform amplitude. During NREM sleep the general trend is for reduced body function, and during REM sleep there is increased body function with the exception of muscle tone, which is decreased (hypotonia).

Through a normal night's sleep, a person's sleep fluctuates between the various stages. Stages III and IV are more frequent early in the night, and REM sleep is more common later in the night and toward morning. Several short nocturnal awakenings per night are normal. The general pattern of sleep changes throughout life; this is important to realize when counseling patients. Infants spend 50% of the night in REM sleep, but by age 20 this drops to 20% and stays at that percentage throughout life. In general, sleep lightens with age, total sleep time decreases, nocturnal awakenings increase, and stage IV deep sleep decreases substantially by age 60.

Other than the normal change in sleep patterns with age, it is important to realize that each person has a rather specific sleep need before he or she feels refreshed and can perform efficiently. In some persons (short sleepers) this may be only 3 or 4 hours, whereas in others (long sleepers) 10, 12, or even more hours a day are required. Also, some people's biologic clocks are set so that they function better at night and prefer to sleep when it is light; the reverse is also true.

The neural substrate of the sleep-wake cycle is complex. Wakefulness is maintained via the ascending reticular activating system (ARAS) and the thalamic projection system as they stimulate the cortex. If the ARAS activity is high, sleep is not possible. If ARAS activity is reduced, the transition to sleep state is possible. NREM sleep (stages I to IV) requires reduced ARAS activity and involvement of the serotonergic system of pontine raphe nuclei. For REM sleep to occur there must be interaction between the adrenergic (norepinephrine) nucleus ceruleus and cholinergic pontine gigantocellular tegmental field. Insomnia can be induced by lesions of the serotonergic cells of the raphe nuclei and by inhibition of serotonin synthesis and reversed by administration of substances that enhance serotonin synthesis.

▓ SLEEP HISTORY

History taking in patients with sleep disturbance is quite specialized and requires detailed inquiry into specific areas. The sleep disorders per se have many unique symptoms that must be pursued in the history. Medical illness, psychiatric difficulties, and environmental factors can also produce or contribute to sleep disturbances and must be carefully reviewed both with the patient and, if possible, family members.

Specific Complaint

Most patients complain of either insomnia (difficulty with onset or maintenance of sleep) or excessive daytime sleepiness. The physician should carefully outline the complaint.

- *Duration.* A sleep disturbance of short duration can mean recent emotional or medical problems, whereas a long-term problem usually indicates a constitutional sleep disorder.
- *Age at onset.*
- Is the complaint daily or intermittent?

For a complete profile of the 24-hour sleep-wake pattern, see Box 23-1.

▓ LABORATORY EVALUATION

The laboratory evaluation is based on the following:

- General medical evaluation: diabetes, thyroid, hypoglycemia, and other endocrine disease
- Psychiatric evaluation or at least the Minnesota Multiphasic Personality Inventory
- Polysomnography (requires special sleep laboratory)
- HLA typing for HLA-DR2 and DQw6 in suspected narcoleptics

BOX 23-1   Complete Profile of 24-Hour Sleep-Wake Pattern

1 *Presleep routine.* Exercise, coffee, food, alcohol, or mental strain before retiring will often prolong sleep onset. What is the role of daily or weekend naps? The importance of the bed partner to the sleep pattern and possibly any recent change in routine or bed partner should be stressed.

2 *Sleep onset time.* How long after getting in bed does the patient fall asleep?

3 *Character of sleep.* It is usually necessary to question the bed partner as well if there is one.
   a Number of nocturnal awakenings
   b Restlessness or jerking of the legs
   c Snoring and its character—are there very loud snorts?
   d Presence of apnea or breath holding spells—are they terminated with respiratory effort and snorting?
   e Sleepwalking, nightmares, or terrors—is there self-injury or injury to bed partner during any of these?
   f Time and ease of awakening in the morning
   g Total length of sleep
   h Is sleep refreshing?
   i Any morning symptoms (e.g., headache, confusion, hallucinations, wet bed, or total transient paralysis)?

4 *Character of waking period*
   a Refreshed
   b Tired during the day
   c Sleep attacks (uncontrollable attacks of actual sleep when sitting, driving, or in any situation with decreased environmental stimulation)
   d Naps
   e Cataplexy (sudden loss of muscle tone with or without falling when experiencing sudden strong emotion, such as fear, anger, or amusement). This can affect hands, masseters, and eyelids as well as antigravity muscles—consciousness is usually preserved unless the attack is prolonged if the patient enters directly into REM sleep.
   f Does the patient use substances (e.g., caffeine, amphetamines) to maintain wakefulness?

BOX 23-1—cont'd

Life Routine and Environmental Factors

1 Does the patient have a very irregular routine, such as doing shift work or excessive traveling?

2 Is the bedroom too hot (above 75° decreases sleep efficiency)?

3 Is environmental noise or light excessive?

4 Is there a new job, house, baby, or other factor?

Emotional Situation

1 Recent or long-term emotional problems, especially depression or anxiety

2 Marital difficulty

3 Death of family member or friend

4 Sexual problems producing anxiety about going to bed

5 History of abuse, a very common problem in sleep disorders patients

Medical History

1 Medications (especially the use of sleeping pills or pschotropic drugs).

2 Alcohol use. Alcohol makes falling asleep easier, but causes frequent nocturnal awakenings as the alcohol is metabolized.

3 Drug abuse or withdrawal. This markedly disrupts sleep patterns.

4 Medical illness (e.g., heart failure or chronic pulmonary disease can cause nocturnal dyspnea and disturbed sleep; thyroid disease and hypoglycemia are also known to disturb sleep).

Family History

A family history of sleep disorder—particularly narcolepsy, restless legs, sleepwalking, night terrors, and hypersomnolence—is obtained in some cases.

CLINICAL SYNDROMES

In 1990, the American Sleep Disorders Association, in conjunction with the European, Japanese, and Latin American Sleep Societies, developed an International Classification of Sleep Disorders (Box 23-2), which is a slightly different classification system and includes many more disorder subcategories. This classification is presented here because it may become the standard taxonomy in the near future.

 BOX 23-2   Clinical Syndromes of Sleep Disorders

1 Dyssomnias
   a Intrinsic sleep disorders (e.g., psychophysiological insomnia, narcolepsy, sleep apnea, restless legs syndrome)
   b Extrinsic sleep disorders (e.g., environmental insomnia, insufficient sleep disorder, alcohol-dependent sleep disorder)
   c Circadian rhythm sleep disorders (e.g., jet lag [time zone change], shift work sleep disorder, delayed sleep phase syndrome)

2 Parasomnias
   a Arousal disorders (e.g., sleepwalking, sleep terrors)
   b Sleep-wake transition disorders (e.g., sleep-talking)
   c Parasomnias with REM sleep (e.g., nightmares, sleep paralysis)
   d Other parasomnias (e.g., bruxism, enuresis, sudden infant death, snoring)

3 Sleep disorders associated with medical/psychiatric disorders
   a Mental disorders (e.g., psychosis, mood disorders, anxiety, panic, or alcoholism)
   b Neurological disorders (e.g., dementia, parkinsonism, sleep-related epilepsy)
   c Medical disorders (e.g., chronic obstructive pulmonary disease, asthma, gastric-reflux, fibrositis)

4 Proposed sleep disorders (e.g., short/long sleeper, menstrual/pregnancy-associated sleep disorder, hypnagogic hallucinations)

In this chapter we have used the Classification of Sleep and Arousal Disorders published by The Association of Sleep Disorder Centers in 1979. This classification requires clinical information as well as data obtained from the sleep laboratory. Two terms should be defined: (1) *dyssomnias* are disturbances in the amount, quality, or timing of sleep (difficulty initiating and maintaining proper sleep or wakefulness) and (2) *parasomnias* are disturbances relating to abnormal events occurring during sleep, such as sleepwalking, night terrors, and nightmares.

I. Disorders in initiating or maintaining sleep (insomnia)
   A. Psychophysiologic: These are disorders of somatized tension and learned sleep.
      1. Transient and situational. The person who is currently undergoing an acute emotional upset will experience (a) difficulty falling asleep, (b) multiple nocturnal arousals, (c) early morning awakening, and (d) subsequent daytime fatigue (not sleepiness). The condition is usually short-lived and resolves as the crisis passes. Treatment should be emotional support and possibly mild tranquilization or sedation at night with a benzodiazepine. These situations are more frequent in highly emotional people. On occasion acute or subacute insomnia is the initial symptom of more serious psychiatric illness or a physical illness such as a metabolic encephalopathy, early cardiac or pulmonary failure, and so on.
      2. Persistent. If symptoms continue for more than three weeks after crisis resolution,

either the disorders discussed below or the possibility that the patient has conditioned himself or herself to the insomnia should be considered.

B. Psychiatric disorders

1. These include personality disorders such as obsessive, hypochondriacal, or neurotic personality in which anxiety is prominent.

2. Affective disorders. Depression and mania are common affective disorders.

   a. Depression. The patient easily falls asleep but has frequent arousals and early morning awakening.

   b. Mania. These patients have trouble falling asleep (sleep-onset insomnia) and sleep only a short time.

3. Schizophrenia. With psychotic decompensation there is severe sleep-onset insomnia as well as difficulty maintaining sleep.

For the emotionally based insomnias it is useful to review the sleeping environment carefully and help the patient establish a regular time of retiring; set proper temperature for the room; decrease noise and light; perform light exercise in the evening; have a warm drink at bedtime (noncaffeinated and nonalcoholic); and possibly intermittently use a benzodiazepine medication such as temazepam (30 mg), choral hydrate (500 to 1000 mg), or others. In chronic cases relaxation therapy or biofeedback training can be helpful.

C. Insomnia associated with drugs or alcohol (hypnotic-dependent sleep disorder)

1. Tolerance. Depressant drugs (e.g., barbiturates) produce tolerance very shortly and

usually lose their effectiveness as a night-time hypnotic within 2 weeks. Increased dosages are ineffective, and sleep actually becomes less satisfactory than before starting the drug. Long nocturnal awakenings occur, and sleep-onset time lengthens.

2. Withdrawal. On withdrawal of sleeping medication there is a distinct withdrawal insomnia unless the dosage is tapered slowly over several nights. Also, because some drugs suppress REM sleep, patients can experience REM rebound with increased dreaming and nightmares.

3. Sustained use of central nervous system stimulants. Coffee, cola and other soft drinks, tea, chocolate, nicotine, and the caffeine found in many analgesic preparations can all be culpable.

4. Other Drugs. Corticosteroids, β-blockers, birth control pills, theophylline, phenytoin, antidepressant medication, and tranquilizers can cause insomnia.

5. Alcohol. This substance acts like other central nervous system depressants in decreasing total sleep, producing persistent interruptions, and acutely suppressing REM sleep. Sleep-onset time is usually shortened in the occasional drinker and lengthened in the alcoholic.

D. Sleep-induced respiratory impairment

1. Sleep apnea syndrome. This syndrome constitutes 5% to 10% of all insomnia cases. The basic problem is that breathing literally stops during sleep. This apnea causes partial or full arousal, and the patient begins to

breathe again. Sleep is repeatedly interrupted during the night, in some patients more than 100 times. There are two principal mechanisms: central apnea, in which the respiratory centers in the central nervous system fail to function, and obstructive apnea, in which the pharynx relaxes and obstructs the free flow of air. In central apnea the patient usually does not complain of difficulty getting to sleep but has a major problem maintaining sleep. There can be some daytime sleepiness, but this is not the principal complaint. The obstructive apnea patient has considerable daytime sleepiness but may be unaware of the sleepiness.

A combined form of central and obstructive sleep apnea has the physiologic and clinical features of both. The most accurate way to document and diagnose sleep apnea is to have the patient studied for several nights in a sleep laboratory; this is obviously not always possible. The alternative is to have the spouse or another person sit with the patient throughout the night and record the patient's sleep pattern. Specifically noted should be long periods of apnea (10 seconds); multiple awakenings after apnea; leg movements; and loud snoring or evidence of obstruction of respiration.

Treatment for central apnea has not been very successful, but fortunately central apnea is less common than obstructive apnea (it can be more serious, depending on the cause).

2. Alveolar hypoventilation not caused by primary pulmonary disease occurs when there is insufficient air exchange at night but no apnea. Causes include obesity with compression of the chest cavity and central nervous system damage from polio, tumor, encephalitis, or high spinal cord lesions, amyotrophic lateral sclerosis (ALS), myasthenia gravis, and myotonic dystrophy. In addition, another syndrome presumed caused by hypoexcitability of the brain stem respiratory center is called central hypoventilation. Multiple awakenings can occur, and patients may complain of insomnia. Hypnotics and alcohol should not be used to ensure sleep because these can worsen the hypoventilation.

E. Sleep-related spontaneous movement disorders

1. Nocturnal myoclonus. Ten percent of middle-aged and older insomniacs are found to exhibit an unusual episodic movement disorder in which the patient experiences frequent (every 20 to 40 seconds, sustained 0.5 to 10 seconds) contractions of the anterior tibial muscles and hip flexors. These jerks interrupt sleep patterns and may awaken the patient. The symptoms are usually far more distressing to the bed partner than to the patient. There is sometimes a family history of sleep disorder. Treatment with clonazepam (1 mg at bedtime) or temazepam (Restoril) has been successful.

2. Restless-legs syndrome. This is a syndrome in which patients feel a deep disagreeable

sensation in the legs that drives the person to move the legs. Many of these patients have nocturnal myoclonus as well. One third of the cases are familial. Patients with painful neuropathies (e.g., diabetes and uremia) or radiculopathy from nerve root impingement can also experience similar problems. Treatment is most successful with mild to moderate leg exercise in the evening and medications at bedtime (Box 23-3).

F. Medical and environmental. As a cause for insomnia, medical and environmental factors have been noted. Medical and neurologic diseases may interrupt sleep and must be considered. Environmental factors such as noise, heat, light, or a bed partner with nocturnal myoclonus may also be incriminated in some cases.

G. Abnormal sleep architecture. In some patients a diagnosis can be made only by use of all-night EEG recordings. Some patients display various patterns such as inability to sustain

---

 BOX 23-3   Medications for the Treatment of Restless Legs Syndrome

Clonazepam 0.5 to 2 mg

Temazepam 30 mg with or without codeine 30 mg

Sinemet 25/100 to 50/200 CR

Carbamazepine 200 mg

Other benzodiazepines such as diazepam

Bromocriptine 2.5 mg

Permax

stage IV or REM patterns and alpha (waking) intrusions into sleep. These abnormalities render the patient unable to sustain an uninterrupted, restorative night's sleep.

H. Short sleeper. This refers to the person who requires only 3 to 4 hours of sleep a night. It is usually more disturbing to other members of the family or the bed partner than it is to the patient.

I. No objective insomnia (sleep state misperception). There are always patients who complain of insomnia who in fact sleep quite soundly. Reassurance of this fact is sometimes but not always successful in answering the complaint.

II. Disorders of Excessive Somnolence

This is the second major syndrome of the sleep disorders. Patients complain of inappropriate and excessive sleepiness, decreased mental and physical performance during the day, unavoidable napping, increased total sleep time, and difficulty achieving full arousal on awakening. This diagnosis should be restricted to patients who have actual sleep attacks or who fall sleep or are drowsy when sedentary and should not be applied to persons who complain of fatigue after inadequate sleep. These disorders cause considerable emotional stress for the patient, and the constant sleepiness interferes with work, socializing, and family relationships.

A. Psychophysiologic. As in insomnia, emotional factors can play a major role in producing daytime fatigue and sleepiness. This may be acute, for example, in depression where the patient feels drained and may withdraw to the bed during a crisis.

B. Psychiatric disorders. Particularly in bipolar depression the patients tend to sleep long hours, take naps, and awake unrefreshed despite adequate sleep.

C. Drugs and alcohol. Tolerance to or withdrawal from stimulant drugs may produce daytime sleepiness. Constant overuse of depressants will do the same.

D. Sleep-induced respiratory impairment

1. Sleep apnea (primarily obstructive). This is a potentially fatal disorder in which the soft tissues of the throat collapse during sleep onset and actually cause partial or complete upper airway obstruction. The patient attempts to breathe but cannot. Respiratory efforts increase, and finally the effort partially arouses the patient, and he or she emits a loud choking snort. Significant anoxia may occur during this time to produce a generalized seizure. Obstructive episodes may be repeated hundreds of times each night. Patients awaken in the morning mentally fuzzy, unrefreshed, and often with headaches. They then complain of excessive sleepiness during the day and may actually have microsleeps in which they literally fall asleep on their feet for a few seconds. Automatic behavior may be seen during this time (e.g., fumbling with clothes, staring around, and mumbling). Because of the strain on the heart and increased intrathoracic pressure, many of these patients become hypertensive and develop pulmonary hypertension, cardiac arrhythmias, and finally cardiac failure.

The initial treatment includes having the patient avoid the following: alcoholic drinks, sedatives, narcotics, diuretics that induce metabolic alkalosis, propranolol (this drug may decrease the ventilatory response to oxygen), and corticosteroids (which may increase body weight and fat deposition). Because the majority of these patients are obese, weight reduction should be undertaken; however, it is not possible to predict those patients who will improve with weight loss. Unfortunately, sleepy overweight individuals have trouble losing weight because they are unable to be very active and do not burn calories very effectively during their frequent naps. Careful assessment by an otolaryngologist is essential; if tonsils are enlarged, tonsillectomy may be indicated; if there is deviated nasal septum or turbinates, corrective surgery is considered; and if there is oropharyngeal obstruction due to soft palate or uvula enlargement, a uvulopalatopharyngoplasty is considered. The jaw is assessed for abnormalities (retrognathia or micrognathia) that may warrant mandibular surgery to enhance air movement. The use of continuous positive airway pressure (CPAP) with a mask in which a compressor delivers air at positive pressure to the upper respiratory tract may help correct snoring or obstructive respiratory depression. If these are not effective, elective tracheostomy is the most effective surgical treatment for obstructive apnea.

2. Alveolar hypoventilation. Interruption of sleep in these patients will also lead to daytime sleepiness. This condition can also be treated with CPAP.

E. Nocturnal myoclonus and restless legs. If sleep is sufficiently disturbed, these patients will complain of daytime sleepiness.

F. Narcolepsy. This is the most celebrated of the sleep disorders, constituting 20% of the patients with sleep disorders. Narcolepsy is a syndrome in which attacks of excessive daytime sleepiness are the primary symptom. These can occur while driving, standing, or working but are particularly prone to occur when the person is relaxed. The patients often drop into REM sleep in less than 10 minutes. The second symptom in the narcolepsy syndrome—cataplexy—is also common and may be partial, such as the jaw dropping or a weak feeling in the knees. Cataplexy is defined as the pathologic loss of muscle tone that develops as a response to an intense affective emotional stimulus (e.g., crying, laughing). Vivid, often frightening hallucinations in the drowsy period (hypnagogic hallucinations) and sleep paralysis (total muscular flaccidity) on awakening in the morning are the final two features of the syndrome. Some patients also develop complex automatic behavior such that, during narcoleptic attacks in which consciousness is impaired and for which they have no memory, they may carry out automatic behavior (writing, speaking, washing). In cases with automatic behavior an EEG may be considered to exclude partial complex seizures. Only 10% to 15% of patients have all four of the above symptoms. This condition has a slight familial tendency (6 to 7 times normal in relative of the proband). Onset is usually during teenage years, and the condition persists throughout life.

The diagnosis can often be made on the history alone, particularly if cataplexy is present, but supportive evidence from the EEG is helpful. The multiple sleep latency test is a useful diagnostic procedure that can be performed in a regular EEG laboratory; however, this should be done after a full polysomnogram, which will rule out other sleep disorders. The patient is brought to the EEG laboratory every 2 hours during the day. The patient has 20 minutes to fall asleep. If this occurs, he or she is allowed to sleep 15 minutes. If the patient enters REM sleep during two of these periods in the absence of other possible explanations, the diagnosis of narcolepsy can be made. The narcoleptic usually enters sleep in 3 to 5 minutes. If sleep onset is greater than 10 minutes, pathologic sleepiness is unlikely. Although the narcoleptic exhibits a short sleep-onset time, the patient does not have very sound sleep.

Nocturnal myoclonus and other sleep problems are routinely present in narcoleptics and tend to interrupt their sleep. There are normal persons with very short sleep onset latency (less than 5 minutes); they are differentiated from the narcoleptic by the otherwise normal sleep and paucity of other symptoms.

HLA typing can be helpful in assisting in the diagnosis of narcolepsy; most whites are HLA-DR2 positive (29% of normals are also positive). In blacks 66% have HLA-DR2 present and a high percentage HLA-DQw6. The EEG is also warranted to exclude seizure discharges. Because narcolepsy is rarely associated with structural brain disease, computed tomography and magnetic resonance imaging are usually not necessary.

Treatment for the daytime sleepiness in the narcoleptic is most effective with methylphenidate (Ritalin). The starting dose is usually 5 mg in the morning and at noon, but considerably higher doses are often needed. Most patients benefit from taking medication on demand (e.g., when about to drive or take a test). The cataplexy is best controlled with Imipramine (25 mg three times a day), protriptyline (5 mg two to three times a day to start with a maximum dosage of 50 to 60 mg/day), or Anafranil (25 to 75 mg h.s.). Short naps (20 minutes) spaced throughout the day may also help to prevent the sleep attacks.

G. Idiopathic hypersomnolence (hypersomnia). This condition is characterized by recurrent sleepiness and irresistible sleep and at times sleep attacks. These patients do not fall asleep while talking or standing but do have sleep episodes. Daytime automatic behavior is common however. Lengthy nonrefreshing naps are taken, and long, sound nighttime sleep is the rule. Morning arousal is often very difficult, and periods of sleep drunkenness (staggering around with automatic behavior) may last up to 2 hours after arising. The etiology of the hypersomnias is not known, but genetic studies indicate a familial incidence. Rarely hypersomnia is secondary to a pathologic process involving the posterior hypothalamus (encephalitis, head injury, brain hemorrhage).

The amphetamines, which are helpful in treating narcolepsy, are far less effective in idiopathic hypersomnolence. Cyproheptadine (Periactin), methysergide (Sansert), and other drugs that suppress serotonin are more effective. Clonazepam (0.5 to 2 mg at night) has also been somewhat successful.

H. Medical, toxic, and environmental factors. As discussed previously, these factors will also cause sleepiness during the day.

I. Periodic syndromes. These are uncommon yet very interesting syndromes of periodic hypersomnolence that seem almost akin to hibernation. The most common is the Klein-Levin syndrome. A condition most common in young (10 to 20 years) males, this syndrome is characterized by periods (hours to days) of sleepiness, increased appetite, abnormal emotional states (dysphoria, aggressive behavior), decreased libido, and irritability. Between attacks, patients show normal sleep-wake cycles. The syndrome is occasionally seen in females when it is related to menstrual cycles. Etiology is unknown, but some type of episodic hypothalamic or diencephalic disturbance is postulated.

J. No objective findings. Some of these are merely long sleepers who complain of needing extra sleep.

III. Disorders of sleep-wake schedule (circadian rhythm sleep disorders)

These are situations in which the normal circadian rhythm is disturbed:

A. Jet lag. This is usually a minor problem for most persons, but individuals who must make frequent long trips over many time zones (worse going west to east) experience considerable difficulty resetting their biologic clocks.

B. Shift work. A common problem for service personnel such as nurses, pilots, ship captains, bus/truck drivers, police, some industrial workers, and busy house officers. Both work and sleeping efficiency are decreased under these circumstances. There is no satisfactory medical solution; occasionally a mild sleeping pill used a day or two after a change may help to ensure sleep onset. Some persons tolerate this better than others, but it is not easy for anyone. Bright light therapy is becoming more commonly used in shift work. If a severe problem exists, the patient simply must change jobs or find some way that shift schedules can be changed to gradually accommodate to the time change.

C. Non–24-hour circadian rhythm. These persons have 25-hour biologic clocks. They drift in and out of phase with the rest of the world in 24-day cycles.

IV. Parasomnias

A. Sleepwalking (somnambulism). This is a problem most often seen in children ages 6 to

12. The nocturnal walk is usually in the early part of the night and may be quite elaborate including opening doors, stepping over furniture, and opening windows. Speech, when present, is mumbled. Occasionally the children awaken during the peregrination but usually do not. It is important to differentiate sleepwalking from partial complex seizures and psychiatric disorders (hysteria, fugue states). The psychiatric disorders are not always distinguishable from pure somnambulism. Seizures are rarely only reported at night; the EEG is helpful in excluding this condition. The problem is usually self-limited, and the first treatment is aimed at protecting the patient from hurting himself or herself (lock windows, etc.). The problem may recur in the 20s or 30s when the person is under unusual emotional stress. Some adolescents or young adults develop somnambulism de novo, which is usually associated with emotional stress. Benzodiazepines may be used in severe cases.

B. Sleep or night terrors. This is a rather frightening although usually benign condition seen in children between the ages of 4 and 15. The children scream or cry out, sit up in bed, and exhibit the look of panic or terror. Some may sleepwalk as well. An autonomic (sympathetic) reaction occurs, with dilated pupils, diaphoresis, tachycardia, and tachypnea. The patients usually have little or no memory for the event, cannot be consoled directly after the event, and do not report vivid dreams. Night terrors may be differentiated from nightmares. The latter are frightening dreams in which there is usually no anxiety or heightened sympathomimetic discharge and the patient has excellent recall of the dream content. Nightmares occur during REM sleep, whereas night terrors occur during initial hours of sleep as part of slow-wave (stage III or IV) sleep. The condition has been known to come on in the 20s or 30s and become chronic. Such patients have a high incidence of chronic anxiety. Temporal lobe seizures and the hypnagogic hallucinations of the narcolepsy syndrome must be considered in the diagnosis. Treatment with diazepam at night is helpful in some patients.

C. REM behavior disorder. This was first described in humans in 1987. It is common in patients with degenerative neurological disease—dementia/CVA/SAH/Parkinson's disease/OPCA—but is also seen in healthy young patients. Incomplete maintenance of REM atonia may affect the arms, legs, and face and permit dream enactment resulting in severe injury to patient or bed partner. This disorder can be clinically indistinguishable from sleepwalking, nocturnal seizure, and psychiatric states. Treat with Clonazepam or other benzodiazepine, and rarely with Tegretol.

V. Enuresis. In primary enuresis the child has not been able to control nocturnal urination to remain dry for a period of 1 month. This is not a rare problem; in fact 3% of children remain enuretic by age 12 (1% to 2% by age 18). There is the occasional adult who has never obtained nocturnal continence and continues to be plagued by enuresis.

This disorder most commonly occurs in boys. There is usually a positive family history of bedwetting, and urologic studies demonstrate a small functional bladder capacity. In secondary enuresis the child has controlled nocturnal urination for months to years before the episodes of bedwetting recur. In evaluating patients with primary enuresis a careful developmental history should be obtained. Psychological factors including the parent's attitude toward the bedwetting and toilet training and specific life stresses at the time bedwetting developed must be considered. Urologic evaluation should be carried out to exclude genitourinary abnormalities. In older patients with secondary enuresis a nocturnal seizure should be considered as the possible mechanism for enuresis. Sleep studies should be performed to exclude nocturnal seizures, obstructive apnea, night terrors, and sleepwalking as being associated with enuresis. Enuresis may occur in any sleep stage but is most common in non-REM sleep and occurs early in the night. Imipramine has been used to reduce the frequency of bedwetting; however, behavioral modification and enuresis alarms (conditioning technique in which the child awakens to a bell that is triggered by urine on the sheet) are also effective.

▣ SUMMARY

Problems getting to sleep and problems staying awake are occasionally experienced by all of us; there are, however, some patients whose sleep problems constitute a major controlling aspect in their lives—these are pathologic sleep disorders. Through the use of special all-night sleep recordings and knowledge of the various sleep syndromes, the physician can usually classify the type of sleep disorder. The cause of these conditions is not understood, but we now recognize the syndromes clinically and can outline a treatment regimen for the specific disorder.

Suggested Readings

Diagnosis and Classification

American Sleep Disorders Association: International Classification of Sleep Disorders, Rochester, Minn, 1990.

Association of Sleep Disorder Centers: Diagnostic classification of sleep and arousal disorders, *Sleep* 2:1, 1979.

Culebras A: The neurology of sleep, *Neurology* 42 (suppl 6): 6, 1992.

Kales A, Soldatos CR, Kales JD: Taking a sleep history, *Am Fam Pract* 22:101, 1980.

Kales A, Vela-Bueno A, Kales JD: Sleep disorders, *Ann Intern Med* 106:434, 582, 1987.

Kales JD, Kales A: Evaluation and diagnosis of sleep disorders patients, *Semin Neurol* 7:243, 1987.

Richardson JW: Symposium on sleep disorders: Mayo sleep disorders update, *Mayo Clin Proc* 65:857, 1990.

Williams RL, Karacan I, editors: Sleep disorders: diagnosis and treatment, New York, 1978, John Wiley & Sons.

Narcolepsy

Aldrich MS: Narcolepsy, *Neurology* 42 (suppl 6):34, 1992.

Manfredi RL, Brennan RW, Cadreux RJ: Disorders of excessive sleepiness: narcolepsy and hypersomnia, *Semin Neurol* 7:250, 1987.

Parkes JD: Daytime drowsiness, *Lancet* 2:1213, 1981.

von den Hoed J, et al: Disorders of excessive daytime somnolence: polygraphic and clinical data for 100 patients, *Sleep* 4:23, 1981.

Insomnia

Gillen JC, Byerley WF: The diagnosis and management of insomnia, *N Engl J Med,* 322:239, 1990.

Parasomnias

Cohen MW: Enuresis, *Pediatr Clin North Am* 22:545, 1975.

Coleman R, Pollak CP: Periodic movements in sleep, *Ann Neurol* 8:416, 1980.

Vela-Bueno A, Soldatos CR: Episodic sleep disorders, *Semin Neurol* 7:269, 1987.

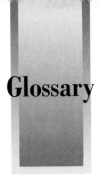

Glossary

abscess encapsulated circumscribed collection of pus located within the brain parenchyma.

absence type of seizure in which patient stares blankly for brief period of time.

abulia apathy and failure to respond verbally (akinetic mutism) because of bilateral frontal lobe dysfunction.

Adie's pupil dilated pupils, which show tonic accommodative and absent light reaction. Indicates cholinergic hypersensitivity.

afferent pupillary defect pupillodilatation when light source is rapidly moved from normal to defective pupil. If positive, indicates unilateral optic nerve lesion.

ageusia loss of sensation of taste usually due to dysfunction of seventh cranial nerve.

agnosia inability to recognize a complex stimulus or object even though the basic sensory system is normal (e.g., visual agnosia is present when a patient can see an object, but cannot recognize it visually).

agraphia inability to formulate ideas into written words and phrases not associated with paralysis of the dominant hand.

akathisia motor restlessness, or the inability to sit still, with constant limb or trunk movements; usually caused by antipsychotic medication.

akinetic mutism patient appears awake, looks at environment but is unresponsive and does not move. Usually due to bifrontal lesions.

alexia acquired failure of visual recognition of written words as a result of structural left hemisphere disease. This is contrasted with dyslexia, which is a developmental reading abnormality without known brain lesion.

amaurosis   loss of vision that can be permanent or temporary, partial or complete (e.g., the unilateral temporary blindness that occurs with carotid artery disease—amaurosis fugax).

amnesia   inability to learn or remember recent events. In neurology this refers to an organic memory dysfunction such as that seen in dementia or Korsakoff's syndrome.

amyloid angiopathy   infiltration of amyloid material into intracranial blood vessels. May cause brain hemorrhage or infarction. May occur without systemic amyloidosis.

amyotrophy   severe muscle atrophy frequently associated with fasciculations due to lesions of lower motor neurons (e.g., amyotrophic lateral sclerosis), roots, or peripheral nerves (e.g., diabetic neuropathy).

aneurysm   localized abnormal dilatation of the cerebral arteries. Aneurysms can be saccular (berry or "congenital") found at bifurcations mainly in the circle of Willis, atherosclerotic fusiform, dissecting, infectious (mycotic), posttraumatic (pseudoaneurysms or arteriovenous fistula), and miliary (microaneurysms).

anisocoria   inequality of pupillary size that may be physiological or due to pathological process. The abnormally sized pupil is the one that reacts less well to light.

anosmia   abnormality of sensation of smell.

aphasia   language disturbance (i.e., abnormal comprehension or expression of spoken language, errors of syntax, and word choice) secondary to brain damage or dysfunction.

aphonia   inability to phonate, but articulation is intact. Usually due to vocal cord lesion.

apoplexy   sudden loss of consciousness or neurological dysfunction due to rupture or occlusion of blood vessel; strokelike.

apraxia   difficulty in carrying out complex motor acts as a result of a defect in motor planning and not weakness, incoordination, or sensory loss.

Argyll-Robertson pupil   miotic irregular pupils that accommodate, but are poorly reactive to, light. Indicative of neurosyphilis.

arousal   the more primitive component of consciousness that is defined as wakefulness and controlled by activity within the brain stem, diencephalon, and most specifically the ascending reticular activating system.

arteriovenous malformations congenital developmental abnormalities of blood vessels caused by persistence of the vascular patterns found in fetal brain (i.e., direct communication between arteries and veins without intervening capillary beds).

astereognosia inability to recognize an object by touching and feeling it but without seeing it. Usually occurs in patients with parietal lesions.

asterixis sign of motor dysfunction seen in certain metabolic encephalopathies (e.g., liver and renal). There is rapid palmar flapping downward movement when the wrist is initially dorsiflexed and the fingers are extended.

ataxia loss of coordination. It can be *sensory* as a result of a lesion in the posterior columns of the spinal cord, posterior roots, or sensory peripheral nerves, or it can be *cerebellar* as a result of focal (midline) or diffuse cerebellar disease.

athetosis slow coarse irregular and nonrhythmical writhing movement of the distal extremities, face, or trunk muscles.

atrophy decrease of tissue mass (wasting) as a result of shrinkage of tissue, or failure to grow as a result of several causes (e.g., disuse atrophy and denervation).

aura beginning of a partial (focal) seizure. Never part of primary generalized seizure.

automatisms semipurposeful movements carried out in complex partial seizures.

awareness the component of consciousness that allows integration of the environment. This is controlled by sensory integrative pathways in the cerebral cortex.

Babinski sign abnormal superficial reflex characterized by dorsiflexion of the great toe together with separation or fanning of the other toes as a response to stimulation of the plantar surface of the foot. It indicates a corticospinal tract (upper motor neuron) lesion.

Battle sign bruises or ecchymoses over mastoid area due to basilar skull fracture.

Bell's palsy lower motor neuron paralysis involving the upper and lower portion of the face.

bitemporal hemianopsia visual field defect confined to lateral peripheral field of vision. Usually due to chiasmal suprasellar mass lesion.

blepharospasm   constant blinking and closing of the eyes that may interfere with patient's ability to see.

bradykinesia   slowness of initiation and performance of motor activities; one of the characteristic features of parkinsonism.

Broca aphasia   expressive type of aphasia characterized by agrammatic and dysfluent speech with severe word finding difficulty and intact comprehension.

bruit   abnormal vascular sound heard over an artery usually indicating arterial stenosis.

bulbar palsy   paralysis caused by lesions of the motor nuclei of the medulla oblongata (bulb) and manifested by atrophy and fasciculations of the tongue and inability to swallow and talk.

caloric testing   stimulating the labyrinth by hot or cold water to assess patients with vertigo or abnormal nystagmus.

carpal tunnel syndrome   an entrapment neuropathy in which the median nerve is compressed by the flexor retinaculum ligaments at the wrist.

cataplexy   sudden loss of muscle tone precipitated by strong emotion (laughing, excitement, crying).

cauda equina syndrome   weakness in the legs (paraparesis) with impaired sphincter tone due to compression of lumbosacral nerve roots by herniated disk or mass lesion.

causalgia   burning persisting pain that radiates distal to an injured nerve trunk.

cerebral infarction   death of region of brain tissue due to occlusion of artery or arteriole. When this occlusion occurs, oxygenation and glucose needs of the tissue are not sufficient to maintain electrical and metabolic needs of brain tissue.

cerebritis   nonencapsulated suppurative infectious-inflammatory reaction within the brain parenchyma.

Cheyne-Stokes respiration   alternating periods of hyperventilation that diminish to periods of hypoventilation and then to short apnea spells. Due to bilateral cerebral hemispheric dysfunction.

choked disc   congestive changes in the optic nerve (e.g., loss of spontaneous venous pulsations, blurring of disc margins, hemorrhages, and exudates) caused by increased intracranial pressure.

chorea   rapid, coarse, semipurposeful, random, nonrhythmic dancelike movements of extremities, trunk, or face.

clonus   rhythmical muscle contractions induced by muscle tension. This is sign of upper neuron lesion.

completed stroke   permanent (fixed) neurologic deficit as a result of thromboembolic cerebral infarction.

concussion   transient and immediate loss of consciousness produced by a non-penetrating blunt impact to the head.

conduction aphasia   language disturbance characterized by impaired repetition and naming but normal comprehension.

confusion   inability to maintain content or stream of coherent mental processing. Inattention is equivalent to confusion, and there is an abnormality of arousal and awareness.

constructional apraxia   disability in constructional skills such as difficulty in drawing to copy block designs, stick patterns, and three-dimensional constructions and difficulty in performing spatial analysis.

contusion   area of hemorrhagic brain necrosis (bruise) produced by a blunt impact to the head frequently associated with neurologic deficit.

convulsion   violent involuntary contraction or a series of contractions of a group (focal) or most (generalized) voluntary muscles with or without loss of consciousness.

cramps   painful involuntary contractions of skeletal muscles.

decerebrate rigidity   postural reflex seen in comatose patients that occurs spontaneously or in response to stimulation and is manifested by clenched jaw, retracted neck, and extended and internally rotated arms and legs. It indicates a diencephalic or midbrain lesion.

decorticate rigidity   postural reflex manifested by flexion and adduction of the arm and wrist and extension of the leg as a result of a hemispheric lesion. It can be unilateral (frequently post stroke) or bilateral in comatose patients.

delirium   acute mental disturbance, usually reversible and characterized by confusion, incoherence, hallucinations, restlessness, and hyperactivity. It is frequently caused by toxic-metabolic disorders.

dementia   progressive deterioration in intellectual, emotional, and social functioning.

diffuse axonal injury a shearing or tearing of the cerebral hemisphere white-matter axons due to traumatic brain injury.

diplegia uni- or bilateral motor disturbances involving two extremities. Lesion involves upper motor neuron and is usually seen in cerebral palsy.

diplopia double vision due to malalignment of the visual images on the retina. This symptom results from impairment of the extraocular muscle mobility.

doll's head movement contralateral conjugate horizontal eye movements when head is rapidly turned.

dysarthria abnormality in speech production secondary to dysfunction in the muscles of articulation or their neural connections, either peripheral or central. No deficit in language.

dysesthesia unpleasant feeling triggered by any ordinary stimuli, usually seen after a partial nerve injury or during recovery from some neuropathies.

dyskinesia abnormal involuntary movements usually due to basal ganglia or cerebellar disorders.

dyslexia severe reading disability with a discrepancy in the ability to recognize and recall words.

dysmetria inability to judge accurately the distance to an object when reaching for it.

dysphagia difficulty swallowing.

dystonia slow, coarse, sustained muscle contraction leading to abnormal postures (e.g., spasmodic torticollis and writer's cramp).

dystrophin muscle protein that is absent in patients with Duchenne dystrophy.

dystrophy group of diseases of undetermined cause, usually hereditary, characterized by weakness as a result of progressive degeneration of muscles.

Eaton-Lambert syndrome a paraneoplastic syndrome usually associated with small-cell lung carcinoma. Patient has muscle weakness and abnormal fatigue. This is due to impaired transmission at the neuromuscular junction. It is similar, but not identical, to myasthenia gravis.

embolism thrombus may form in the heart (cardiogenic cerebral embolism) or from the extra- or intracranial vessels (artery-to-artery embolism) to propagate into an intracranial artery. This artery is then occluded and this may cause a completed stroke.

empyema encapsulated collection of pus in a preformed potential space (e.g., epidural and subdural).

encephalitis inflammation of the brain parenchyma of an infectious origin.

encephalopathy nonspecific term for any noninfectious, generalized cerebral disorder (e.g., traumatic, metabolic, or toxic encephalopathy).

endarterectomy surgical procedure to remove atherosclerotic plaque from the arterial wall. Procedure is usually performed on extracranial portion of the carotid artery.

epidural lesion in the potential space between the dura and the skull or vertebral bodies; often involved in traumatic (epidural hematoma) or infectious processes (epidural abscess).

epilepsy a group of diseases of the central nervous system in which the patient has *recurrent* seizures.

extrapyramidal not primarily involving the pyramidal or corticospinal tract; usually used to describe abnormal involuntary movements (dyskinesias) caused by basal ganglion abnormalities.

fasciculation brief twitches of groups or bundles of muscle fibers seen through the skin in superficial muscles or through mucosa as in the tongue, which usually result from active degeneration of anterior horn cells or occasionally from nerve root damage or anticholinesterase drugs.

fibrillation short contractions of single muscle fibers detectable only by electromyography.

flaccid absence or decrease of muscle tone.

fortification migraine visual delusion or hallucination. This appears as an angular pattern or zigzag luminous bands of broken lines to suggest the view of fortified walls.

gait apraxia walking pattern in which feet appear stuck to floor (as caused by magnetic force). This is seen in patients with normal pressure hydrocephalus.

glioma any tumor of glial origin either histologically benign (astrocytoma, ependymoma, oligodendroglioma) or malignant (glioblastoma multiforme).

habit spasm rapid stereotyped movement that involves eyelid, mouth, shoulder.

hallucinations a sensory perception without a source in the external environment. They can be auditory, visual, olfactory, and tactile.

hemianesthesia absence or significant decrease in sensation over one side of the body.

hemiballism irregular, random, nonrhythmic violent flinging (flailing) movements of the arm or leg on one side of the body; associated with a lesion in the subthalamic nucleus.

hemiparesis weakness of one side of the body.

hemiplegia complete paralysis of one side of the body.

hemisection syndrome pathological process confined to one side of the spinal cord. There is motor weakness with impaired proprioception-vibration ipsilateral to the lesion and impaired pain and temperature sensation contralateral to the lesion (Brown-Sequard syndrome).

herniation shift in intracranial structures due to differential pressure within brain compartments caused by brain mass lesion. Lesions in posterior fossa may force cerebellar tonsils through foramen magnum (tonsillar herniation). Hemispheric mass may force the ipsilateral temporal lobe (uncus) through the tentorial incisura (uncal herniation).

homonymous hemianopia visual defect in one side of the visual field that is present in both eyes. It is due to a lesion in the contralateral cerebral hemisphere.

Horner's syndrome caused by a lesion in the sympathetic system above or at the level of the cervical spine; characterized by miosis, partial ptosis, enophthalmos, and anhidrosis on the face on the side of the lesion.

hydrocephalus pathologic condition characterized by increased cerebrospinal fluid volume manifested by enlargement of part or the entire ventricular and/or subarachnoid system.

hyperesthesia burning sensation produced by a moving stimulus.

hyperpathia exaggerated response to sensory stimulus.

hypnagogic hallucinations frightening nightmares on awakening as occur in patients with narcolepsy.

incontinence loss of neurogenic control of bladder or bowel function usually due to spinal cord dysfunction but may be due to brain or peripheral nerve disease.

intracerebral hemorrhage bleeding that occurs within the brain parenchyma usually due to ruptured blood vessel. Most common in hypertensive patients due to ruptured miliary (Charcot-Bouchard) aneurysms.

lacunae small (less than 15 mm) infarcts often seen in the basal nuclei and pons and frequently caused by small artery disease produced by hypertension, microatheroma, microembolism, and so forth.

locked-in syndrome quadriplegia with cranial nerve paralysis such that the patient can not communicate by speaking. The patient's consciousness is normal. The patient is de-efferented and can communicate only by utilizing eye movements. Due to lesion involving ventral pons.

long tract sign see upper motor neuron.

lower motor neuron lesion lesion of the motor nuclei of the brain stem or anterior horns of the spinal cord; characterized clinically by flaccid paralysis, marked atrophy, and areflexia. Fasciculations are frequent.

Marcus-Gunn pupillary defect see **afferent pupillary defect.**

meningioma neoplasm that originates from arachnoidal cells and dural fibroblasts and is frequently attached to the dura. The neoplasm is usually benign and displaces rather than invades brain tissue.

meningitis inflammatory reaction of the pia and arachnoid and the cerebrospinal fluid that they enclose.

mental retardation group of disorders of childhood characterized by faulty development of intelligence and manifested by inability to learn and to react appropriately to the daily activities.

migraine general term for any vascular headache (literally a pain of half of the head).

miosis constriction of the pupil as a result of increased parasympathomimetic tone or decreased sympathomimetic tone.

mononeuropathy involvement of a single nerve usually due to entrapment or vascular ischemia. If multiple nerves are involved, referred to as "mononeuropathy multiplex."

multiple sclerosis inflammatory-demyelinating disorder involving CNS myelin sheath. Symptoms disseminated in time and space. Diagnosis usually established by MRI or CSF findings.

myasthenia gravis disorder characterized by weakness and abnormal fatigue due to neuromuscular junction transmission defect. Usually due to thymic abnormalities and characterized by presence of acetylcholine receptor antibodies and positive Tensilon test.

myasthenic syndrome   see **Eaton-Lambert syndrome.**

mydriasis   pupillary dilatation as a result of decreased parasympathomimetic tone or increased sympathomimetic tone.

myelopathy   disease that affects partially or completely (transverse) a segment or segments of the spinal cord (e.g., traumatic myelopathy, ischemic myelopathy).

myoclonus   rapid, coarse, random nonpurposeful contraction of a muscle group that is sufficient to move the joint.

myopathy   primary disease of muscle characterized by symmetrical proximal muscle weakness, normal sensation, and normal stretch reflexes (if inflammatory, *polymyositis*; if dystrophic, *myotonic dystrophy*; etc.).

myotonia   involuntary painless delay in relaxation of skeletal muscles after contraction, associated with high-frequency and high-amplitude electrical discharges.

narcolepsy   multiple brief periods during which the patient falls asleep during the day.

neuralgia   stabbing or throbbing pain in the course or distribution of a nerve (e.g., trigeminal neuralgia).

neuropathy   lesion affecting peripheral nerves. If isolated to one nerve, *mononeuropathy;* if symmetrical bilateral, *polyneuropathy*; if multiple isolated scattered individual nerves, *multiple mononeruopathy*; and so forth.

nystagmus   rhythmic oscillating movement (horizontal, vertical, or rotary) of the eyeball in which there is an initial slow movement in one direction followed by rapid movement back to the initial position.

oculocephalic reflex   see **doll's head movement.**

ophthalmopathy   paralysis or restriction of eye muscles as may occur in thyroid disease.

optic atrophy   pallor of the optic nerve head usually caused by inflammatory disease (neuritis) or intracranial hypertension (papilledema).

optic neuritis   inflammatory disease of the optic nerve characterized by impaired vision, defective pupillary reactivity to light, and blurring of the optic nerve head margins.

organic brain syndromes group of diseases in which brain damage or dysfunction results in a change in behavior.

oscillopsia visual sensation of movement, blurring of vision, or constant movement of the objects within the field of vision in patients with nystagmus.

otorrhea leakage of CSF from the ear due to basilar skull fracture.

papilledema see choked disc.

paraparesis partial loss of strength (weakness) of both lower extremities.

paraplegia total loss of strength (paralysis) of both lower extremities.

paresthesia abnormal sensations in the absence of specific stimulation—feelings of tingling, itching, numbness, heaviness, and so on.

peripheral facial (infranuclear) palsy paralysis of half (one side) of the face—both upper (forehead) and lower face—caused by any lesion affecting the seventh cranial nerve, from the brain stem nucleus to the nerve terminal.

Phalen sign symptoms produced with forced wrist flexion in the distribution of median nerve as seen in patients with carpal tunnel syndrome.

phantom limb pain persistent pain in the distribution of an amputated extremity.

polyneuropathy neurological condition due to impaired function of peripheral nerve with damage to the myelin sheath and/or axon. Characterized by sensory, motor, and/or automatic dysfunction beginning initially in feet and then extending to proximal portion of the extremity.

postictal neurological dysfunction that persists following seizure. This may be generalized (impaired consciousness) or focal (hemiparesis). This deficit usually resolves within 24 hours.

progressive muscular atrophy slowly progressive wasting of muscles frequently associated with fasciculations and caused by degeneration of anterior horn cells. It can be a manifestation of motor neuron disease or a familial disorder (Werdnig-Hoffman or Kugelberg-Welander).

progressive stroke also known as stroke in evolution is focal ischemia in which neurologic symptoms progress or fluctuate within 12 to 24 hours while the patient is under observation.

pseudoathetosis abnormal involuntary extremity movements occurring in outstretched hands due to impaired proprioception.

pseudobulbar palsy clinical state in which there is weakness of the lower face, swallowing mechanisms, phonation, and tongue as a result of bilateral damage of the upper motor neurons or the corticobulbar tracts.

pseudoseizure an apparent seizure characterized by an alteration of consciousness and motor manifestations but no change in EEG pattern during the episode. Also referred to a "hysterical" or "psychogenic" seizure.

ptosis drooping of the upper eyelid usually caused by levator palpebral muscle weakness.

pyramidal tract signs clinical signs such as Babinski sign and clonus that are seen in upper motor neuron lesions.

quadriplegia (same as tetraplegia) paralysis of all extremities.

rachischisis group of disorders produced by lack of fusion of the dorsal midline structures of the primitive neural tube (e.g., spina bifida anencephaly).

radiculopathy lesion affecting the spinal nerve roots.

reflex sympathetic dystrophy pain of a burning causalgic nature due to dysfunction of the sympathetic nervous system.

reversible ischemic neurological deficit Strokelike syndrome in which neurological deficit persists for longer than 24 hours but resolves within several days.

rhinorrhea leakage of CSF from the nose due to basilar skull fracture.

rigidity increased muscle tone that is equal throughout the entire range of muscle movement. It is usually seen in patients with parkinsonism.

Romberg sign clinical sign to evaluate balance, primarily proprioceptive loss (posterior column of spinal cord). A positive Romberg sign is diagnosed when the patient who is standing with feet together falls on closing his or her eyes.

sciatica pain and/or paresthesia which extends from low back to posterolateral thigh and leg to the foot.

scintillation bright flashing lights such as sparklers as seen in migraine aura or visual seizures.

scotoma central area of decreased visual acuity surrounded by normal peripheral vision.

seizure episodic attack of abnormal neurologic function during which consciousness is altered and motor or sensory disturbances are present.

sleep apnea syndrome characterized by recurrent episodes of cessation of breathing during sleep with preservation of thoracoabdominal respiratory efforts (obstructive type) or without (central type).

spasmodic torticollis (wryneck) localized form of dystonia that involves mainly the sternocleidomastoid, trapezius, semispinalis, splenius capitis, and posterior muscles of the neck.

spasticity state of hypertonicity secondary to a lesion in the corticospinal or corticobulbar tracts. Increased tone in the antigravity muscles, increased muscle stretch reflexes, and presence of pathologic reflexes (Babinski and Hoffman signs).

spinocerebellar degenerations group of disorders (Friedreich's ataxia, hereditary spastic ataxia, and hereditary spastic paraplegia) of undetermined cause that affects the corticospinal and spinocerebellar tracts.

spondylosis, cervical general term for degenerative disease of the intervertebral disks, articular facets, and supporting soft tissues of the cervical spine causing radiculopathy or myelopathy.

squint term that is used synonymously with strabismus; it refers to an imbalance of the extraocular muscles.

status epilepticus repeated recurrent seizures from which the patient does not fully recover consciousness between individual seizures.

stereognosis ability to appreciate the shape of an object using tactile sensation alone. A defect in the ability is termed *astereognosia.*

straight-leg raising test (Lasegue's test) pain and symptoms of sciatica that can be elicited by raising the affected leg with the patient in the prone position. In normal subjects, the leg can be raised to 90 degrees without inducing pain.

stroke   rapidly developing focal neurologic deficit seen in any cerebrovascular disease regardless of the cause (ischemic or hemorrhagic).

subarachnoid hemorrhage   bleeding due to head trauma or ruptured berry aneurysm. Symptoms include severe headache, photophobia and meningeal signs.

subdural hematoma   collection of blood that forms between the dura and arachnoid membrane, usually over the cerebral hemispheres.

syncope   brief period of loss of consciousness due to impaired brain metabolism. Usually due to systemic or cardiovascular etiologies and rarely due to neurological illness.

syringomyelia   cavitation (cyst) of the central part of the spinal cord and manifested by amyotrophy of upper extremities and segmental sensory loss of dissociated type (loss of pain and temperature and preservation of touch).

tabes dorsalis   form of ataxia caused purely by sensory deficit produced by lesions of the dorsal root ganglia and dorsal columns of the spinal cord.

tic   sudden, stereotyped, irresistible spasm, usually a motor twitch; can be used to describe the response to a sudden pain, as in tic douloureux.

tilt table test   utilized to evaluate patients with unexplained episodes of loss of consciousness in whom neurocardiogenic (vasovagal) syncope is considered most likely diagnosis.

Tinel sign   to illicit tingling, or paresthesias, in the distribution of a specific nerve by tapping lightly over the nerve.

tinnitus   unwanted noise (usually with ringing, buzzing, or roaring nature) experienced by the patient that has no source in the environment.

Todd's postictal paralysis   neurological deficit that is present immediately following a seizure and resolves within 24 hours.

tonic pupil   see **Adie's pupil**.

transient ischemic attacks (TIA)   isolated episode of focal neurologic dysfunction of vascular origin that lasts less than 24 hours (usually a few minutes) and leaves no permanent neurologic deficit.

tremor rhythmic involuntary shaking or trembling.

trigeminal neuralgia also known as tic douloureux; consists of paroxysms of lightninglike, excruciating unilateral facial pain that shoots down one or a combination of the branches of the trigeminal nerve.

upper motor neuron lesion lesion that involves the tract that originates in the large (Betz) neurons of the motor cortex and terminates in the motor nuclei of the brain stem or anterior horns of the spinal cord (corticospinal tract). Characterized clinically by spastic paralysis, hyperreflexia, and Babinski sign.

vascular malformation abnormal formation of arteries, capillaries, or veins supplying the brain and/or spinal cord. These vessels are fragile and may rupture to cause intracerebral hemorrhage.

vegetative state these patients appear awake, have normal sleep-wake states, and maintain spontaneous cardiovascular and respiratory function but are able to respond to stimulation only in reflex manner. When this condition persists for longer than 1 month, it is chronic. Pathologically, there is extensive bilateral cerebral hemispheric damage with brain stem sparing.

venous pulsations pulsations of the central retinal vein seen with funduscopic examination. Their presence indicates that intracranial pressure is *not* elevated at the time they are visualized.

venous sinus thrombosis hypercoagulability within the draining venous system that may lead to impaired circulation of CSF (hydrocephalus, increased intracranial pressure), and/or venous infarcts.

vertigo subjective feeling of movement of the environment or the body that does not correspond to actual movement, but is internally generated. Vertigo is usually a sensation of rotating or spinning.

Wernicke aphasia language disorder characterized by fluent speech and impaired comprehension.

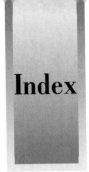

Index